	DATE DUE		
JAN 0 7 2002			

SCIENCE AND MEDICINE IN THE OLD SOUTH

SCIENCE AND MEDICINE IN THE OLD SOUTH

EDITED BY

Ronald L. Numbers and Todd L. Savitt

LOUISIANA STATE UNIVERSITY PRESS

Baton Rouge and London

Copyright © 1989 by Louisiana State University Press
All rights reserved
Manufactured in the United States of America
First printing

98 97 96 95 94 93 92 91 90 89   5 4 3 2 1

Designer: Laura Roubique Gleason
Typeface: Palatino
Typesetter: The Composing Room of Michigan, Inc.
Printer: Thomson-Shore, Inc.
Binder: John H. Dekker & Sons, Inc.

Library of Congress Cataloging-in-Publication Data

Science and medicine in the Old South.

   Consists primarily of papers from the first and
second Barnard-Millington symposia, sponsored by
the University of Mississippi Center for the Study
of Southern Culture, held at Oxford, Miss. in 1982
and at Jackson, Miss. in 1983.
   Includes index.
   1. Medicine—Southern States—History—19th century—
Congresses.   2. Science—Southern States—History—19th
century—Congresses.   I. Numbers, Ronald L.   II. Savitt,
Todd Lee, 1943–   .   III. University of Mississippi.
Center for the Study of Southern Culture.   [DNLM: 1. History of Medicine, 19th Cent.—United States—congresses.
2. Science—history—United States—congresses.
WZ 70 AA1 S46 1982–83]
R154.5.S68S35   1989   610'.975   88-32648
ISBN 0-8071-1464-2 (alk. paper)

For
ANN J. ABADIE
who made this book possible

CONTENTS

CONTENTS

PREFACE AND ACKNOWLEDGMENTS

O ver half a century has passed since the publication of Thomas Cary Johnson's celebratory history *Scientific Interests in the Old South* (1936), a rebuttal to charges that the oppressive intellectual atmosphere of the antebellum South had stifled scientific activity. Although Johnson discovered ample evidence of scientific interests, he neglected to compare the southern record with those of other regions, thus overlooking, as several reviewers pointed out, "the only method which would have given meaning to his ardent research."[1] In recent years a number of quantitative studies of nineteenth-century science have provided clues for assessing the relative achievements of southerners (see Chapter 1), but no comprehensive analysis of science—or medicine—in the Old South has appeared since Johnson's book. Indeed, with a few notable exceptions, southern historians have ignored scientific and medical developments, while historians of American science and medicine have shied away from regional studies. As Sally Gregory Kohlstedt recently pointed out in a historiographical review of science in America, "studies of regional science have been relatively rare and the subject invites investigation."[2]

1. Bert James Loewenberg, Review of Thomas Cary Johnson, Jr.'s *Scientific Interests in the Old South*, in *American Historical Review*, XLIII (1937–38), 166. See also the reviews of Johnson by Carl Bridenbaugh in *Isis*, XXVII (1937), 517; and Charles S. Sydnor, in *South Atlantic Quarterly*, XXXVII (1938), 221.

2. Sally Gregory Kohlstedt, "Institutional History," in Sally Gregory Kohlstedt and Margaret W. Rossiter (eds.), *Historical Writing on American Science*, *Osiris*, 2nd ser., I (1985), 21.

This collection of interpretative essays, most of which were prepared originally for the first (1982) and second (1983) Barnard-Millington symposia on southern science and medicine, represents a significant step in that direction. Unlike Johnson, many of the contributors to
this volume consciously attempt to place the history of antebellum
science and medicine in a comparative context—not because of regional pride or prejudice but to assist in identifying the distinctive aspects
of the Old South's involvement in science and medicine. Only in this
way could they, for example, isolate the possible effects of slavery on
the growth of science or determine the uniqueness of so-called states-
rights medicine. The resulting view, focusing on the period from about
1830 to 1860, highlights some of the ways in which the region's peculiar
institutions and environment influenced the direction of science and
medicine. This perspective also reveals the Old South to have been
less scientifically and medically distinctive than earlier works have
suggested.

The Barnard-Millington symposia, sponsored by the Center for the
Study of Southern Culture at the University of Mississippi, brought
together historians of the Old South and historians of American science and medicine in a collaborative effort to synthesize the results of
recent scholarship, to extend the boundaries of existing knowledge,
and to identify areas for future research. The Center used the occasion
to honor two of the antebellum South's most prominent scientists,
both of whom had ties to the University of Mississippi. Frederick A. P.
Barnard (1809–1889), a Yale-educated northerner, went south in 1837
to teach mathematics and natural history at the University of Alabama.
In 1854 he moved to the University of Mississippi, where he built the
observatory that currently houses the Center for the Study of Southern
Culture and served successively as professor of mathematics and astronomy, as president, and as chancellor. In 1860 he was elected president of the American Association for the Advancement of Science, and
four years later he began a quarter-century tenure as president of
Columbia University in New York City. John Millington (1779–1868)
enjoyed a successful career in England as a scientific lecturer and author before leaving for the New World about 1830. In the mid-1830s he
joined the faculty of the University of Virginia as a professor of chemistry, natural philosophy, and engineering. When the University of
Mississippi opened in 1848, he became its first professor of the natural
sciences, and for a time he headed the state geological survey. In 1853,
at age seventy-four, he resigned from his position at Oxford to become

professor of chemistry and toxicology in the Memphis Medical College.[3]

The Barnard-Millington symposia, which gave birth to this volume, owed their existence to funding from the National Endowment for the Humanities and to the organizational skills of the staff at the University of Mississippi's Center for the Study of Southern Culture. William Ferris, director of the Center, encouraged us to undertake this project and enthusiastically supported its progress. Ann J. Abadie, associate director of the Center, oversaw arrangements for the symposia from preliminary plans to final report, from travel schedules to side trips to the Delta, from catfish meals to home-style receptions. Her energy, intelligence, and congeniality made the symposia memorable occasions for all participants. In fact, it is no exaggeration to say that without Ann Abadie this book would not exist. She is truly a special person.

At Oxford, which hosted the symposium "Science in the Old South," Sarah Dixon, Sue Hart, and Dottie Abbott provided invaluable assistance. For the symposium "Medicine in the Old South," held in Jackson, the University of Mississippi Medical Center served as co-sponsor and the Department of Continuing Education coordinated the arrangements. The Mississippi State Department of Archives and History graciously opened the House Chamber of the Old Capitol Museum for our meetings. Patti Carr Black, director of the State Historical Museum, mounted a special exhibit entitled "Medicine in Antebellum Mississippi" to coincide with the symposium. To all we are most grateful.

The conferences in Oxford and Jackson were devoted entirely to the discussion of previously circulated papers, many of which benefited substantially from criticisms and suggestions offered by participants.

3. William J. Chute, *Damn Yankee! The First Career of Frederick A. P. Barnard: Educator, Scientist, Idealist* (Port Washington, N.Y., 1978); T. C. J. [Johnson], Jr., "John Millington," in *Dictionary of American Biography,* XII, 647.

For contributing to these scholarly exchanges, we thank, in addition to the contributors to this volume, the following invited participants:

Michele L. Aldrich, American Association for the Advancement of Science
John C. Boles, Rice University
James O. Breeden, Southern Methodist University
Blaine A. Brownell, University of Alabama in Birmingham
Catherine Clinton, Harvard University
John K. Crellin, Duke University
A. Hunter Dupree, Brown University
John Duffy, University of Maryland
Paul D. Escott, University of North Carolina at Charlotte
Drew Gilpin Faust, University of Pennsylvania
Neal C. Gillespie, Georgia State University
John C. Greene, University of Connecticut
Wayland D. Hand, University of California at Los Angeles
Robert J. Haws, University of Mississippi
Martin Kaufman, Westfield State College
Kenneth F. Kiple, Bowling Green State University
Sally Gregory Kohlstedt, Syracuse University
Judith Walzer Leavitt, University of Wisconsin-Madison
Ronald L. Lewis, University of Delaware
Anne Millbrooke, United Technologies
John H. Moore, Florida State University
Lawrence N. Powell, Tulane University
Albert J. Raboteau, Princeton University
Nathan Reingold, Smithsonian Institution
Charles E. Rosenberg, University of Pennsylvania
Henry D. Shapiro, University of Cincinnati
Dale C. Smith, Uniformed Services University of the Health Sciences
Merritt Roe Smith, Massachusetts Institute of Technology
Charles Reagan Wilson, University of Mississippi
Richard A. Wines, Fisher Junior College
James Harvey Young, Emory University

We gratefully acknowledge Beverly Jarrett, at the Louisiana State University Press, for her interest and encouragement; Barbara Phillips, for her assistance; and Mary Hester, for her fine editorial work.

PART I

SCIENCE IN THE OLD SOUTH

INTRODUCTION

No issue has dominated discussions of science in the Old South more than the influence of slavery, the region's most distinctive antebellum institution. As Ronald L. Numbers and Janet S. Numbers show in Chapter 1, the debate over science and slavery has engaged historians since the early decades of this century, when Samuel Eliot Morison accused the cotton kingdom of killing "practically every germ of creative thought," and Thomas Cary Johnson, Jr., responded with his chauvinistic *Scientific Interests in the Old South* (1936).[1] Drawing on recent quantitative studies by other historians of science and using their own statistical analyses, the Numberses suggest that the failure of the Old South to keep pace with the Northeast "resulted more from demographic and environmental factors"—particularly the absence of a strong urban culture—than from slavery itself. They find that "the presence or absence of slavery has no predictive value in locating American scientists" during the antebellum period and that support for science in the South grew rather than declined as proslavery sentiment hardened in the years after 1830.

The Numberses do concede, however, that slavery may have produced "secondary effects inimical to science," a point emphasized by William K. Scarborough in Chapter 4, "Science on the Plantation." Scarborough argues that despite the presence of considerable scientific activity on southern plantations, "slavery saddled the region with an overwhelmingly rural agricultural economy" and contributed to the

---

1. For a recent discussion, see Robert V. Bruce, *The Launching of Modern American Science, 1846–1876* (New York, 1987), 57–63.

"cult of the country gentleman," which channeled southern talent into agricultural and political careers rather than into science and industry. Moreover, until late in the period, science offered southern planters little of practical value. "In short," observed John H. Moore at the first Barnard-Millington symposium, "prior to 1860 southern planters did more to promote the advancement of science than science did for the antebellum southern plantation."

The strongest indictment of slavery appears in Chapter 5 by Charles B. Dew, "Slavery and Technology in the Antebellum Southern Iron Industry," which argues that the conservative influence of slavery helps to explain why "technological innovation largely bypassed the South's iron industry." Using the example of William Weaver's ironworks at Buffalo Forge, Virginia, Dew illustrates how slave labor discouraged the adoption of state-of-the-art industrial technology. Although other factors, such as the location of anthracite coal beds in eastern Pennsylvania and Weaver's limited entrepreneurial skills, undoubtedly contributed to the decline of Buffalo Forge, Dew provides a convincing example of how cultural factors affected technological development. Science, it seems, played even less of a role in southern industries than it did on southern plantations; according to Dew, industrialization in the Old South was "almost totally unaffected" by early nineteenth-century science.

The other chapters in this section say little about slavery, but nevertheless challenge a number of common preconceptions about the history of science in the Old South. In contrast to such historians as Richard Hofstadter, who described the late antebellum college as suffering from "severe general intellectual paralysis," and E. Merton Coulter, who accused the University of Georgia of sticking "to the beaten track of the classics," Thomas G. Dyer in "Science in the Antebellum College" (Chapter 2) shows that southern colleges followed their northern counterparts in giving science an increasingly prominent place in the curriculum.[2] In a case study focusing on the University of Georgia, Dyer questions "widely held assumptions concerning the sterility of the so-called classical curriculum" and the reputed educational conservatism of the region, showing that support for science in Athens compared favorably with that in the better colleges of the North.[3]

2. Richard Hofstadter and Walter P. Metzger, *The Development of Academic Freedom in the United States* (New York, 1955), 259; E. Merton Coulter, *College Life in the Old South* (New York, 1928), 48, and 254–55 regarding the contempt of the trustees for science.
3. Stanley M. Guralnick's *Science and the Ante-Bellum American College* (Philadelphia,

In Chapter 3, "Scientific Societies in the Old South," Lester D. Stephens examines the less successful efforts of urban southerners to create scientific institutions that might rival the distinguished societies of Boston and Philadelphia.[4] Drawing from the experiences of the Old South's two most prosperous societies, the Elliott Society of Natural History in Charleston and the New Orleans Academy of Sciences, both founded in 1853, Stephens explores the contributions of these organizations to the professionalization of science in the region, as well as the reasons why they failed to win national recognition.

In the only essay in Part I to look at how science influenced antebellum southern thought, E. Brooks Holifield explores the relationship between science and theology in the Old South (Chapter 6). In contrast to historians such as Samuel Eliot Morison and Clement Eaton, who have stressed the conflict between science and religion in the nineteenth century, Holifield emphasizes the positive attitudes toward science of the South's "gentlemen theologians," who pledged allegiance to what T. Dwight Bozeman has called "doxological science."[5] Despite the appearance of signs of strain in the 1850s, throughout most of the antebellum period the elite town clergy of the South optimistically developed a "theology of natural science" that harmonized perfectly with the theology of the Bible.

Although the essays in this volume help to clarify the place of science in the culture of the Old South and to identify the extent and importance of regional distinctiveness, much historical work remains to be done. In the area of science and religion, for example, Holifield's pioneering research on the "gentlemen theologians" needs to be sup-

---

1975) includes no southern colleges in the sample of fifteen institutions upon which the study is based. For a recent look at the teaching of science in one border state, see Eric H. Christianson, "The Conditions for Science in the Academic Department of Transylvania University, 1799–1857," *Register of the Kentucky Historical Society*, LXXIX, no. 79 (1981), 305–25.

4. For an earlier, sketchier survey, see Joseph Ewan, "The Growth of Learned and Scientific Societies in the Southeastern United States to 1860," in Alexandra Oleson and Sanborn C. Brown (eds.), *The Pursuit of Knowledge in the Early American Republic* (Baltimore, 1976), 208–18.

5. Samuel Eliot Morison, *The Oxford History of the United States, 1783–1917* (2 vols.; London, 1927), II, 16; Clement Eaton, *The Civilization of the Old South: Writings of Clement Eaton*, ed. Albert D. Kirwan (Lexington, Ky., 1968), 181–86; Theodore Dwight Bozeman, *Protestants in an Age of Science: The Baconian Ideal and Antebellum American Religious Thought* (Chapel Hill, 1977). For a recent historiographical critique, see Ronald L. Numbers, "Science and Religion," in Sally Gregory Kohlstedt and Margaret W. Rossiter (eds.), *Historical Writing on American Science, Osiris*, 2nd ser., I (1985), 59–80.

5

plemented by parallel studies of the attitudes of southern scientists and of nonelite groups. We also need further exploration of the apparent deepening concern among religious leaders in the 1850s about the negative effects of science.

Of particular importance for southerners was the scientific debate in the 1840s and 1850s over the unity of the human race. In *The Leopard's Spots: Scientific Attitudes Toward Race in America, 1815–59* (1960), William Stanton has argued that the theologically orthodox South "turned its back on the only intellectually respectable defense of slavery it could have taken up" (*i.e.*, the polygenist theory, according to which blacks and whites represented separately created species) in favor of the biblical stories of Adam and Eve and the curse on Noah's son Ham, who allegedly fathered the Negro race. Stanton, however, devoted relatively little attention to the opponents of polygenism and dismissed the clergyman-naturalist John Bachman, one of its most outspoken critics, as "half theologian, half scientist, lost and confused between the hemispheres of his own personality." Bachman and like-minded southerners deserve better, and Thomas Virgil Peterson has taken a first step toward a deeper understanding of them in his monograph *Ham and Japheth* (1978), which shows the social and religious functions served by the traditional story of Ham.[6] The relationship between polygenism and racism also demands further attention. Stanton suggested that most of the polygenists were motivated by scientific rather than social concerns—an interpretation that both William Henry Longton and Hamilton Cravens have recently challenged.[7]

The practical uses of science in the Old South have also been neglected. We still know little about the teaching of applied science in southern colleges, and the history of technology in the Old South, whether science-based or otherwise, merits an entire volume of its own. William K. Scarborough has demonstrated that science and slavery could coexist on the southern plantation, but we know little about the specific ways in which the plantation system encouraged or retarded science. During the first Barnard-Millington symposium,

6. William Stanton, *The Leopard's Spots: Scientific Attitudes Toward Race in America, 1815–59* (Chicago, 1960), 194; Thomas Virgil Peterson, *Ham and Japheth: The Mythic World of Whites in the Antebellum South* (Metuchen, N.J., 1978). See also H. Shelton Smith, *In His Image, But . . . : Racism in Southern Religion, 1780–1910* (Durham, 1972), 152–65.

7. William Henry Longton, "The Carolina Ideal World: Natural Science and Social Thought in Ante-Bellum South Carolina," *Civil War History*, XX (1974), 118–34; Hamilton Cravens, "History of the Social Sciences," in Kohlstedt and Rossiter (eds.), *Historical Writing on American Science*, 183–207, esp. 188–89. See also Reginald Horsman, *Josiah Nott of Mobile: Southerner, Physician, and Racial Theorist* (Baton Rouge, 1987).

Robert J. Haws surmised that antebellum state governments in the South promoted science only when it promised practical results, such as the economic benefits expected from agricultural and geological surveys. Indeed, southern states, beginning with North Carolina in 1823 and South Carolina the following year, led the nation in organizing state geological surveys.[8]

The chapters in this section demonstrate that the level of scientific activity in the Old South compared favorably with that found in other primarily nonurban regions of the nation. And they suggest that in many settings, such as colleges, scientific societies, and churches, this activity closely paralleled developments elsewhere. What they do not show is the extent to which southern scientists collectively shared a regional identity and created a distinctive scientific community, or the extent to which they relied on northern-based institutions for sustenance and on nonsouthern scientists for advice and encouragement.

Several essays suggest that southerners displayed a greater interest in natural history than in natural philosophy, but the precise ways in which the plants, animals, and rocks of the region affected the scientific roles played by southerners merit further study.[9] Biography would be one way to approach these issues, but to date only a few of the forty leaders of the American Association for the Advancement of Science who lived in the antebellum South (see Chapter 1) have been the subjects of book-length studies,[10] and this list does not even in-

8. Of all the sciences pursued in the Old South, geology has received the most attention. See, for example, Charles S. Sydnor, "State Geological Surveys in the Old South," in David Kelly Jackson (ed.), *American Studies in Honor of William Kenneth Boyd* (Durham, 1940), 88–109; James X. Corgan (ed.), *The Geological Sciences in the Antebellum South* (University, Ala., 1982); and James X. Corgan (ed.), *History of Geology and Geological Education in the Southern and Border States,* a special issue of *Earth Sciences History,* IV, no. 1 (1985), which includes considerable material on the antebellum period.

9. Harold L. Burstyn has recently described the work of William Ferrel, a school teacher in Nashville, who in 1856 published "the first modern account of the general circulation of atmosphere and ocean" and gave the science of geophysical fluid dynamics "its major impetus in the nineteenth century" ("William Ferrel and American Science in the Centennial Years," in Everett Mendelsohn [ed.], *Transformation and Tradition in the Sciences: Essays in Honor of I. Bernard Cohen* [Cambridge, England, 1984], 337–51). For an additional example of southern interest in mathematics and natural philosophy, see James W. Montgomery, Jr., and W. Porter Kellam, "Mathematical Backwoodsman of the West: Charles Francis McCay," *Georgia Historical Quarterly,* LXVII (1983), 206–14.

10. See, for example, Horsman, *Josiah Nott;* Lester D. Stephens, *Joseph LeConte: Gentle Prophet of Evolution* (Baton Rouge, 1982); William J. Chute, *Damn Yankee! The First Career of Frederick A. P. Barnard: Educator, Scientist, Idealist* (Port Washington, N.Y., 1978); John Hebron Moore, *Andrew Brown and Cypress Lumbering in the Old Southwest* (Baton Rouge,

clude such prominent southern scientists as Moses Ashley Curtis, an Episcopal minister and botanist from Hillsboro, North Carolina, who distinguished himself as a mycologist. Scholarly biographies of John L. Riddell, John Lawrence Smith, and John Bachman, to name only a few of numerous possibilities, would contribute greatly to our understanding of the relationship between science and southern society and would shed welcome light on such matters as motives, patronage, and the social uses of science. Collective biographies of the Charleston naturalists and of the New Orleans Academy circle would be especially valuable.[11] The contributions to this volume should thus be seen as an intermediate point in the study of antebellum southern science, not as the final word.

1967); John S. Lupold, "From Physician to Physicist: The Scientific Career of John Le-Conte, 1818–1891" (Ph.D. dissertation, University of South Carolina, 1970); and Tamara Miner Haygood, *Henry William Ravenel, 1814–1887: South Carolina Scientist in the Civil War Era* (Tuscaloosa, Ala., 1987). For an insightful shorter treatment, see Richard M. Jellison and Phillip S. Swartz, "The Scientific Interests of Robert W. Gibbes," *South Carolina Historical Magazine,* LXVI (1965), 77–97.

11. For a cursory introduction to the Charleston naturalists, see G. Edmund Gifford, Jr., "The Charleston Physician-Naturalists," *Bulletin of the History of Medicine,* XLIX (1975), 556–74. Lester D. Stephens is currently studying the Charleston group during the late antebellum period while simultaneously preparing a biography of John Bachman.

CHAPTER 1

SCIENCE IN THE OLD SOUTH: A REAPPRAISAL

Ronald L. Numbers and Janet S. Numbers

In 1927 Harvard's Samuel Eliot Morison touched off a heated historical debate on science in the Old South when he charged that "by 1850 the cotton kingdom had killed practically every germ of creative thought," including science.[1] Stung by this undocumented snub, Thomas Cary Johnson, Jr., of the University of Virginia rose to his region's defense, accusing the Harvard scholar of unforgivable arrogance and inexcusable sloppiness. To refute Morison's claim, Johnson compiled two hundred pages documenting scientific activity in the Old South in lecture halls and classrooms, on plantations and in towns, among gentlemen as well as "Sweet Southern Girls," to whom he devoted an entire chapter. On the basis of largely anecdotal evidence, he concluded that "between 1801 and 1861, the people of the Southern States in common with those of the North and of Western Europe were intensely interested in the exploration and mastery of the forces of nature."[2] In other words, the cotton kingdom had *not* destroyed creative thought in the Old South.

Although some historians, such as Fletcher M. Green, rejoiced that Johnson had disproved the common notion "that slavery and its defense stifled intellectual interests" in the antebellum South, others, including Bert James Loewenberg, Carl Bridenbaugh, and Charles

This essay originally appeared, in slightly different form, in the *Journal of Southern History,* LXVIII (1982), 163–84.

1. S. E. Morison, *The Oxford History of the United States, 1783–1917* (2 vols.; London, 1927), II, 15, 24 (quotation).
2. Thomas Cary Johnson, Jr., *Scientific Interests in the Old South* (New York, 1936), 10.

Sackett Sydnor, faulted the Virginian for failing to compare the record of the South with that of the North—"the only method," according to Loewenberg, "which would have given meaning to his ardent research."[3] Despite this crucial limitation, Johnson's work apparently convinced its intended target. In his new Oxford history, published in 1965, Morison atoned for his previous offense by describing scientific achievement as "the fairest cultural flower of the South before the Civil War."[4]

Ironically, by the time of this belated recantation nonchauvinistic southern historians, led by Kentucky's Clement Eaton, were beginning to confirm much of Morison's earlier negative judgment. In *The Mind of the Old South*, first published in 1964, Eaton concluded that "the southern mind of the antebellum period was, on the whole, essentially unscientific." During "the 1820's and early 1830's," he said, "the South was a favorable place for the pursuit of pure science," but the subsequent rise of "religious and proslavery orthodoxies" and the pervasive influence of romanticism destroyed "the detachment and bold imagination essential to scientific discovery." James O. Breeden endorsed these conclusions in his biography *Joseph Jones, M.D.: Scientist of the Old South*, the most important recent contribution to the historiography of antebellum science.[5] Neither Eaton nor Breeden, however, compared science in the North and South.

While these southern historians wrestled verbally with the problem of science in the Old South, historians of science in America, concerned with the broader picture, approached the issue statistically and provided the regional comparisons Johnson and others had failed to make. From these studies it is now possible to evaluate the South's scientific record in a concrete way by comparing its performance with those of other regions and determining whether or not southern science declined with the rise of proslavery sentiment in the 1830s.

3. Fletcher M. Green, *North Carolina Historical Review*, XV (1938), 88–89; Bert James Loewenberg, *American Historical Review*, XLIII (1937–38), 166–67; Carl Bridenbaugh, *Isis*, XXVII (1937), 517–19; Charles S. Sydnor, *South Atlantic Quarterly*, XXXVII (1938), 221. These comments all appeared in reviews of Johnson's *Scientific Interests*.

4. Samuel Eliot Morison, *The Oxford History of the American People* (New York, 1965), 513. We are indebted to Susan Schnitzer for bringing this source to our attention. Merle Curti also acknowledged the scientific accomplishments of the antebellum South (*The Growth of American Thought* [3rd ed.; New York, 1964], 427–28).

5. Clement Eaton, *The Mind of the Old South* (Rev. ed.; Baton Rouge, 1967), 243 (first quotation), 224 (second and third quotations), 244 (fourth quotation); James O. Breeden, *Joseph Jones, M.D.: Scientist of the Old South* (Lexington, Ky., 1975), xi. Eaton's influence is also evident in Sally Gregory Kohlstedt, *The Formation of the American Scientific Community: The American Association for the Advancement of Science, 1848–1860* (Urbana, 1976), 222.

TABLE 1.
BIRTH AND EMPLOYMENT OF FIFTY-FIVE LEADING AMERICAN
SCIENTISTS, 1815–1845

Region	Birthplace	Primary Place of Employment
South	1 (1.8%)	6 (10.9%)
Border	2 (3.6%)	1 (1.8%)
New England	21 (38.2%)	15 (27.3%)
Middle Atlantic	22 (40.0%)	29 (52.7%)
North Central	0 (0.0%)	4 (7.3%)
Foreign	9 (16.4%)	0 (0.0%)

SOURCE: Adapted from George H. Daniels, *American Science in the Age of Jackson* (New York, 1968), 201–28; Clark A. Elliott, *Biographical Dictionary of American Science: The Seventeenth Through the Nineteenth Centuries* (Westport, Conn., 1979).

Judged by almost every measurable criterion—publication, participation in national associations, inclusion in the *Dictionary of American Biography*, and the founding of scientific journals and societies—the Old South lagged markedly behind the Northeast in promoting science. In *American Science in the Age of Jackson*, George H. Daniels listed the fifty-five most prolific contributors to sixteen scientific journals from 1815 to 1845. Among these "leading American scientists," only one, the physician-chemist John Lawrence Smith, was born in the South; and only six worked primarily in the South: John Bachman (Charleston), John Patten Emmet (Charlottesville), Nicholas Marcellus Hentz (Alabama, North Carolina, and South Carolina), Charles Grafton Page (Fairfax County, Virginia), Gerard Troost (Nashville), and Smith (Charleston).[6] A comparison of the South with New England and the Middle Atlantic region suggests that antebellum southerners lacked the enthusiasm for science displayed by the North (Table 1).[7]

The Old South fares somewhat better in studies covering the entire period from 1800 to the Civil War. Among the more than five hundred

6. George H. Daniels, *American Science in the Age of Jackson* (New York, 1968), 201–28.

7. Unless otherwise specified, regional classifications are as follows: *South*—Alabama, Arkansas, Florida, Georgia, Louisiana, Mississippi, North Carolina, South Carolina, Tennessee, Texas, and Virginia; *Border*—Delaware, Kentucky, Maryland, Missouri, and the District of Columbia; *New England*—Connecticut, Maine, Massachusetts, New Hampshire, Rhode Island, and Vermont; *Middle Atlantic*—New Jersey, New York, and Pennsylvania; *North Central*—Illinois, Indiana, Iowa, Michigan, Minnesota, Ohio, and Wisconsin; and *West*—California, Oregon, and the western territories.

TABLE 2.
BIRTH AND RESIDENCE OF AMERICAN SCIENTISTS, 1800–1863

Region	Birthplace	Adult Residence
South	36 (7.4%)	79 (11.9%)
Border	20 (4.1%)	88 (13.2%)
New England	193 (39.5%)	183 (27.5%)
Middle Atlantic	160 (32.7%)	241 (36.2%)
North Central	8 (1.6%)	58 (8.7%)
West	0 (0.0%)	16 (2.4%)
Foreign	72 (14.7%)	0 (0.0%)

SOURCE: Adapted from Clark A. Elliott, "The American Scientist, 1800–1863: His Origins, Career, and Interests" (Ph.D. dissertation, Case Western Reserve University, 1970), 59–60, 142–43.

NOTE: Each scientist is counted for each residence during adult life.

Americans identified by Clark A. Elliott as having published three or more articles in American journals indexed by the *Royal Society Catalogue of Scientific Papers* (1800–1863), 7.4 percent were born in the South and 11.9 percent worked in the region, an achievement far inferior to that of the Northeast (Table 2).[8] South Carolina ranked at the top of the southern states as the birthplace of fifteen scientists and the adult residence of twenty; Virginia claimed second place as the birthplace of nine and residence of eleven.[9]

The activities of the American Association for the Advancement of Science (AAAS), "the first truly national voluntary organization in the United States in which the leading persons in all fields of science took

8. Clark A. Elliott, "The American Scientist, 1800–1863: His Origins, Career, and Interests" (Ph.D. dissertation, Case Western Reserve University, 1970), 59–60, 142–43. For a summary of this study without regional comparisons, see Elliott, "The American Scientist in Antebellum Society: A Quantitative View," *Social Studies of Science*, V (1975), 93–108.

9. In another analysis of the antebellum scientific community, Donald deB. Beaver devised a methodology to select the 138 American scientists "most productive" between 1800 and 1860. Omitting six whose places of birth were unknown, the regions of birth were the South, four (3.0 percent); Border, five (3.8 percent); New England, fifty-six (42.4 percent); Middle Atlantic, forty-six (34.8 percent); North Central, one (0.8 percent); foreign, twenty (15.2 percent) ("The American Scientific Community, 1800–1860: A Statistical-Historical Study" [Ph.D. dissertation, Yale University, 1966], 350).

an active interest," provide another means of identifying the antebellum scientific community, one based on participation rather than publication. In her history of the AAAS from its founding in 1848 to its suspension during the Civil War, Sally Gregory Kohlstedt labels as "leaders" those members who held at least one office or presented at least one paper.[10] In 1850, the year the association held its spring meeting in Charleston, the South contributed 16.2 percent of the leaders and 22.3 percent of the nonslave population of the United States. Ten years later the figures had dropped to 11.6 percent and 20.3 percent, respectively. Although the South trailed the Border, New England, and Middle Atlantic regions, it far outdistanced the North Central and West (Table 3). As Kohlstedt has shown, the regional distribution of the association's 2,068 members closely parallels that of its leaders.[11]

The same pattern of southern "backwardness in science" emerges in Robert V. Bruce's statistical profile of American scientists who were active between 1846 and 1876 and subsequently honored by inclusion in the *Dictionary of American Biography* (Table 4).[12] Even during this relatively late period, the South continued to employ more scientists than it produced, although the gap had narrowed substantially (compare Tables 1 and 4).

As we might expect, the Old South also failed to support scientific journals and societies at a level comparable to that of the North. Of the 337 American publications begun before 1849 that "made a regular practice of including scientific material," only 24 (7.1 percent) were edited in the South (Table 5). Similarly, the South (including most of the Border states) accounted for only five of the thirty-five scientific societies in America in 1855 (Table 6).

From these various comparative studies we now know that the antebellum southern mind was only relatively—not essentially—un-

---

10. Kohlstedt, *Formation of the American Scientific Community*, 192–93.

11. *Ibid*, 203.

12. Robert V. Bruce, "A Statistical Profile of American Scientists, 1846–1876," in George H. Daniels (ed.), *Nineteenth-Century American Science: A Reappraisal* (Evanston, Ill., 1972), 79. The South's relatively inferior position during this period is confirmed in Amos J. Loveday, Jr., "A Statistical Study of the American Scientific Community, 1855–1860" (M.A. thesis, Ohio State University, 1970), a work based on data from 377 individuals "who averaged publishing at least one article or pamphlet every five years or one book every seven years." According to Loveday (p. 12), the South (including Kentucky, Delaware, Maryland, and the District of Columbia) produced only "7.9 percent of the scientists, while accounting for 45.14 percent of the nonslave population in 1820."

TABLE 3.

REGIONAL DISTRIBUTION OF AAAS LEADERS, 1850 AND 1860

Region	No. AAAS Leaders	% AAAS Leaders	% U.S. Pop. (nonslave)	Science Index[1]
1850				
South	27	16.2	22.3	.73
Border	22	13.2	10.0	1.32
Slave	49	29.3	32.3	.91
New England	59	35.3	13.6	2.60
Middle Atlantic	50	29.9	29.5	1.01
North Central	9	5.4	23.6	.23
West	0	0.0	0.9	.00
Free	118	70.6	67.7	1.04
U.S.A.	167	100.0	100.0	1.00
1860				
South	19	11.6	20.3	.57
Border	31	18.9	10.1	1.87
Slave	50	30.5	30.4	1.00
New England	58	35.4	11.4	3.10
Middle Atlantic	42	25.6	27.2	.94
North Central	14	8.5	28.3	.30
West	0	0.0	2.7	.00
Free	114	69.5	69.6	1.00
U.S.A.	164	100.0	100.0	1.00

SOURCE: U.S. Census, 1850, 1860; AAAS, *Proceedings*, 1850, 1860. AAAS leaders are identified in Sally Gregory Kohlstedt, *The Formation of the American Scientific Community: The American Association for the Advancement of Science, 1848–1860* (Urbana, 1976).

[1]Science Index = the percentage of AAAS leaders in a region divided by the percentage of the nonslave U.S. population in that region.

scientific.[13] Although the Old South failed to keep pace with the Northeast, it generally outperformed the more recently settled North Central region. But did it also, as Clement Eaton has argued, reduce its

13. Additional statistical evidence supporting this conclusion can be found in Robert Siegfried, "A Study of Chemical Research Publications from the United States Before 1880" (Ph.D. dissertation, University of Wisconsin, 1952), 134–35; and William Browning, "The Relation of Physicians to Early American Geology," *Annals of Medical History*, n.s., III (1931), 563. According to Siegfried, only one of the sixty-two "major producers" in chemistry (John Lawrence Smith of Charleston) came from the South.

TABLE 4.
BIRTH AND RESIDENCE OF *DAB* SCIENTISTS, 1846–1876

Region	Birthplace	Primary Residence
South	30 (7.2%)	8.3%
Border	12 (2.9%)	3.3%
New England	170 (41.0%)	27.2%
Middle Atlantic	173 (41.7%)	44.4%
North Central	30 (7.2%)	11.4%
West	0 (0.0%)	5.4%

SOURCE: Robert V. Bruce, "A Statistical Profile of American Scientists, 1846–1876," in George H. Daniels (ed.), *Nineteenth-Century American Science: A Reappraisal* (Evanston, Ill., 1972), 74–79.

NOTE: Bruce includes Delaware, Maryland, and District of Columbia with the Middle Atlantic states; his Border region comprises Kentucky, Tennessee (therefore not included in the South), and Missouri.

support for science as "the religious and proslavery orthodoxies" hardened after the mid-1830s?[14] The answer is no. If anything, southerners *increased* their commitment to science during the decades immediately preceding the Civil War.

With one possible exception,[15] none of the quantitative studies of American science supports Eaton's hypothesis. After examining the birthplaces by decade of over five hundred antebellum scientists, Elliott concluded that "the number or percentage of scientists born . . . [in the South] did not decline as the nineteenth century proceeded and the cult of slavery assumed a greater importance in their regional outlook."[16] Of Bruce's *DAB* scientists, 5.5 percent of those active in 1846 were born in the South; by 1861 the number had climbed to 9.3.[17] The South's sponsorship of scientific journals also increased markedly, rising from zero in the decade following 1810, to 1.9 percent

14. Eaton, *Mind of the Old South*, 224. Charles S. Sydnor raised this question in his review of Johnson's *Scientific Interests* in the *South Atlantic Quarterly*, XXXVII (1938), 221.

15. The South's production (by birth) of AAAS leaders declined from 11.9 percent in the 1800s, to 9.7 percent in the 1810s, to 6.6 percent in the 1820s, and to zero in the 1830s (Kohlstedt, *Formation of the American Scientific Community*, 209). Because those born from 1810 through the 1820s matured in the 1830s and 1840s, the significance of these figures is difficult to determine.

16. Elliott, "American Scientist," 66. Beaver found the number of scientists born in the South to remain virtually constant from 1810 through the 1840s (Beaver, "American Scientific Community," 351).

17. Bruce, "Statistical Profile," 76.

TABLE 5.

REGIONAL DISTRIBUTION OF SCIENTIFIC JOURNALS FOUNDED FROM 1771 TO 1849

Region	Journals
South	24 (7.1%)
Border	37 (11.0%)
New England	77 (22.8%)
Middle Atlantic	162 (48.1%)
North Central	36 (11.0%)

SOURCE: Adapted from George H. Daniels, *American Science in the Age of Jackson* (New York, 1968), 229–30.

in the 1820s, to 8.0 percent in the 1830s, and to 11.0 percent in the 1840s.[18]

Clearly, the notion of a golden age of southern science during the 1820s and early 1830s has little substance. As the Virginian John Holt Rice discovered in 1824 during a tour of the Northeast, his state already lagged woefully behind its northern neighbors in fostering science. In contrast to what he saw, Virginia had "no extensive philosophical apparatus . . . no great collections of subjects in natural history; no splendid cabinets of minerals; no botanical gardens; no anatomical preparations for the benefit of young citizens, for the excitement of their curiosity, and the aid of their researches."[19] Fortunately for the Old South, the situation got better, not worse.

What factors explain the Old South's failure to cultivate science at a level comparable to that of New England and the Middle Atlantic region, or even of the Border states? We can gather some clues by looking at the correlations between regional characteristics (for example, slavery, urbanization, education and literacy, wealth, and occupational patterns) and the residences of AAAS leaders, who, according to Kohlstedt, reflected the composition of the active scientific community in the United States during the last decade before the Civil War.[20]

18. Daniels, *American Science*, 229–30.

19. Quoted in Richard B. Davis, *Intellectual Life in Jefferson's Virginia, 1790–1830* (Chapel Hill, 1964), 177. Davis (p. 180) concedes that "Rice was right in observing that Virginia was behind in these matters."

20. Kohlstedt, *Formation of the American Scientific Community*, 190. AAAS participation does, however, seem to have been influenced by accessibility to meetings, a factor that

16

TABLE 6.
REGIONAL DISTRIBUTION OF SCIENTIFIC SOCIETIES IN AMERICA,
1855

Region	Societies
South	5 (14.3%)
New England	13 (37.1%)
Middle Atlantic	12 (34.3%)
North Central	4 (11.4%)
West	1 (2.8%)

SOURCE: Adapted from Ralph S. Bates, *Scientific Societies in the United States* (3rd. ed.; Cambridge, Mass., 1965), 51.

NOTE: Bates's North Central region includes Missouri, and his South includes Delaware, Maryland, Kentucky, and District of Columbia.

These correlations indicate that while neither slavery nor wealth greatly affected scientific activity, antebellum scientists tended to concentrate in urban areas that possessed libraries and a large commercial class (Table 7).

The reasons why slavery and science do not correlate become apparent when we consider the data presented in Table 3. If we look not only at the South, but at all slaveholding states, we see that the percentage of AAAS leaders in the slave states nearly equals the percentage of the nation's nonslave population in those regions. In fact, in 1860 the two are virtually identical: 30.5 percent of AAAS leaders and 30.4 percent of the nonslave population of the United States lived in slave states. In contrast, the North Central region, which had no slaves, supported far fewer AAAS leaders than its large population would suggest. Even in New England, the states of Maine, Vermont, and New Hampshire failed to produce scientists in proportion to their populations. Thus, the presence or absence of slavery has no predictive value in locating American scientists.

Although slavery may produce secondary effects inimical to science—for example, wasted time and energy devoted to its defense, an antipathy toward centralized government, and a predominantly agri-

---

may partially explain the underrepresentation of the South's largest city, New Orleans. The development of cultural institutions in New Orleans may also have suffered as a result of conflict between the English and French segments of the population and because of the city's large transient population.

TABLE 7.

CORRELATIONS BETWEEN REGIONAL CHARACTERISTICS AND AAAS LEADERS

Regional Characteristic	1850	1860
Slave population	−.166	−.226
Population density	.329	.406*
Urbanization: cities above 100,000	.438*	.482**
Urbanization: cities above 25,000	.376*	.614***
Urbanization: cities above 2,500	.499*	.659***
College students in population aged 15–24	.254	.044
College income per student	.295	.326*
Wealth per capita (nonslave)	.244	.000
Illiteracy (nonslave)	−.240	−.143
Persons per library volume (nonslave)	−.334	−.359*
Adult males in commerce (nonslave)	.365*	NA
Adult males in agriculture (nonslave)	−.408*	NA
Adult males in the professions (nonslave)	−.067	NA

*$p < .05$.
**$p < .01$.
***$p < .001$.

cultural economy—there are few historical or logical reasons for suspecting that slavery per se inhibits science. As Roger Hahn has argued in his study of the Paris Academy of Sciences, the pursuit of science depends less on specific social and political settings than on scientists being provided with "a modicum of financial support and intellectual independence."[21] The slave societies of ancient Greece gave birth to science as we know it today; it flourished under the despots of Ptolemaic Egypt, the absolute monarchs of early modern Europe, and the Communist rulers of the Soviet Union. A century and a half ago Alexis de Tocqueville thought that a democratic society like America's, which lacked an aristocratic leisure class, could not support theoretical science. "Permanent inequality of lot leads men to confine themselves to the proud and sterile search for abstract truths," he wrote, "while

21. Roger Hahn, *The Anatomy of a Scientific Institution: The Paris Academy of Sciences, 1666–1803* (Berkeley, 1971), 316 (see also p. x).

the institutions of democratic society tend to make them look only for the immediate practical applications of science."[22]

Slavery, instead of inhibiting science, could encourage it by giving slaveholders the leisure and wealth to pursue their scientific interests. In the late seventeenth century Virginia's leading botanist, John Banister, asked friends in London to send him "4 or 6 young negroes" so that he could achieve the financial independence needed to continue his botanizing.[23] Similarly, in the 1820s the University of Virginia provided its professor of chemistry, John Patten Emmet, with a personal slave to free the professor from mundane chores.[24]

The number of prominent southern scientists who owned slaves undercuts the argument that slaveholding led to habits of mind incompatible with rigorous scientific thought. Among slaveowning scientists were planters like Henry William Ravenel and James Hamilton Couper, southern-born college professors like John and Joseph LeConte, transplanted northerners like John Bachman and Frederick A. P. Barnard, and foreign immigrants like Andrew Brown, the lumber baron of Natchez, Mississippi.[25] Young Oscar Lieber, who lost his life in the Civil War, identified with the extreme secessionists in South Carolina and acquired a reputation as an outspoken defender of slavery.[26] These individuals represented the cream of the Old South's scientists. Ravenel was widely recognized as the country's leading authority on fungi. Barnard served as the antebellum South's only

22. Alexis de Tocqueville, *Democracy in America,* ed. Jacob P. Mayer and Max Lerner (New York, 1966), 427, 430 (quotation).

23. Joseph and Nesta Ewan, *John Banister and His Natural History of Virginia, 1678–1692* (Urbana, 1970), 75.

24. Stanley M. Guralnick, *Science and the Ante-Bellum American College* (Philadelphia, 1975), 103; Philip A. Bruce, *History of the University of Virginia, 1819–1919* (5 vols.; New York, 1920–1922), II, 16–17. Robert V. Bruce alleges that "several scientists deputized slaves as collectors in the field—a grotesque and barren forced marriage of oppression to enlightenment." Bruce, "Statistical Profile," 79.

25. Arney R. Childs (ed.), *The Private Journal of Henry William Ravenel, 1859–1887* (Columbia, S.C., 1947); Robert P. Brooks, "James Hamilton Couper," *Dictionary of American Biography,* IV, 468–69; John S. Lupold, "From Physician to Physicist: The Scientific Career of John LeConte, 1818–1891" (Ph.D. dissertation, University of South Carolina, 1970); William D. Armes (ed.), *The Autobiography of Joseph LeConte* (New York, 1903); [John B. Haskell and Catherine L. Bachman], *John Bachman, D.D., LL.D., Ph.D.: The Pastor of St. John's Lutheran Church, Charleston* (Charleston, S.C., 1888); William J. Chute, *Damn Yankee! The First Career of Frederick A. P. Barnard: Educator, Scientist, Idealist* (Port Washington, N.Y., 1978); John Hebron Moore, *Andrew Brown and Cypress Lumbering in the Old Southwest* (Baton Rouge, 1967). Joseph Jones, a physician-physiologist, also owned slaves (see Breeden, *Joseph Jones,* 7–8).

26. Lupold, "From Physician to Physicist," 93.

president of the AAAS and went from the presidency of the University of Mississippi to the presidency of Columbia University. John LeConte went from South Carolina College to the presidency of the University of California. Joseph LeConte, who followed his brother west, became a prominent geologist and ardent reconciler of science and religion.

An explanation much more plausible than slavery for the South's scientific record is its agricultural orientation, which discouraged the growth of urban centers of all sizes. Table 7 shows a significant negative correlation between agricultural employment and AAAS leaders; urbanization is by far the most accurate index of scientific ability. These results agree with all other statistical studies of the antebellum scientific community, which reveal that, despite the predominantly rural composition of American society, a markedly disproportionate number of scientists grew up and worked in urban areas.[27] Thus, as Elliott has previously concluded, "The lack of an urban culture in the South is more likely the reason for the very small number of scientists born there than was any constraint produced by the existence of slavery."[28]

Given the affinity between science and urban settings, we would expect to find the greatest concentration of scientists in the South's two largest cities, New Orleans (168,675 in 1860) and Charleston (40,522). However, during the 1850s only three AAAS leaders made their homes in New Orleans, two fewer than lived in tiny Charlottesville, Virginia (Table 8). The most likely explanation for New Orleans' weak participation in the AAAS was its geographical remoteness, which inhibited

27. See, for example, Kohlstedt, *Formation of the American Scientific Community,* 204, 209–10; Elliott, "American Scientist," 67–68; and Beaver, "American Scientific Community," 155–58, 205.

28. Elliott, "American Scientist," 76. Beaver, it should be noted, questions the value of urbanization in explaining the South's scientific record. "Although throughout this period [1800–1860] the population of the North-East and the South are nearly equal," he says, "by birthplace the North-East produces 91% of the scientists, the South 8.1%. . . . this difference is not strictly proportional to the greater urbanization of the North-East. About 40% of the white population of the United States lives in the South in this period. Supposing it to be entirely rural, it should produce at least 22% of the scientists on the list. That is, even supposing the South to be entirely devoid of the advantage of urbanization, it still underproduces scientists by nearly a factor of 3. Therefore there must be factors other than the urbanization of birthplace which are important in the making of a scientist" (Beaver, "American Scientific Community," 156). Several factors help to explain the difference between his and our conclusions: (1) He is dealing with birthplaces, while we are working with adult residences. (2) His assumption of roughly equal populations in the Northeast and South does not apply to the nonslave population in America (Tables 3 and 4). (3) If we accept the census definition of urban (that is, towns over 2,500), then, according to the data in Tables 3 and 4, the Northeast was over four times more urban than the South in 1850 and over five times more urban in 1860.

TABLE 8.

AAAS LEADERS IN THE SOUTH, 1850–1860

Alabama:
  Mobile
    Josiah Clark Nott
  Tuscaloosa
    Frederick A. P. Barnard
    John William Mallet
    Michael Tuomey
Georgia:
  Athens
    William Louis Jones
    John LeConte
    Joseph LeConte
    Charles F. McCay
  Culloden
    John Darby
  Darien
    James Hamilton Couper
  Macon
    Joseph LeConte
Louisiana:
  New Orleans
    Caleb G. Forshey
    John L. Riddell
    John Lawrence Smith
Mississippi:
  Jackson
    Joseph W. Matthews
    R. Morris*
  Natchez
    Andrew Brown
  Pontotoc
    Richard Bolton*
  Oxford
    Frederick A. P. Barnard
    Eugene W. Hilgard
North Carolina:
  Chapel Hill
    Alexander Fisher Olmsted
  Charlotte
    Daniel M. Barringer
    John Heysham Gibbon*

South Carolina:
  Charleston
    John Bachman
    Peter C. Gaillard
    Lewis R. Gibbes
    John E. Holbrook
    Francis S. Holmes
    Patrick N. Lynch
    William Middleton Michel
    James Moultrie
    Henry William Ravenel
    St. Julien Ravenel
  Columbia
    Robert W. Gibbes
    John LeConte
    Joseph LeConte
    Oscar M. Lieber
    Charles F. McCay
Tennessee:
  Knoxville
    Henri Erni
  Lebanon
    James M. Safford
  Nashville
    William Ferrel
    Benjamin C. Jillson
    Gerard Troost
Texas:
  Rutersville:
    Caleb G. Forshey
Virginia:
  Charlottesville
    Edward H. Courtenay
    William B. Rogers
    Robert E. Rogers
    John Lawrence Smith
    Francis H. Smith
  Portsmouth
    Nathan B. Webster

NOTE: Asterisks indicate that biographical information was not available.

communication with other cities and made attendance at AAAS meetings difficult.[29] We know from other sources that New Orleans supported a lively scientific community, even though few of its members joined national organizations like the AAAS. When twenty-seven residents founded the New Orleans Academy of Sciences in 1853, *De Bow's Review* crowed that "There is no city in the Union, of its size, containing a greater number of scientific men than New-Orleans; and no other city affording greater facilities for scientific research."[30]

Charleston, less remote geographically and more attuned culturally to the rest of the nation, presents a different story.[31] Dr. Augustus Addison Gould of Boston declared at the 1850 meeting of the AAAS in Charleston that South Carolina ranked "among the first in scientific inquiry, few States having preceded her in such efforts. . . . In Science, South-Carolina has stood almost alone in the South."[32] This was not a hollow compliment. In 1850 South Carolina's percentage of AAAS leaders was nearly five times greater than its percentage of the nonslave population in America, a mark surpassed only by the District of Columbia and Massachusetts. Ten years later its ratio had dropped to about four to one, but still it trailed only the District of Columbia, Massachusetts, and Connecticut. Although South Carolina had only

29. See Allan R. Pred, *Urban Growth and the Circulation of Information: The United States System of Cities, 1790–1840* (Cambridge, Mass., 1973), 55, 93.

30. "The New-Orleans Academy of Sciences," *De Bow's Review*, XVII (1854), 606; Johnson, *Scientific Interests*, 161–62.

31. Much has been written about Charleston's scientific community. See, for example, William M. Smallwood, *Natural History and the American Mind* (New York, 1941), 102–19; Raymond P. Stearns, *Science in the British Colonies of America* (Urbana, 1970), 593–619; G. Edmund Gifford, Jr., "The Charleston Physician-Naturalists," *Bulletin of the History of Medicine*, XLIX (1975), 556–74; and Joseph Ewan, "The Growth of Learned and Scientific Societies in the Southeastern United States to 1860," in Alexandra Oleson and Sanborn C. Brown (eds.), *The Pursuit of Knowledge in the Early American Republic: American Scientific and Learned Societies from Colonial Times to the Civil War* (Baltimore, 1976), 208–18.

32. American Association for the Advancement of Science, *Proceedings, Third Meeting . . . 1850* (Charleston, 1850), 214–15. The influence of the 1850 AAAS meeting in Charleston on South Carolina's scientific standing is difficult to assess. Although this session allowed a number of Charlestonians to become AAAS "leaders," we do not feel that it significantly skews the evidence. First, comparative studies based on other criteria (e.g., Elliott, "American Scientist") confirm South Carolina's leadership in the Old South. Second, the AAAS chose to meet in Charleston because it had already become the scientific center of the South. Third, the AAAS held only one of its twelve meetings from 1850 to 1860 in a southern city, thus giving host cities in the North a decided advantage in recruiting. Fourth, although several Charlestonians apparently participated only in 1850, not one of these became a leader solely on the basis of an honorary appointment to the Local Committee.

half the population of Virginia, it supported two and a half times as many scientists. Fifteen (34.9 percent) of the South's forty-three AAAS leaders in the 1850s lived in South Carolina, and ten of these (23.2 percent of the total) resided in Charleston (Table 8). Thus, when visitors complimented South Carolina on its scientific accomplishments, they were actually paying tribute to Charleston, which, to paraphrase Gould, stood almost alone in the antebellum South.

Away from Charleston and New Orleans, southern scientists languished in intellectual isolation. As early as 1773 a correspondent in the *Virginia Gazette* attributed the slow progress of science in the Old Dominion "to the Want of that Intercourse and Association which is necessary to the Perfection of every Power of Man, whether mental or bodily." The greatest need, he continued, was for "populous Cities, where Men of genius, from Motives of Amusement or Business reside together; of these we have a very distant Prospect Indeed."[33] The writer's pessimism was not unwarranted. Nearly seventy years later William Barton Rogers, the University of Virginia geologist who later served as the first president of the Massachusetts Institute of Technology, described life in the largely rural South as being "as dull as a mill-pond in a deep hollow where no breeze can touch it."[34] In 1856 Barnard wrote from Oxford, Mississippi, that "I have in reality been reduced to idleness and intellectual stagnation by the atmosphere of mental apathy which surrounds a devotee of science here. There is so little attention of mind with mind—there are so few who are intellectually active."[35] It is true, as Thomas Cary Johnson, Jr., concluded years ago, that "for the most part the scientists of the Old South led lonely lives, separated by many miles from fellow-workers in their chosen fields."[36] Science as a consequence suffered. As Rogers discovered in Charlottesville, "Solitude is, after all, no friend to Science."[37]

Deprived of colleagues at home, isolated southern scientists attached great value to contacts with friends in the scientific centers of the North. Men like Barnard and Rogers belonged to a transregional

33. Quoted in Carl Bridenbaugh, *Cities in Revolt: Urban Life in America, 1743–1766* (New York, 1955), 408–409.

34. [Emma Rogers (ed.)], *Life and Letters of William Barton Rogers* (2 vols.; Boston, 1896), 1, 181.

35. Chute, *Damn Yankee*, 159.

36. Johnson, *Scientific Interests*, 175. For additional complaints of scientific isolation, see *ibid.*, 61; Richard M. Jellison and Phillip S. Swartz, "The Scientific Interests of Robert W. Gibbes," *South Carolina Historical Magazine*, LXVI (1965), 81; and Charles S. Sydnor, *A Gentleman of the Old Natchez Region: Benjamin L. C. Wailes* (Durham, 1938), 171.

37. [Rogers (ed.)], *Life and Letters*, 1, 149.

scientific community, sustained by regular correspondence and occasional visits. "My chief stimulus of a truly exciting kind is received from your letters," Rogers wrote to his brother Henry Darwin Rogers, a geologist at the University of Pennsylvania; "they impart new life to me, and really make me happy in scientific ardour and hope."[38] During his years in Athens and Columbia, John LeConte relied on letters from Joseph Henry of the Smithsonian Institution, Alexander Dallas Bache of the Coast Survey, and especially Harvard's Benjamin Peirce to maintain "regular contact with the inner-workings of the scientific community."[39]

One of the many advantages of urban living was the availability of libraries, which, as is shown in Table 7, correlates with the presence of scientists. In 1850, however, the South possessed the poorest library resources of any region in the country. During the next decade it improved its collections spectacularly but still lagged behind New England by a ratio of one to three (Tables 9 and 10). At times, the absence of scientific books severely curtailed scientific activity. For example, in 1844, while collaborating with John James Audubon on *The Viviparous Quadrupeds of North America*, John Bachman complained to his son-in-law in New York City that "to go ahead with my work, I must have books for reference. Charleston is a poor place for scientific works. I am often sadly at a loss for books I desire to consult. . . . Sometimes, I have to set aside a species, for the lack of specimens and books. The books are to be found in New York and Philadelphia, but are expensive. I would not have you buy them; but could you not copy for me such articles as we need?"[40]

Throughout the antebellum period the South also suffered from relatively high illiteracy rates (Tables 9, 10), and even literate southerners often prided themselves more on their conversational skills than on book learning.[41] Before the British geologist Charles Lyell visited the South in the early 1840s, scientific acquaintances in the North warned him that "the hospitality of the planters might greatly interfere with my schemes of geologizing in the Southern states." To head off this problem, Lyell carried letters of introduction asking to excuse him

38. *Ibid*. See also Chute, *Damn Yankee*, 174.

39. Lupold, "From Physician to Physicist," 102, 105 (quotation).

40. [Haskell and Bachman], *John Bachman*, 202–203, 210. On the unavailability of books in Savannah, see Richard H. Shryock (ed.), *Letters of Richard D. Arnold, M.D., 1808–1876* (1929; rpr. New York, 1970), 19.

41. Clement Eaton, *The Freedom-of-Thought Struggle in the Old South* (New York, 1964), 57.

from "dinners and society," a request "every where kindly and politely complied with."[42]

The role of colleges in promoting science remains ambiguous. Table 7 shows no significant correlation between number of AAAS leaders and the percentage of young people age fifteen to twenty-four in college. Generally, the Old South compiled an enviable record in higher education. In 1850, for example, 0.38 percent of its youth were enrolled in college, compared with 0.36 percent in New England and the Middle Atlantic (Tables 9 and 10). But despite the South's commitment to higher education, it trained relatively few scientists, while the colleges in the Northeast trained more than three-fourths of all scientists in the country. As Kohlstedt has shown, Harvard and Yale alone educated 32 percent of the scientific leaders in America. Among the top ten scientist-producing schools, the South had only one: South Carolina College, which had five alumni that tied it for ninth place.[43]

Why, with its numerous colleges and ample financial support, did the South turn out so few scientists? The answer is far from clear, although we can suggest several contributing factors. Even though southern colleges routinely offered instruction in the various scientific disciplines, the sciences failed to dislodge the classics from their curricular pedestal.[44] Matthew Fontaine Maury, one of the Old South's most famous scientists, blamed the lack of scientific training on "the humbuggery of the Learned Languages." "When our young men leave college," he wrote in 1836, "most of them (some exceptions) are prepared as little for entering upon the world as they were when they entered college, the reason of this is that every young man is taught to believe Latin and Greek of the first importance; consequently everything that is solid & practical, such as mathematics, chemistry, & the like, is made to occupy a subordinate place & only a smattering of them is obtained."[45]

F. A. P. Barnard, the scientist-president of the University of Mis-

42. Charles Lyell, *Travels in North America, in the Years 1841–42* (2 vols.; New York, 1845), I, 123–24.

43. Kohlstedt, *Formation of the American Scientific Community*, 210–11. South Carolina College should be tied for eighth place because of six former students: Peter Cordes Gaillard, Lewis Reeves Gibbes, Robert Wilson Gibbes, Oscar Lieber, Josiah Clark Nott, and Henry William Ravenel.

44. Eaton, *Freedom-of-Thought Struggle*, 216–19. At the University of Virginia more students elected to study science than ancient languages, but its elective system was atypical (Johnson, *Scientific Interests*, 9).

45. Quoted in Eaton, *Mind of the Old South*, 239–40.

TABLE 9.
REGIONAL CHARACTERISTICS, 1850

Regional Characteristic	South	Border	Slave[1]	New England	Middle Atlantic	North Central	West	Free[2]	USA[3]
% Slave	38.6	16.5	33.2	0.0	0.0	0.0	0.0	0.0	13.8
Inhabitants per sq. mi.	9	21	10	42	59	16	0.1	6	7
% Urban (> 100,000)	1.6	7.1	3.0	5.0	14.5	2.4	0.0	8.2	6.0
% Urban (> 25,000)	2.6	13.8	5.3	7.8	20.3	3.1	18.8	11.7	9.1
% Urban (> 2,500)	5.8	16.9	8.5	28.7	25.5	8.9	[25.9]	20.4	15.4
% College students in pop. 15 to 24	0.38	0.61	0.44	0.36	0.36	0.42	0.00	0.37	0.40
College income per student in dollars	80	84	82	72	79	36	0	62	70
Wealth per capita in									

dollars (nonslave)	513	347	462	414	340	210	180	307	357
% Illiterate (nonslave)	9.2	8.2	8.9	1.9	3.3	4.3	16.9	3.6	5.3
Persons per library book (nonslave)	12.5	5.0	8.6	2.2	2.7	10.4	NA	3.5	4.3
% Adult males in commerce (nonslave)	19.2	26.4	21.4	36.8	36.9	22.4	69.4	33.1	29.5
% Adult males in agriculture (nonslave)	58.7	45.5	54.7	34.5	32.6	58.0	13.2	40.7	44.7
% Adult males in professions (nonslave)	2.3	1.9	2.2	1.6	1.5	1.7	1.0	1.6	1.8

SOURCE: U.S. Census, 1850.

[1]Figures in the Slave column represent the South and Border regions combined.

[2]Figures in the Free column represent the New England, Middle Atlantic, North Central, and West regions combined.

[3]Figures in the USA column represent the slave and free regions combined.

TABLE 10.
REGIONAL CHARACTERISTICS, 1860

Regional Characteristic	South	Border	Slave[1]	New England	Middle Atlantic	North Central	West	Free[2]	USA[3]
% Slave	38.7	13.5	32.1	0.0	0.0	0.0	0.1	0.0	12.6
Inhabitants per sq. mi.	12	28	14	46	74	21	0.5	9	10
% Urban (> 100,000)	1.9	11.6	4.4	5.7	22.1	3.5	0.0	11.0	8.4
% Urban (> 25,000)	3.0	15.6	6.3	14.7	27.9	5.2	7.8	15.7	12.0
% Urban (> 2,500)	6.9	20.2	10.3	36.6	35.4	13.5	15.1	25.9	19.8
% College students in pop. 15 to 24	0.74	0.86	0.77	0.41	0.33	0.76	0.47	0.52	0.62

College income per student in dollars	60	65	62	98	63	35	75	52	56
Wealth per capita in dollars (non-slave)	932	587	817	594	500	440	423	488	588
% Illiterate (nonslave)	7.4	6.8	7.2	2.7	3.0	3.2	8.1	3.2	4.4
Persons per library book (nonslave)	2.4	3.3	2.6	0.8	1.8	3.8	3.6	1.9	2.1

SOURCE: U.S. Census, 1860.

[1]Figures in the Slave column represent the South and Border regions combined.

[2]Figures in the Free column represent the New England, Middle Atlantic, North Central, and West regions combined.

[3]Figures in the USA column represent the slave and free regions combined.

sissippi, believed that the reluctance of southern colleges to purchase expensive scientific equipment drove many scientifically inclined students to the North. He estimated in the 1850s that perhaps half of the two hundred Mississippi youth then studying in the North went there because of that region's superior scientific attractions, which included newly created scientific schools at Harvard and Yale, the likes of which the South would not soon see.[46] For whatever reasons, northern colleges did in fact attract numerous students from the South. Nearly half of Princeton's student body in some years came from slaveholding states, and the percentage of southerners at Harvard and Yale often exceeded ten.[47]

Another possibility, suggested by one historian, is that "the standards of education in the South [before the Civil War] were not so high as those of the northern community."[48] Although this charge remains undocumented, it does conform to the findings of Robert H. Knapp and Hubert B. Goodrich for the period 1880 to 1941. The South, they found, ranked lowest of all regions in the production of scientists, in part because it suffered "a distinct liability in terms of the quality of its students," or so it seemed to Knapp and Goodrich.[49]

Finally, the semirural location of many of the South's colleges may have isolated them from the influences most conducive to the growth of science. Or is it merely coincidental that the leading scientist-producing colleges of the North tended to be located in urban, industrial centers?

Religion and climate, two untested factors, may also have retarded the South's scientific growth, though in both cases the evidence is inconclusive. Beginning at least with the Morison-Johnson exchange decades ago, historians have been speculating on the possible relationship between science and religion in the Old South. Morison argued that an illicit union between evangelical Christianity and the ideology of slavery gave birth to a "bastard puritanism" in the South inimical to science. Johnson responded to this by insisting that "the decaying deism of the South was a much more fertile soil for a time than the insufficiently rotted Calvinism of New England."[50] Clement

46. Chute, *Damn Yankee,* 166. Despite this charge, Barnard in 1858 valued the University of Mississippi's scientific collections and apparatus at nearly double the worth of the university's library (Guralnick, *Science,* x).

47. Charles F. Thwing, *A History of Higher Education in America* (New York, 1906), 254–55.

48. *Ibid.,* 257.

49. R. H. Knapp and H. B. Goodrich, *Origins of American Scientists* (Chicago, 1952), 39.

50. Morison, *Oxford History,* II, 16; Johnson, *Scientific Interests,* 198.

Eaton took Morison's side, maintaining that "by 1830 the deism and skepticism of the eighteenth-century Enlightenment had virtually disappeared in the South," leaving the field clear for the unimpeded growth of anti-intellectual sects, which flourished in the South in the decades just before the Civil War. More recently, however, E. Brooks Holifield has emphasized the "rationality" of the urban clergy in the Old South and their fondness for science.[51]

Examples of religious pressures adversely affecting science in the Old South are not difficult to find, though their significance should be assessed cautiously. In the early 1830s orthodox South Carolinians sought to remove Thomas Cooper from the presidency of the state college, in part because he taught that Genesis and geology did not agree.[52] Nearly three decades later Henry Hammond, professor of geology at the University of Georgia, created a stir in Athens by teaching that it took 22,000 years "to bring the earth to the present condition."[53] And, as William Stanton has shown, some southerners turned their backs on a politically attractive and scientifically respectable theory of human origins at least in part because it threatened to undermine the Scriptures.[54]

Although the North did not escape occasional skirmishes between clergy and scientists, such clashes seem to have persisted longer in the South. When Robert Wilson Gibbes, a physician-geologist from Columbia, attempted to vindicate "geology from suspicion of leading to infidelity" at the AAAS meetings in Charleston in 1850, Alexander Dallas Bache, the shocked northern president of the association, could scarcely believe at first that such assurances were still necessary. He learned, however, that "a lesser wave of the same class with that which rose to overwhelm geology some twenty years since, sweeps with

51. Clement Eaton, *The Civilization of the Old South: Writings of Clement Eaton*, ed. Albert D. Kirwan (Lexington, Ky., 1968), 181–82,185–86, quotation on 182; E. Brooks Holifield, *The Gentlemen Theologians: American Theology in Southern Culture, 1795–1860* (Durham, 1978), 77–85.

52. Dumas Malone, *The Public Life of Thomas Cooper, 1783–1839* (New Haven, 1926), 352, 356.

53. Edward J. Thomas, *Memoirs of a Southerner, 1840–1923* (Savannah, Ga., 1923), 31–32. E. Merton Coulter, *College Life in the Old South* (New York, 1928), 255, also refers to this incident. In the mid-1850s rumors alleged that John LeConte had led students at the University of Georgia into infidelity by teaching heretical ideas about the antiquity of the earth (E. Merton Coulter, "Why John and Joseph LeConte Left the University of Georgia, 1855–1856," *Georgia Historical Quarterly*, LIII [1969], 26).

54. William Stanton, *The Leopard's Spots: Scientific Attitudes Toward Race in America, 1815–59* (Chicago, 1960), 194. On the southern commitment to biblical anthropology, see also Thomas V. Peterson, *Ham and Japheth: The Mythic World of Whites in the Antebellum South* (Metuchen, N.J., 1978).

considerable force over the Southern portion of our Union, and requires to be stayed with judgment to subsidence."[55] During the 1850s the University of Virginia offered lectures "on the evidences of Christianity to counteract the tide of infidelity threatened by the new scientific investigations," and the Presbyterians of Mississippi voted to endow professorships on the connection of the natural sciences with revealed religion to defend against "the most insidious attacks [that] are made upon revealed religion, through the Natural sciences."[56] Such reactions suggest, at best, a defensive posture on the part of some southerners toward science and scientists.

The southern climate may also have taken a toll on science. In the eighteenth century, the physician-naturalist Alexander Garden of Charleston graphically described to an English correspondent why he did not pursue natural history with more enthusiasm:

> Our long & hot summers enervate & unbrace the whole System, so that our nervous system must convey fainter & duller representations of the External Beauties of nature that surround us, to our Souls than what you possibly can conceive. . . . [W]ere you to sweat out, for two or three summers, the finer parts of your good English blood and Animal spirits & have every Fibre & Nerve of your Body weakened, relaxed, enervated, & unbraced by a tedious Autumnal Intermittant under a sultry, suffocating & insufferable sun, you would then be made in some manner a judge of the reason of our want of taste or Fire. . . . [I]nstead of Fire & life of imagination, indifference and a gracefull despondency would overwhelm your mind.[57]

Such conditions not only sapped zeal for science and inconvenienced would-be investigators, but bred diseases that resulted in premature death. As Charleston's part-time resident Charles Upham Shepard explained to his friend Benjamin Silliman, "The shuttle seems to fly faster in the loom of human life within the tropics than in the temper-

---

55. A. D. Bache, "Remarks upon the Meeting of the American Association at Charleston, S. C., March, 1850," American Association for the Advancement of Science, *Proceedings, Fourth Meeting . . . 1850* (Washington, D.C., 1851). For Gibbes's views on geology and theology, see Jellison and Swartz, "Scientific Interests of Robert W. Gibbes," 88–89.

56. Eaton, *Freedom-of-Thought Struggle*, 326 (first quotation); Clement Eaton, "Professor James Woodrow and the Freedom of Teaching in the South," in George B. Tindall (ed.), *The Pursuit of Southern History: Presidential Addresses of the Southern Historical Association, 1935–1963* (Baton Rouge, 1964), 439 (second quotation).

57. Edmund Berkeley and Dorothy Smith Berkeley, *Dr. Alexander Garden of Charles Town* (Chapel Hill, 1969), 125. See also Abraham Vicker's complaint in Ewan, "Growth of Learned and Scientific Societies," 210.

ate zone."[58] The southern climate did not, however, always affect science adversely. We know, for example, that the comparative anatomist Jeffries Wyman, who suffered from tuberculosis, spent several winters in the 1840s teaching in Richmond in order to escape the harsh Massachusetts winters.[59]

What kind of scientist, then, worked in this land of slavery and plantations, small towns and inadequate libraries, oppressive summer heat, and evangelical preachers? Our profile of forty AAAS leaders (those listed in Table 8) who lived in the South between 1850 and 1860 indicates that the typical antebellum scientist was the son of a planter or farmer (39.1 percent) born in 1812 in a slaveholding state (52.5 percent).[60] South Carolina was the birthplace of 27.5 percent of southern scientists; 20.0 percent of the total came from Charleston alone. Thirty percent came from the North, 17.5 percent from abroad. Only two, both planters, attended neither college nor medical school. Sixteen (40.0 percent) of the scientists held M.D. degrees. Two, Eugene Woldemar Hilgard (Heidelberg) and John William Mallet (Göttingen), had earned Ph.D.s.[61]

Over three-fourths of the AAAS leaders in the South lived either in the cities of Charleston and New Orleans or in college towns. Half earned their living as college professors, while nearly a fourth (22.5

58. Gloria Robinson, "Charles Upham Shepard," in Leonard G. Wilson (ed.), *Benjamin Silliman and His Circle: Studies on the Influence of Benjamin Silliman on Science in America* (New York, 1979), 97. Stephen S. Visher in *Scientists Starred, 1903–1943, in "American Men of Science"* (Baltimore, 1947), 58, suggests that science suffered in the South because its climate attracted blacks and "the easy-going types of whites." On the southern climate, see also Bruce, "Statistical Profile," 79; and Robert V. Bruce, *The Launching of Modern American Science, 1846–1876* (New York, 1987), 62–63.

59. George E. Gifford, Jr., "Twelve Letters from Jeffries Wyman, M.D.: Hampden-Sydney Medical College, Richmond, Virginia, 1843–1848," *Journal of the History of Medicine,* XX (1965), 309–33.

60. In 1850 twenty-seven AAAS leaders listed a southern residence; in 1860 nineteen (including nine carryovers from 1850) did so. In addition, six leaders who were not members in 1850 or 1860 lived in the South during the 1850s. This gives a total of forty-three southern AAAS leaders, of whom we could find biographical data for forty. Notably absent from this group is Matthew Fontaine Maury, perhaps the Old South's best-known scientist; the explanation is that he lived in Washington, in the Border region.

61. The most popular northern colleges among southern AAAS leaders were Yale (4), West Point (3), Williams (2), and Rensselaer Polytechnic Institute (2). South Carolina College (6) led in the South, followed by the University of Georgia (4). For medical school, southern scientists favored the Medical College of South Carolina (6), the University of Pennsylvania (4), and the College of Physicians and Surgeons in New York City (3).

percent) practiced medicine.[62] Because there were fewer native southerners than there were academic positions, the South offered better
employment opportunities than New England, for example, which
produced more scientists than it could employ. "You will grow in the
south much faster than in the north," F. A. P. Barnard advised his
friend Edward Claudius Herrick, of New Haven.[63] Similarly, William
Barton Rogers passed up an opportunity to move to Philadelphia in the
mid-1830s, partly because his reputation in Virginia was rising so
rapidly that he believed he would "soon have no competition among
the scientific men of the State."[64] In Philadelphia he would be just one
of many fish in a large pond.

Southern scientists, as Clark Elliott has observed, tended to focus
their interests on the biological and geological sciences, commonly
called natural history, rather than on the physical sciences and mathematics.[65] Among the southern AAAS leaders whose scientific interests
are known, 21 (58.3 percent) specialized in natural history, including
geology, 7 (19.4 percent) in chemistry, 4 (11.1 percent) in physics and
astronomy, 3 (8.3 percent) in mathematics, and 1 (2.8 percent) in ethnology. Finally, southern scientists were more often Presbyterians and
Episcopalians than members of the larger, but less cerebral, Baptist and
Methodist churches.

Although science may not have been "the fairest cultural flower of
the South before the Civil War," it did grow on southern soil. If the
antebellum South did not give birth to an Asa Gray in botany, a Joseph
Henry in physics, or a Louis Agassiz in zoology, it did produce the
country's leading mycologist, Henry William Ravenel, its foremost
herpetologist, John Edwards Holbrook, and its most famous oceanog-
rapher, Matthew Fontaine Maury—to say nothing of J. Lawrence
Smith, William Barton Rogers, John Leonard Riddell, Joseph LeConte,
and others who made significant, if not seminal, contributions to nine-

62. In addition to the professors and physicians, there were four planters, two teachers, two ministers (or three if we count the unidentified Reverend R. Morris of Jackson,
Mississippi), one lawyer, one industrialist, and one engineer.

63. Chute, *Damn Yankee*, 76.

64. [Rogers (ed.)], *Life and Letters*, I, 112–13. See also Rogers's comments, I, 288.

65. Elliott, "American Scientist," 179. Richard Beale Davis has detected the same
emphasis among southern scientists during the colonial period (*Intellectual Life in the
Colonial South, 1585–1763* [3 vols.; Knoxville, Tenn., 1978], II, 986). On geology in the Old
South, see Charles S. Sydnor, "State Geological Surveys in the Old South," in David K.
Jackson (ed.), *American Studies in Honor of William Kenneth Boyd* (Durham, 1940), 86–109;
and James X. Corgan (ed.), *The Geological Sciences in the Antebellum South* (University, Ala.,
1982).

teenth-century science. Thomas Cary Johnson did not err in claiming to have discovered evidence of scientific interests in the Old South; his mistake lay in implicitly trying to prove equality with the North. The Old South failed to keep pace with the regions to its north, but this failure resulted more from demographic and environmental factors than from slavery-related mental attributes.

CHAPTER 2

SCIENCE IN THE ANTEBELLUM COLLEGE: THE UNIVERSITY OF GEORGIA, 1801–1860

Thomas G. Dyer

F ew aspects of the southern experience have been studied less systematically than the history of higher education. In the purportedly national surveys of the development of higher learning, the reader searches in vain for more than occasional reference to southern colleges and universities. Those interested in the history of southern higher education will find only slightly more in the major syntheses of southern history. By and large, these have leaned heavily on histories of individual colleges and universities, a genre unencumbered by excessive attention to historical context, critical analysis, or factual accuracy. Although a few institutional histories make real contributions to an understanding of southern higher education, most are ardently filiopietistic and represent unabashed paeans to the college allegedly under study.[1]

Thus, to begin even tentatively to address a complex and important topic such as science in the antebellum college requires more than a little foolhardiness in the absence of very much scholarship. Fortunately, however, a few articles and books provide insight into the role of science in southern institutions.

Although Stanley Guralnick has concentrated on the Northeast, he has laid very important groundwork with his study of science in fifteen

1. For recent national surveys of the history of American higher education, see John Brubacher and Willis Rudy, *Higher Education in Transition* (3rd ed.; New York, 1976); and Frederick Rudolph, *The American College and University: A History* (New York, 1962). Older studies include Charles F. Thwing, *A History of Higher Education in America* (New York, 1906).

36

antebellum colleges. Guralnick demonstrates that though the various sciences developed at slightly different paces throughout antebellum American colleges, they generally grew in importance. He couches his arguments in a criticism of traditional interpretations of antebellum higher education, which have perpetuated numerous hoary myths concerning the nineteenth-century college. His criticism is part of a recent reevaluation of antebellum higher education that confronts many of the assumptions and arguments of an older group of scholars.[2]

According to the older school of interpretation, the college of the colonial and Revolutionary period developed in a most positive fashion and showed great promise during the immediate post-Revolutionary years. After the turn of the century, however, colleges proliferated excessively, paid little heed to the needs of society, and became prisoners of "classical" higher education, denominationalism, or both. Richard Hofstadter, who adopted this view, labeled the antebellum years as the period of the "Great Retrogression" in American higher education. In his opinion, most of the nation's colleges stagnated during this time, awash in an outmoded and undesirable adherence to the classical tradition and forgetful of responsibilities to society at large. Hofstadter and other like-minded historians have pointed to southern colleges as the worst offenders during the "Great Retrogression" because of their attachment to the classical tradition and have adduced the allegedly large migration of southerners to northern schools as

2. Stanley M. Guralnick, *Science and the Ante-Bellum American College* (Philadelphia, 1975); Guralnick, "Sources of Misconception on the Role of Science in the Nineteenth Century American College," *Isis*, LXV (1974), 352–66; Guralnick, "The American Scientist in Higher Education, 1820–1910," in Nathan Reingold (ed.), *The Sciences in the American Context: New Perspectives* (Washington, D.C., 1979), 99–141. For a sampling of the scholarship that reevaluates antebellum higher education, see James Axtell, "The Death of the Liberal Arts College," *History of Education Quarterly*, XI (1971), 339–52; Hugh Hawkins, "The University Builders Observe the Colleges," *ibid.*, 353–62; David B. Potts, "American Colleges in the Nineteenth Century: From Localism to Denominationalism," *ibid.*, 363–80; and Natalie A. Naylor, "The Ante-Bellum College Movement: A Reappraisal of Tewksbury's Founding of American Colleges and Universities," *History of Education Quarterly*, XIII (1973), 261–74.

For an enthusiastic and somewhat polemical account of the importance of science in antebellum southern colleges, see Thomas Cary Johnson, Jr., *Scientific Interests in the Old South* (New York, 1936), 11–45. For a recent article that probes the influence of science at Transylvania University, see Eric H. Christianson, "The Conditions for Science in the Academic Department of Transylvania University, 1799–1857," *Register of the Kentucky Historical Society*, LXXIX (1981), 305–25.

conclusive evidence of the substantial inferiority of colleges below the Mason-Dixon Line.[3]

All of this has considerable relevance to the place of science in the antebellum college. If science received little or no serious emphasis in the colleges, then the argument that the classics and classical tradition dominated education would have merit. If, however, the sciences were alive and well in southern colleges, then it would appear that these schools might not have been so conservative and tradition bound as is generally thought.

Whether we examine northern, midwestern, or southern colleges, most of the important questions remain the same: How did science develop within the antebellum collegiate curriculum? To what extent were institutional resources allotted to the sciences? How was science taught in the colleges? How strongly were scientists represented on college faculties? Did colleges engage in scientific activity outside the classroom? Of what importance was the use of scientific instruments and apparatus? Who were the professors of science and how able were they? How did the colleges respond to societal needs for scientific instruction?

Although it will not be possible to provide complete answers to these questions here, an examination of the importance of the sciences in one southern institution may provide some important clues. The University of Georgia, chartered in 1785 and opened in 1801, is an apt subject for such an analysis because its history spans the entire first half of the nineteenth century and because it typifies, in many respects, the emergent state universities of the post-Revolutionary and antebellum periods.[4]

During the colonial period the only college south of the Potomac was the College of William and Mary, established in 1696. The Revolution-

3. This explanation appears in George P. Schmidt, "A Century of the Liberal Arts College," in William Brickman and Stanley Lehrer (eds.), *A Century of Higher Education: Classical Citadel to Collegiate Colossus* (New York, 1962); Allan Nevins, *The State Universities and Democracy* (Urbana, 1962); Frederick M. Mumford, *The Land Grant College Movement* (Columbia, Mo., 1940); Richard Hofstadter, *Academic Freedom in the Age of the College* (New York, 1961); and Richard Hofstadter, "The Revolution in Higher Education," in Arthur M. Schlesinger, Jr., and Morton White (eds.), *Paths in American Thought* (Boston, 1963), 269–90.

4. The best history of the antebellum University of Georgia is E. Merton Coulter, *College Life in the Old South* (Athens, Ga., 1973). Less satisfactory is Robert P. Brooks, *The University of Georgia Under Sixteen Administrations* (Athens, Ga., 1955). See also Thomas G. Dyer, *The University of Georgia: A Bicentennial History, 1785–1985* (Athens, Ga., 1985), from which portions of this paper are derived.

ary era witnessed the foundings of several tiny institutions in the South, including the College of Charleston and Hampden-Sydney College, which at first struggled to survive. Soon after the war they were joined by numerous other institutions in the South, the Northeast, and the Midwest. By 1800, therefore, higher education in the South, like higher education in the Midwest and the more rural reaches of New England and the Middle Atlantic states, had barely begun. Over the ensuing sixty years before the outbreak of the Civil War, colleges would proliferate throughout the United States. In the South and the Midwest in particular, numerous institutions would be established that would lend credence to the traditional disparagement of the character of antebellum higher education, but other institutions would appear that would make creditable, even significant, contributions to the development of American higher education.

The proliferation of "colleges" in the South and in every other settled region of the country would mislead later historians to conclude that hundreds of institutions of higher education had been established in the South and elsewhere. In fact, the term "college" was used broadly to encompass a variety of institutions, ranging from what would be termed primary schools today through those that did offer collegiate-level instruction. The number of institutions offering collegiate-level instruction was actually quite small. Probably fewer than one hundred schools offered a level of instruction and degree of rigor that would permit them to claim status as institutions of higher learning.

In the South, as in the Midwest, the state university movement developed gradually. Before the Civil War, state universities were established in eight southern states, Georgia (chartered 1785, opened 1801), North Carolina (chartered 1789, opened 1796), Tennessee (1794), South Carolina (1801), Virginia (1819), Alabama (1831), Mississippi (1848), and Louisiana (1860), and in seven midwestern states, Ohio (1804), Michigan (1817), Indiana (1820), Missouri (1839), Iowa (1847), Wisconsin (1849), and Minnesota (1851). The founding dates of the universities in these states reflect the gradual and nearly parallel development of public higher education in the two regions.

Although chartered in 1785 in the first blush of post-Revolutionary fervor as the first state university in the new nation, the University of Georgia had neither students, professors, nor physical facilities until 1801, five years after the University of North Carolina opened its doors. During the hiatus, however, the governing board of the phantom college devised a six-year curriculum that included four years of standard collegiate fare but had only a slight emphasis on science. When the college did open, it had a president who took a different view of collegiate education.[5]

A mathematician and scientist with a strong interest in meteorology and physics, Josiah Meigs would be the only noncleric to head the college until the late 1890s. For six years prior to his appointment, Meigs had been a professor of natural philosophy at Yale College, but was chased from Yale because of his Jeffersonian views. The course of study that Meigs designed for the new college had clear elements of Jeffersonian educational philosophy imbedded in it. Weary of the heavy religious atmosphere at Yale, the new president gave a pronounced secular character to the college and was encouraged by Jefferson, who wrote of his hope that the example being set in the new colleges of the middle and southern states would ultimately break the "clerical chains" that bound New England colleges.[6]

Meigs's curriculum contained the standard ingredients of the traditional four-year liberal arts program of the late eighteenth century, including an emphasis on Latin and Greek, the classics, moral philosophy, mental philosophy, and the sciences. The first curriculum provided no scientific studies for freshmen and only a little more for sophomores. Juniors studied natural philosophy and astronomy "with the application of its principles to the determination of Geographic longitudes and latitudes by observations of solar eclipses, by the eclipses of Jupiter's satellites and by the lunar observations." Science, in all possible cases, would be taught by experiment. Chemistry, new to the college curriculum, would include "actual experiments demonstrative of its principles." Meigs selected botany for study during the junior year and required students to learn the Linnaean system of classification. During the senior year, Georgia had very little science in its course of study. Thus, despite Meigs's strong personal interest in the sciences, the initial curriculum at Georgia conformed largely to the liberal arts curriculum at the better American colleges.[7]

Meigs's selection of texts included Ferguson's *Astronomy,* Ewing's *Practical Astronomy* and the well-known natural philosophy text by

5. Minutes of the Senatus Academicus of the University of Georgia, 1799–1872, pp. 16–17, in the University of Georgia Archives.

6. Coulter, *College Life,* 14–16; Minutes of the Board of Trustees of the University of Georgia, June 17, 1801, pp. 33–36, in the University of Georgia Archives (hereinafter cited as Trustee Minutes); Thomas Jefferson to Josiah Meigs, May 20, 1802, in William Meigs, *Life of Josiah Meigs* (Philadelphia, 1887), 125–26.

7. Trustee Minutes, June 17, 1801.

Enfield. In ordering the first books for the college library, Meigs selected a much wider range of scientific treatises, including Vaello on electricity, Priestley on air, Chaptal's *Chemistry*, Fourcroy's *Chemistry*, and Erasmus Darwin's *Zoonomia*. Of the thirty books Meigs ordered, twenty had a strong mathematical or scientific orientation and included works on botany, hydrostatics, fluxions, mechanics, and other branches of natural philosophy. Meigs insisted that the institution acquire philosophical apparatus and also ordered a mercurial thermometer and a barometer.[8]

President Meigs's orientation to the scientific extended beyond curriculum design and text selection into a primitive type of research. Although he considered himself a mathematician, he often undertook decidedly scientific experiments and especially delighted in measuring the flow of water from springs. In addition, he took it upon himself to instruct the local populace in the science of meteorology and occasionally wrote letters to newspapers in Georgia explaining meteorological phenomena. Evidence of some community interest in the scientific appeared when the trustees of the institution required nonmembers of the college to pay $10 for the privilege of attending Meigs's lectures in natural philosophy.[9]

In his first written report to the Board of Trustees, President Meigs seemed generally optimistic but complained to the trustees of the delay in procuring philosophical apparatus, noting that upperclassmen had been "subjected to peculiar inconveniences and embarrassments in their progress, from want of Books and Instruments." When word came that the scientific equipment had left London on its way to Athens, Meigs rejoiced and reported to the board that the apparatus "will be at least equal in real utility to any . . . belonging to any literary institution in the United States." The trustees, who appeared to share Meigs's enthusiasm for scientific matters, authorized the president to purchase whatever additional equipment he thought necessary for the university.[10]

Relations between Meigs and the Board of Trustees did not remain amicable for long. Increasingly, the conservative Federalists who made

8. *Ibid.*

9. Coulter, *College Life,* 16; Trustee Minutes, May 31, 1805. Meigs measured the flow of the campus spring in gallons, investigated the formation of hail, and also conducted a study of the magnetic needle for the United States Congress. By using formulas for measuring the speed of falling bodies, he determined that the fallen angels of the Bible fell 1,832,308,363+ miles in nine days and inferred that this indicated the depths of Hell.

10. Trustee Minutes, November 11, 1803, and May 31, 1804.

up the board believed that they would prefer a more conventional college president, one of their own political stripe and one who could project a more pious image to the state's denominationalists, who were then attacking the university. Within a short time, the board decided that it would no longer tolerate the iconoclastic Meigs, who had also incurred the wrath of an influential local cleric, and first reduced him in rank to professor of natural philosophy and then fired him. One of Meigs's enemies on the board quoted him as saying that "they [the trustees] had made him Professor of Natural Philosophy and Chemistry, and given him a poor pitiful salary of twelve hundred dollars—damn them, he reckoned they would make him next Professor of Cabbages and Turnips."[11]

During the next five years the University of Georgia came perilously close to extinction as enrollments dropped dramatically. Gradually, however, the institution gathered strength under its new president, Moses Waddel, a Presbyterian minister, and remained relatively stable throughout the antebellum period. Under Waddel and his clerical successor, Alonzo Church, the importance of science grew steadily as curriculum and faculty expanded, and the college acquired some of the accoutrements that indicated a commitment to scientific study.

Until the early 1830s, the curriculum underwent little change, but by the middle years of the decade, an exfoliation of the program in science had begun. A professor of natural history joined the faculty, bringing the total to three professors of science and mathematics in a faculty of six. By 1834, botany had entered the sophomore course of study, and the junior year, traditionally heavy with scientific subjects, included navigation, engineering, fluxions, natural philosophy, natural history, and additional mathematics. Seniors continued studies of natural philosophy and added astronomy and physics. Of the thirteen subjects covered during the junior year, seven were in science or mathematics.[12]

By 1839, both curriculum and faculty reflected additional change. Now the seven-member faculty included three professors of natural philosophy and allied subjects and a newly appointed professor of civil engineering and natural philosophy, Charles McCay. At the request of the trustees, the faculty presented in the annual catalog a detailed description of the course of study that revealed the emphasis on science at Georgia. Hydrostatics, hydraulics, pneumatics, acoustics, elec-

11. Trustee Minutes, August 4, 1811, August 8, 1811, and August 22, 1811.
12. *Catalog of the Officers and Students of Franklin College, 1834–35.*

tricity, magnetism, and optics all crowded under the capacious umbrella of "natural philosophy." Taught over a two-year span, the course rested in part on Olmsted's text, which had replaced the venerable but badly outdated Enfield. Chemistry, taught in the junior year, involved the study of the elements, "application of chemistry to the arts; the phenomena of caloric, radiant, sensible, and latent [heat]; [and] galvanic electricity." Astronomy students concentrated on the study of gravity, refraction, nutation, aberration, eclipses, occultation, comets, "fixed stars," uranographical problems, theories of the sun and moon, and the theory of the planets. Botany emphasized taxonomy and practical lessons in the botanical garden, while geology, taught separately, stressed the fundamental principles of that discipline. By 1839, the college had increased its emphasis on mechanics and offered physics at what would today be considered a basic level. More significantly, the arrival of Professor McCay permitted the addition of both differential and integral calculus, and in 1840, McCay taught the institution's first course in civil engineering. The curriculum remained virtually unchanged until 1855, when a benefactor endowed a chair in agriculture. A yearlong series of lectures in that subject did not, however, become a part of the regular curriculum.[13]

The early concern that adequate philosophical apparatus be acquired persisted throughout the period, and the trustees repeatedly made significant appropriations for the purchase of scientific instruments. Even during the interim between the administrations of Meigs and Waddel, the college continued to show concern for the scientific side of the curriculum and especially for the deteriorating state of the apparatus. When a donor gave the college $1,000, its first sizable gift, the board quickly appropriated the money for the purchase of additional apparatus. And remarkably, during a time of great institutional stress, the new professor of natural philosophy, Henry Jackson, received "discretionary power to extend his purchases to the sum of two thousand dollars more." Within a few years $4,000 more had been allotted for purchase of apparatus and an additional $1,000 to make alterations in the "apparatus room."[14]

The purchase of so much expensive equipment made the guardians of the institution concerned about its care and maintenance. The apparatus seemed especially liable to injury from unsupervised use by the

13. *Catalog, 1839–40.* See also the catalogs for 1841 through 1855. Guralnick suggests that the four-of-seven proportion was typical of the more progressive northern colleges (Guralnick, *Science,* 42–43).

14. Trustee Minutes, July 25, 1816, December 10, 1817, and November 23, 1820.

undergraduates, so the college declared that only juniors and seniors could use the various pieces of equipment and then only with professorial permission. In addition, the college purchased a number of airtight and dust-free cases to house the sensitive instruments. The financial outlay also made the trustees concerned about whether the faculty used the apparatus to the fullest extent. Consequently in 1822, the board complained strongly that they "were unequivocally dissatisfied" with the annual examination of seniors "and especially the part of which would require the use of the philosophical apparatus for demonstration." The board investigated further and determined that the apparatus had not been "sufficiently used in the Course of Instruction" and resolved that "in all the demonstrative sciences connected with the Collegiate Course in which the Philosophical Apparatus is necessary for illustration that it on no occasion be dispensed with." Although a desire for enhanced institutional status doubtless moved the trustees to place such a heavy emphasis on the acquisition of scientific apparatus, they may have valued it most for its presumed effectiveness in improving instruction by moving science from the abstract to the demonstrable.[15]

Concerns about the apparatus crowd the pages of the institutional records for the remainder of the antebellum period. More often than not, these concerns focused on the need for new equipment to prevent the college from falling behind sister institutions. In 1822, when the popular science professor Henry Jackson declared the chemical apparatus deficient, the trustees quickly responded with an appropriation of $1500 for new equipment and established a permanent fund of $300 per year for the purchase of chemicals and the hire of a laborer and a slave to assist in maintenance. Although no complete list of the equipment survives, orders for individual items indicate that the science professors at Georgia sought to acquire the latest available instruments. In 1827, Professor Jackson purchased a deflagrator, and by 1829 the collection housed two ediometers and a calorimeter. The trustees also ordered additional unnamed equipment from France during that year. By 1832, the college had acquired its own telescope at a cost of $800 and had begun to discuss the construction of an observatory.[16]

During the early 1850s a growing interest in applied science derived in part from the depletion of southern soil and an awakening interest in industrialization led to the purchase of scales and weights for analyz-

15. Trustee Minutes, June 19, 1821, and April 10, 1822.
16. Trustee Minutes, November [?], 1822, August 1, 1827, August 4, 1829, and August 1, 1832.

ing soils and mineral waters. In addition, the guardians of the college directed that "Mr. Mellon's instrument for illustrating the Laws of Radiant Heat" be purchased. Soon, more sophisticated meteorological instruments joined the collection, as did a compound microscope. The trustees noted the "high place" that microscopes occupied in scientific investigation and declared that one should be acquired to enable professors to repeat experiments for classes and "to aid in original researches." When the much-desired instrument arrived, the committee charged with inspection of philosophical apparatus nearly swooned over this "very superior instrument," noting "the solidity of the frame, the ingenuity of the accessory of apparatus and the perfection of the lenses." To enhance the instrument even further, orders went out for more lenses of higher power. Two years later, a polarizing apparatus, a stuescope (?) and tools to maintain the equipment became a part of the apparatus.[17]

At various times during the 1850s the college acquired other instruments, including a magnito electrical machine, a gyroscope, surveying equipment, a "new and improved" air pump, and instruments for "experiments on the earth, vibrations, electricity and sounds, also on light and one or two instruments connected with hydraulics." In addition, the trustees purchased two skeletons and diagrams for use in scientific instruction. Before the Civil War broke out, the collection included instruments for the study of acoustics, pneumatics, and electricity; a "sans bath"; and a table for blowing glass. In the late 1850s, ventilation problems developed in the chemical laboratory requiring "means to carry off noxious vapors and gases generated during performance of experiments." Installation of ventilators would prevent the "stampedes of the class from the room [which] often occur."[18]

The college also began very early to collect mineralogical specimens, and like most antebellum colleges, provided for a special cabinet in which to house the collection. The trustees appropriated $500 for acquisition of specimens in 1831 and made smaller appropriations throughout the remainder of the period. Institutional records do not make clear the extent of the collection, but an atmosphere of self-congratulation infused the annual reports of the committee charged with its supervision. Occasionally, related items were added to the collection, including shells and fossils, and in one instance the college

17. Trustee Minutes, August 27, 1850, August 5, 1851, July 31, 1854, and August 2, 1853.

18. Trustee Minutes, July 31, 1854, July 25, 1855, August 3, 1856, August 2, 1853, August 8, 1857, August 3, 1858, and August 5, 1858.

made provisions for acquiring casts of rare fossils. Considerable interest in mining and geology existed in Georgia, and the college responded by giving the mineralogical collection a local flavor. Thus, in 1848 the trustees established a "Georgia Department" in the collection.[19]

While interest in the mineral cabinet and apparatus remained high throughout the antebellum period, the adjunct to the scientific curriculum that most often occupied the trustees, the faculty, and the president was the botanical garden established in 1833. From the outset the garden captured the interest of the college community and local citizens. If contemporary accounts are to be believed, its fame spread throughout the nation, even to distant New York, where a newspaper carried a glowing account of its wonders.[20]

Enthusiasm for the garden persisted for some time. A group of trustees returned from an inspection in 1834 full of confidence about the garden's future and with warm congratulations for Malthus Ward, the professor of natural science who inspired the garden's foundation. The committee recommended a much-increased appropriation for the next year with the observation that "these objects . . . furnish of themselves a wide field of study and Science. Their importance in the business of life and interests of society are daily becoming more manifest." "A taste for such pursuitts [sic]," the group's spokesmen observed, would "more and more be regarded as a necessary part of a liberal education." Four hundred dollars went to the improvement of the garden and the "sun house." Throughout the life of the garden, college officials argued that it would prove to be an important instructional resource, an important vehicle for horticultural experimentation, and an aesthetically pleasing adjunct to the university. The garden did prove to be an attractive and popular place, and some unsuccessful efforts were made to convert it into an experimental plot, but whether it contributed in any significant way to instruction in the botanical and horticultural sciences is unclear since no faculty or student commentary on this point has survived.[21]

By 1835, the trustees had grown even more convinced of the utility and importance of the garden and suggested enlarging the total area to 2.5 acres. The garden was expanded and a gardener hired at a total cost of $450. Appropriations for the plot gradually climbed over the next

19. Trustee Minutes, August 4, 1831, August 1, 1837, August 3, 1841, August 2, 1848, and passim.
20. Coulter, College Life, 41–43.
21. Trustee Minutes, August 5, 1834.

few years, but with expenses rising, the trustees decided to establish an "experimental fruit garden" that would make the entire operation self-sustaining through the sale of fruit trees. "At the same time," the board observed, "dissemination of fruit trees suited to our soil and climate would confer an important benefit on the state." The gardener set out fruit trees, but it quickly became apparent that revenues would not cover the expense of garden maintenance.[22]

Criticism of the garden evoked another justification for the enterprise from university officials, who argued that students derived important benefits that made it well worth the expense. The garden would continue to provide "tempting and stimulating investigation into natural Sciences, leading to useful and manly exercises having a fine effect in morals and health."[23]

By 1842, the garden had become so expensive and consumed such a significant percentage of the institution's scarce funds that the board contemplated abandonment but ultimately decided to continue it at a reduced rate of support under the supervision of a group of local trustees, the prudential committee. This group, which acted for the board between meetings, thought that the garden should possibly be abandoned, but an improved financial picture soon allowed for a slight increase in the appropriation.[24]

The garden's supporters subsequently hit on another device for saving it and argued that a "rapidly increasing taste for ornamental gardening should insure an income from the sale of plants more than sufficient to defray" the expenses of repairs and cost of plants. In addition, they would mount an effort to convince the residents of Athens of the garden's value and seek contributions for its maintenance.[25]

In the early 1850s, the fortunes of the garden improved when the greenhouse was renovated and a new scaffolding added to the display area. The most significant change, however, came with the introduction of running water into the greenhouse and other parts of the garden "for the purpose of irrigation." The trustees also thought that the garden's ornamental features stood in need of enhancement, so they ordered the installation of "*jets d'eau.*" Such trappings may have worried the science faculty since the trustees felt compelled to add that while the main purpose of instruction in botany should be kept in

22. Trustee Minutes, August 3, 1835, November 12, 1828, and August 5, 1839.
23. Trustee Minutes, August 7, 1839, and August 4, 1841.
24. Trustee Minutes, November 13, 1843, and August 7, 1844.
25. Trustee Minutes, August 5, 1846.

47

view, the garden could be exhibited to the public and "especially to the student as a model garden of taste and beauty."[26]

The botanical garden continued to be a point of contention in the university community for the remainder of the decade, and some evidence suggests that it precipitated a larger dispute over the worth of science in the curriculum. The trustees, in response to the critics, collectively mounted a defense of the study of science that reveals in sharp detail the value they attached to scientific learning.

World history would show, they argued, that the "natural sciences have been cherished in exact proportion to the advance of civilization." In Georgia, the need for scientific investigations of natural phenomena demanded that the state's university heed the advancing importance of systematic scientific study. Doing away with the botanical garden would deal a severe blow to a state where "the study of natural Science is not appreciated properly" and the linkages between higher education and economic development were little understood. The trustees lamented that nearly all of the other states had initiated "inquiries into their Nat. History at the public expense," but nothing had as yet been done in Georgia. "To aid in removing this reproach," they resolved to improve the botanical garden, expand the mineralogical cabinet and "bring up the library in the department of Natural Science by special appropriation to an equality with other departments of Science and learning." A substantial minority of the board objected to further commitment of support to the garden and moved to abandon it altogether. A vote of twelve to seven rejected the motion and showed that the twenty-year-old romance with the botanical garden had not ended. The details of the garden's ultimate fate are obscure; apparently it was sold in 1856, and the $1,000 obtained through its sale was used to construct an iron fence around the campus.[27]

Expensive apparatus and a botanical garden would have amounted to little, of course, without the essentially able faculty members who were responsible for the scientific portion of the curriculum. Josiah Meigs, the first professor of natural philosophy, had solid training at Yale and a good reputation as a mathematician. Henry Jackson, his successor, took responsibility for assembling the apparatus and guided the development of the scientific curriculum in the early days. Other

26. Trustee Minutes, August 5, 1850.
27. Trustee Minutes, August 2, 1853, 229–32; Coulter, *College Life*, 43; W. Porter Kellam (ed.), "Reminiscences of the Original Botanical Garden of the University of Georgia," *Newsletter, University of Georgia, The Friends of the Botanical Garden*, XI (Fall 1982), 20.

professors of science at Georgia developed strong reputations, and during the early and mid-1850s, a first-rate faculty resided in Athens. The LeConte brothers, Joseph and John, both taught in the university, as did William Louis Jones and Charles F. McCay, all recognized leaders in southern scientific circles. Jones and Joseph LeConte were two of the first four graduates of the Lawrence Scientific School and had studied with Louis Agassiz. John D. Easter, the college's first doctor of philosophy, replaced Joseph LeConte in 1858. Although the remoteness of Athens militated against close and frequent contact with leading scientists throughout the nation (similar situations no doubt existed in midwestern colleges), Joseph LeConte did not think the university inconducive to scientific study and intellectual life in general.[28]

At times, science professors enjoyed some advantages not shared by their colleagues in other areas of the college. In the 1820s, for example, Henry Jackson received a higher salary, a precedent only occasionally honored throughout the period but one that guaranteed at least parity with nonscientists. In addition, Jackson sought and won release from performing "police duties" customarily assigned to professors. When the remainder of the faculty objected, the trustees broke their agreement with Jackson, who quickly resigned. A compromise resulted in Jackson's return and his being excused from some disciplinary duties.[29]

Another attempt by science professors to win release from the bothersome task of policing student behavior triggered a significant battle in the university fought at least in part over the place of science in the curriculum and the role of the science professoriat. In the mid-1850s John LeConte registered protests over time spent by faculty in constabulary duties, but the protests did not move the irascible old president of the institution, Alonzo Church. President Church's public criticism infuriated the young professor, who also began to vent his feelings publicly. LeConte complained that the disciplinary duties impeded his ability to prepare adequately for laboratory exercises. Church responded with an attack that suggested that LeConte's scientific inclinations had led him toward "infidel sentiments." Newspapers throughout the state came to LeConte's defense and declared that if the esteemed scientist should leave, it would cause a "state of calam-

28. See the University of Georgia college catalogs, 1845–60; see also William D. Armes (ed.), *The Autobiography of Joseph LeConte* (New York, 1903), 157.
29. Trustee Minutes, August 14, 1822, November 9, 1824, August 3, 1825, and August 5, 1825.

ity." Joseph LeConte soon entered the fray, and sentiment against Church increased. Calls for the president's resignation came from several quarters and by autumn, 1856, the conflict combined with other problems to lower enrollment from nearly two hundred to a pitiful seventy-nine. Soon the Board of Trustees called for the resignation of the entire faculty. Initially all were accepted, but ultimately Church and a professor who had avoided the dispute were rehired.[30]

The trustees responded to the problems of the institution by appointing an investigative commission that devised a plan to restructure the university thoroughly. The plan, first proposed in 1855, won adoption and was partially implemented in 1859. Now the university would be divided into four different schools: a school of modern languages and literature, and by "public demand," schools of law, applied science, and agriculture. The school of applied science was to be frankly utilitarian in its content and organization. Instruction would be provided to young men with the intention of preparing them to be engineers, manufacturers, agriculturalists, chemists, and miners. Mathematical and scientific concepts would be used in the study of masonry, stonecutting, and civil and mechanical engineering. The school would also emphasize the application of mechanics to machinery and engineering, and "the science of construction in all its branches."[31]

In the school of agriculture, a laboratory would be established primarily for the scientific analysis of soils and manures, the assaying of ores and minerals, and "the quantitative and qualitative analysis of mineral waters." In the laboratory budding young chemists would also analyze and test drugs and study food preservation. A "desirable appendage" to the school would be an "experimental farm, where the principles of agriculture could be illustrated by practice." Fears of a South made agriculturally sterile by one-crop agriculture and insuffi-

30. During the dispute, the trustees passed a rule that made it possible for students to rise with their class even if they had not satisfactorily completed prescribed courses in mathematics and science. Coulter interprets this episode as an indication of the hostility of the trustees to science, but it appears to be no more than a temporary aberration in the generally favorable treatment the sciences received at the hands of the board. The politics of the moment no doubt occasioned the trustee action, which may have been related to the rising sentiment for utilitarianism, a doctrine opposed by most of the faculty. E. Merton Coulter, "Why John and Joseph LeConte Left the University of Georgia," *Georgia Historical Quarterly*, LIII (1969), 19–20; Coulter, *College Life*, 27–28, 35–37. The best account of the LeConte-Church episode is in Lester D. Stephens, *Joseph LeConte: Gentle Prophet of Evolution* (Baton Rouge, 1982), 45–52.

31. Trustee Minutes, April 9, 1855, July 30, 1855, and November [?], 1855.

cient attention to conservation moved the trustees to suggest that the state issue bonds for the support of the school.[32]

In justifying the establishment of a school of applied science, the trustees acknowledged that there had been frequent objections to traditional liberal education. Critics charged that the liberal arts did not "sufficiently prepare the mind for the active duties of life" and were simply not practical. The board lamented the absence of a school of applied science in the South and pointed to the technological schools already established in the North. Technological education had been pioneered at the Rensselaer Institute and at West Point in the early 1820s, and in the late 1840s and early 1850s, a few other institutions, including Brown, Dartmouth, Pennsylvania, and Union, had added divisions that emphasized such things as civil engineering, mining, and manufacturing. "The universal experience," the board noted, "is that of success." Georgia's school of applied science would be divided into three departments: engineering, practical chemistry, and practical geology. The trustees showed a special interest in the application of science to textile manufacture and the application of geological principles to mining. In time, after the success of the three original schools had been assured, it would be possible to add departments of "Practical Astronomy, Zoology, and Botany."[33]

The plan became a subject of debate and interest not only on the campus but throughout the state. At least one scientist on the faculty, Joseph LeConte, objected to such plans and as early as 1854 wrote of the increasing national sentiment for "practical education." In an article entitled "Utilitarian Spirit of the Age," published in the *Georgia University Magazine*, LeConte excoriated what he saw as the tendency toward an excessive emphasis on materialism in education at the expense of liberal education. "The utilitarian spirit, like a dreadful vampire," he argued, "is sucking the blood of our spiritual life." The dominant spirit of the age tended toward making "education entirely subservient to material success in life—to the accumulation of wealth . . . [and] to the utter neglect of all other higher objects."[34]

Newspapers like the Milledgeville *Federal Union* gave the design a hearty endorsement. The university had too long lain under the spell of classicism, which regarded the "eis and ous, kou and kous" as "the

32. Trustee Minutes, November [?], 1855.
33. *Ibid.*
34. Joseph LeConte, "Utilitarian Spirit of the Age," *Georgia University Magazine*, VII (March, 1855), 353–62.

tests of college excellence." The new age of "practical utility" demanded "practical men, civil engineers, to take charge of public roads, railroads, mines, scientific agriculture and etc."[35]

Although the 1855 plan did not win approval from the trustees, a similar plan put forward in 1859 was adopted and resulted in the reorganization of the institution into four schools: agriculture, civil engineering and applied mathematics, law, and commerce. With support from the governor of the state, the reorganization began with the division of the institution into the four schools and a preparatory institute and the appointment of a presiding officer who now bore the more imposing title of chancellor instead of president. The Civil War slowed the reorganization, but it was revitalized after the war. In the 1870s, however, a wave of conservatism plunged the school back into a program of study that differed very little from the antebellum curriculum.[36]

With its strong orientation toward applied science, the plan to transform the University of Georgia was a culmination of a trend that had been evident since the Jacksonian era, when a small group of educational reformers had argued for more utilitarian education. The scientific additions to the curriculum in the 1830s reflected this influence and substantially altered the institution. By the late 1850s, crosscurrents of southern nationalism combined with the triumph of the philosophy of utilitarian higher education to produce a plan that had a strongly modern flavor more often associated with the rise of the universities of the post–Civil War period. In fact, the Georgia plan can be seen as a part of an emerging prewar national trend toward a system of state universities whose missions were quite similar to that of the modernized Georgia university.

The Georgia experience with science and with higher learning in general invites comparison with other colleges throughout the South and the nation. The level of instruction; the growth of science in the curriculum; the quality and concomitant increase in the number of faculty primarily concerned with the sciences; and the emphasis on curricular adjuncts such as the philosophical apparatus, the geological cabinet, and the botanical garden all suggest that in its emphasis on science, the University of Georgia compared quite favorably with the fifteen New England and Middle Atlantic colleges studied by Guralnick.

35. Trustee Minutes, April 9, 1855; Coulter, *College Life*, 201.
36. See Dyer, *The University of Georgia*, Chapters 4 and 5.

Comparison of the scientific emphases at Georgia with those of other southern institutions and the state universities of the Midwest is more difficult because of the absence of research on the subject. Some southern institutions had clear and important emphases on science. Transylvania University, which functioned as a state university in Kentucky, expended large sums on philosophical apparatus, had an important medical school, and counted several prominent scientists among its faculty in the nineteenth century. Similarly, the University of South Carolina seems to have had a scientific orientation similar to that of the University of Georgia and counted among its faculty several distinguished scientists during the early nineteenth century, including Thomas Cooper and Lewis R. Gibbes. Southern state universities founded later in the century included the University of Alabama and the University of Mississippi, both of which profited from the presence of F. A. P. Barnard, who introduced science into the curricula of each institution and pushed each to acquire scientific equipment and some of the other accoutrements of scientific instruction. Historians of institutions like the University of Virginia, the University of North Carolina, and the University of Tennessee have given comparatively little attention to the role of science in those colleges during the antebellum period. Although it is not possible to draw firm conclusions concerning the orientation of those institutions, it can be said that their curricula bore strong resemblances to those of the other southern state universities.[37]

It is similarly difficult to draw comparisons with the state universities of the Midwest, though fragmentary information suggests that strong similarities existed between the way that science developed in those institutions and at the University of Georgia. It appears, however, that Indiana University developed at a slightly more rapid pace than Georgia and some of the institutions studied by Guralnick. Indiana, for example, granted its first bachelor of science degree in 1855,

37. John D. Wright, Jr., *Transylvania: Tutor to the West* (Lexington, Ky., 1975), 34–35, 46–51, 70–71, 74–77, 122–23, 164–65; Daniel Walker Hollis, *University of South Carolina* (Columbia, S.C., 1951), 30–33, 42–49, 76–79, 202–203; James B. Sellers, *History of the University of Alabama, 1818–1902* (University, Ala., 1953), 34–35, 46–47, 50–53, 68–71, 80–87, 148–49, 152–55, 162–63; Allen Cabaniss, *The University of Mississippi: Its First Hundred Years* (Hattiesburg, 1971), 8–11, 16–17, 34–41; Philip Alexander Bruce, *History of the University of Virginia, 1819–1919* (5 vols.; New York, 1920), I, 26–35, 322–23, II, 104–17; Kemp Plummer Battle, *History of the University of North Carolina* (2 vols.; Chapel Hill, 1907), I, 48–51, 54–55, 94–95, 642–43; Stanley J. Folmsbee, "East Tennessee University 1840–1879: Predecessor of the University of Tennessee," *University of Tennessee Record*, LXII (1959), 8–11, 28–29.

and five years later had "lifted it on an even plane" with the bachelor of arts. Fifteen years earlier, however, the scientific elements within the curriculum at Indiana and at Georgia were virtually identical. Both had begun to combine lecture and experimental demonstration, and both possessed significant quantities of scientific equipment. Georgia had erected Philosophical Hall for its scientific classes and laboratories, and Indiana had recently built a chemical laboratory. By 1851, Indiana had established a science department that anticipated by several years Georgia's design for a school of applied science.[38]

By contrast, science appears to have developed a little more slowly at the University of Wisconsin after its founding in 1849 than it did at the University of Mississippi founded the year before. Although the historians of Wisconsin present only scattered information concerning the development of science in that institution prior to the Civil War, they do conclude that Wisconsin did not offer a significant number of scientific courses in its early years. Only two of six professorships established for the new university would be concerned with scientific studies. Mississippi had a stronger scientific orientation and counted two distinguished scientists among its early faculty, Barnard, who joined the faculty in 1854, and John Millington, a member of the original faculty and of the Royal Astronomical Society and the Linnaean Society. In the years just prior to the Civil War, Barnard directed an expansion of the scientific areas of the institution that brought it some visibility for its support of experimental science and gave him increasing prominence as a scientist in his own right.[39]

In short, Georgia seems not to have been sharply different from comparable southern institutions or most northern colleges. Certainly, the active scientific interests and the growth of the importance of science in the curriculum at the Athens institution call into question widely held assumptions concerning the sterility of the so-called classical curriculum. And if the antebellum University of Georgia typifies many other southern institutions, as it appears, then some rethinking will have to be done concerning the importance of the classical tradition to southern society and the reputed conservatism of the region in higher education.

38. Thomas D. Clark, *Indiana University: Midwestern Pioneer* (4 vols.; Bloomington, Ind., 1970), I, 168–69, IV, 117, 148.

39. Merle Curti and Vernon Carstensen, *The University of Wisconsin: A History* (2 vols.; Madison, 1949), I, 84, 72–74; Cabaniss, *The University of Mississippi*, 36–37, 16–17.

CHAPTER 3

SCIENTIFIC SOCIETIES IN THE OLD SOUTH: THE ELLIOTT SOCIETY AND THE NEW ORLEANS ACADEMY OF SCIENCES

Lester D. Stephens

E ven before the American colonies had gained their independence, some American devotees of science had come to recognize the benefits of banding together in learned societies for the common purpose of promoting and advancing scientific knowledge. Among the earliest of these associations were the American Philosophical Society, founded in Philadelphia in 1743, and the Charleston Library Society, established in 1748. Their support of scientific inquiry as an important branch of knowledge came to be shared by other learned societies that sprang up in the new nation. Eventually, however, American scientists recognized a need for special societies to promote and advance their endeavors, and by the 1820s a number of them had succeeded in organizing associations for the express purpose of displaying natural specimens and exchanging scientific information. Quite naturally, such societies were founded in the cities of the young nation, and they tended to flourish best in the largest urban areas. Since the larger cities developed first in the North, the more successful learned societies and scientific associations usually prospered better there than in the predominantly agrarian South. Nevertheless, from the late eighteenth century to the time of the outbreak of the Civil War in 1861, a number of southerners interested in scientific knowledge sought to sustain and promote their efforts through formal associations.[1]

1. Brooke Hindle, *The Pursuit of Science in Revolutionary America, 1735–1789* (Chapel Hill, 1956), *passim;* Ralph S. Bates, *Scientific Societies in the United States* (2nd ed.; New York, 1958), 1–84; Joseph Ewan, "The Growth of Learned and Scientific Societies in the Southeastern United States to 1860," in Alexandra Oleson and Sanborn C. Brown (eds.), *The Pursuit of Knowledge in the Early American Republic* (Baltimore, 1976), 208–18; Thomas

By 1773, the Charleston Library Society had formed a museum of natural history. In 1815 the collections of the Charleston Museum, as it came to be called, were passed over to the care of the South Carolina Literary and Philosophical Society, founded in 1813 for the primary purpose of collecting, arranging, and preserving natural specimens. Led by Stephen Elliott, an accomplished botanist and author of a highly respected work on the flora of South Carolina and Georgia, the Society flourished until the mid-1830s. Meanwhile, scientific activity was progressing in New Orleans, where a Lyceum of Natural History was established in 1825. But it too faded from existence, and by the late 1830s, neither of the two major cities in the lower southern states could claim an active scientific society.[2]

Similar efforts were also made in the border states during the second and third decades of the nineteenth century. In 1827, for example, the Delaware Academy of Natural Sciences was established, and within six years the fledgling organization had created a museum. The Academy was incorporated into the Botanical Society of Wilmington in 1842, which remained active until 1851. The formation of the Virginia Historical and Philosophical Society in 1831 represented another attempt to promote the study of natural history in the border states, as did the establishment of the Columbian Institute for the Promotion of Arts and Sciences some fifteen years earlier in the District of Columbia. The Virginia society survived for only a few years; the Columbian Institute lasted a bit longer and was absorbed, in spirit at least, by the National Institution for the Promotion of Science, founded in 1842, which, although not especially successful, became "the spiritual antecedent of the National Institute and the National Academy of Sciences."[3]

Perhaps the most notable of the scientific societies in the border states prior to the 1850s, however, was the Maryland Academy of Science and Literature, founded in 1822. Although the fact that it declined and was reorganized on several occasions suggests a lack of

Cary Johnson, Jr., *Scientific Interests in the Old South* (New York, 1936), *passim;* William Martin Smallwood and Mabel Sarah Coon Smallwood, *Natural History and the American Mind* (New York, 1941), 101–29.

2. Bates, *Scientific Societies*, 45–63; Ewan, "The Growth of Learned and Scientific Societies in the Southeastern United States to 1860," in Oleson and Brown (eds.), *The Pursuit of Knowledge*, 208–18; Johnson, *Scientific Interests*, 126–75; Albert E. Sanders, "The Charleston Museum and the Promotion of Science in Antebellum South Carolina" (Paper delivered at the Third Citadel Conference on the South, April 25, 1981, Charleston, S.C.).

3. Bates, *Scientific Societies*, 45–63.

sustained activity, the publication of scientific papers in its *Transactions* in 1837 and its cabinet of "several thousand zoological, botanical, and mineralogical specimens" indicate that the Maryland Academy achieved a high degree of respectable progress in the promotion of scientific inquiry.[4] Not until the formation of the Elliott Society of Natural History (ESNH) and the New Orleans Academy of Sciences (NOAS) in 1853, however, did southern scientists succeed in their efforts to establish societies that consistently carried forward programs of a professional nature. That they succeeded where their earlier counterparts had failed was perhaps more due to conditions than to any major shortcomings of their predecessors. By the 1850s Charleston and New Orleans enjoyed the benefits of a large nucleus of scientists and could thus sustain formal scientific societies. No less important was the influence of a regional pride in the 1850s that motivated southern scientists to show the strength of their own culture in the face of increasing condemnations by northern spokesmen.[5] Southern scientists needed only some prompting to organize formal associations in those cities. In the case of Charleston, the impetus came from Louis Agassiz.

From the time of his first visit to Charleston in 1847, Agassiz not only praised local naturalists for advancing science in their city but also encouraged them to develop and enlarge the Charleston Museum. Held in high esteem among southern intellectuals, Agassiz wielded a strong influence upon Charleston's scientists, especially Francis S.

---

4. *Transactions of the Maryland Academy of Science and Literature*, I (1837), iii–xii, 17–190; Bates, *Scientific Societies*, 45–47; Johnson, *Scientific Interests*, 172–74. See also Sally Gregory Kohlstedt, *The Formation of the American Scientific Community: The American Association for the Advancement of Science, 1848–60* (Urbana, 1976), and George H. Daniels, *American Science in the Age of Jackson* (New York, 1968), 6–62.

5. A clear identification of all southerners considered to be scientists in the 1820s in either city is not possible, but available evidence seems to indicate that they were fewer than one half of those known to be engaged in scientific pursuits in the 1840s and 1850s. Although the following publications by John McCrady constitute somewhat indirect evidence, they support the contention that southern pride played a role in the development of the southern scientific societies in the 1850s: "A System of Independent Research, the Chief Educational Want of the South" (Address delivered at the Inauguration of the Charleston College Library, 1856), copy available in the Charleston Library Society Pamphlet Collection; "A Few Thoughts on Southern Civilization," *Russell's Magazine*, I (1857), 225–28, 338–49, 546–56, and II (1857), 212–26; "Home Education: A Necessity of the South" (Oration delivered before the Chrestomathic Society of the College of Charleston, March 2, 1860), copy available in the South Caroliniana Library, University of South Carolina; and "The Study of Nature and the Arts of Civilized Life," *De Bow's Review*, XXX (1861), 579–606.

Holmes (1815–1882), an able and ardent, if not always accurate, student of natural history. Holmes had already received considerable recognition for his collection of fossil specimens, despite his very limited formal training in scientific subjects. In 1850, when the museum was incorporated into the College of Charleston, Holmes was appointed to the post of curator. In the same year the American Association for the Advancement of Science met in Charleston. Thus Holmes, taking advantage of the heightened interest in the professionalization of science in the city and encouraged by Agassiz, set about to establish a scientific society. The effort came to fruition in November, 1853, with the formation of the Elliott Society of Natural History.[6]

As announced in its original circular, the Elliott Society was organized "for developing the Natural History of our Country, especially of our own State; and for promoting and cultivating the science." Named after Stephen Elliott, the Society chose the reputable naturalist and German Lutheran clergyman John Bachman as its first president. But illness and pressing pastoral duties prevented Bachman from taking an active role in the early meetings of the Society, and later, after he got involved in a great controversy with Josiah Nott of Mobile on the subject of racial origins, his activity in the Society declined further. Still, the Society kept him as its president for three years, probably in the belief that his name, like that of Stephen Elliott, would help establish its standing. In 1856 the Society elected Lewis R. Gibbes as its president, but after a year of hard work on behalf of the Society, Gibbes insisted that he was too busy to serve another term. The Society then chose the Charleston physician James Moultrie as its president. The choice was not good; although Moultrie was genuinely interested in chemistry and physiology and had published on those topics, he was also deeply involved in social affairs and thus missed many of the

6. Edward Lurie, *Louis Agassiz: A Life in Science* (Chicago, 1960), 143–44, 184–85; G. Edmund Gifford, Jr., "The Charleston Physician-Naturalists," *Bulletin of the History of Medicine*, XLIX (1975), 556–74; Johnson, *Scientific Interests*, 147–48; *Cyclopedia of Eminent and Representative Men of the Carolinas of the Nineteenth Century* (2 vols.; Madison, 1892), I, 508–10; Robert W. Gibbes to Lewis R. Gibbes, July 11, 1847, and William Stimpson to Lewis R. Gibbes, December 8, 1859, both in Lewis R. Gibbes Papers, Library of Congress; Francis S. Holmes to Henry W. Ravenel, September 26, 1853, in Henry W. Ravenel Papers, Special Collections, Clemson University Library; Francis S. Holmes, L. A. Frampton, and Francis T. Miles to Edmund Ravenel, October 5, 1853, and same to Lewis R. Gibbes on same date, both in Charleston Museum Library; Lester D. Stephens, *Ancient Animals and Other Wondrous Things: The Story of Francis Simmons Holmes, Paleontologist and Curator of the Charleston Museum*, Contributions from the Charleston Museum, XVII (Charleston, S.C., 1988).

Society's meetings. In need of a dedicated president, the Society turned once more to Gibbes, who served as president continuously thereafter until 1889.[7]

The history of the Elliott Society is inextricably linked with the career of Gibbes, who acted as its primary leader for thirty-one of its almost thirty-eight years of existence. Although he was not the central figure behind its founding, Gibbes quickly became the guiding force of the association, and almost single-handedly kept it alive after the Civil War. Born in 1810 in Charleston, Gibbes graduated with honors from South Carolina College in 1829. He later studied medicine in Charleston, taught mathematics at South Carolina College, and attended medical and natural history lectures in France. In 1838 he was appointed professor of mathematics at the College of Charleston, where he remained for fifty-four years. During his career he established himself as an authority in astronomy, botany, chemistry, mathematics, and zoology.[8]

When Gibbes became president of the Elliott Society in 1856, the membership of the Society stood at forty-five, a respectable number that compared favorably with membership enrollments during the formative years of both the Academy of Natural Sciences of Philadelphia (ANSP), founded in 1812, and the Boston Society of Natural History (BSNH), established in 1830. Within two years, the Elliott Society's membership had increased to fifty-eight. In 1859 the Society claimed seventy-nine members, but many of them were inactive and failed to pay their dues. The Society was compelled to suspend its activities during the Civil War, but by that time it had also nearly exhausted the supply of potential members, who were drawn mainly from those groups identified by Nathan Reingold as the scientific "researchers" (individuals who were generally employed in scientific occupations and who devoted most of their time to scientific inquiry) and the scientific "practitioners" (individuals principally "employed in scientific or science-related occupations" and who published fewer and more practical studies than the "researchers"). The Society did little to

7. Circular contained in "Letters of Edmund Ravenel," South Carolina Collection, Charleston Museum Library; Minute Book of the Elliott Society of Natural History, 1853–1867, Charleston Museum Library (hereinafter cited as ESNH Minute Book). The *Proceedings of the Elliott Society of Natural History* are derived from these minutes, but they omit some details.

8. Lester D. Stephens, "Lewis R. Gibbes and Scientific Activity in Charleston" (Paper presented before the Third Citadel Conference on the South, Charleston, South Carolina, April 25, 1981).

encourage the support and activity of scientific "cultivators," that is, those individuals who held nonscience occupations but maintained a strong interest in scientific discoveries and supported the efforts of the "researchers."[9] Since the population of Charleston was much smaller than that of Boston, the ESNH clearly had fewer scientific cultivators available, but this was perhaps all the greater reason why it should have gladly welcomed them as members. By encouraging the support of cultivators, the BSNH was able in its first ten years to acquire an active membership of 285.[10] But the ESNH was founded to promote science as a professional discipline, and its members apparently believed that they could not achieve this purpose if they admitted those who lacked personal commitment to sustained scientific pursuits.

Of the seventy-nine members of the ESNH in 1859, some 33 percent were medical doctors, and 10 percent were college professors. But these categories overlap somewhat inasmuch as some of the professors were also medical doctors associated with the local medical college, and at least two of the men listed as medical doctors were employed at the College of Charleston. Nevertheless, the number of members trained in medicine clearly represented a sizable portion of the membership of the ESNH just before the Civil War. They had played an even larger role in the founding of the Society, constituting slightly over 50 percent of the original membership. The same was true of the professors, who made up nearly one fourth of the charter membership. Only one of the original members was a clergyman, John Bachman, but he was equally well known as a zoologist. By 1859, however, the number of clergymen admitted had grown to 8 percent, and the number of others (of whom most of the identifiable ones were lawyers, journalists, businessmen, city officials, or planters) had increased to 51 percent.[11]

9. ESNH Minute Book; Nathan Reingold, "Definitions and Speculations: The Professionalization of Science in America in the Nineteenth Century," in Oleson and Brown (eds.), *The Pursuit of Knowledge*, 33–69. Reingold's terms are used throughout this paper.

10. On the BSNH, see Sally Gregory Kohlstedt, "The Nineteenth-Century Amateur Tradition: The Case of the Boston Society of Natural History," in Gerald Holton and William A. Blanpied (eds.), *Science and Its Public: The Changing Relationship* (Dordrecht, Holland, 1976), 173–90. See also "Constitution and By-Laws of the Boston Society of Natural History" and "List of Members," *Boston Journal of Natural History*, III (1840–41), 454–511. On the ANSP, see Patsy A. Gerstner, "The Academy of Natural Sciences of Philadelphia, 1812–1850," in Oleson and Brown (eds.), *The Pursuit of Knowledge*, 174–93.

11. *Constitution and By-Laws of the Elliott Society of Natural History of Charleston, S.C., as Adopted by the Society in Convention, February, 1857* (Charleston, S.C., 1857). A copy in the Special Collections Division, College of Charleston Library, contains handwritten additions to the list of members. Information on other members added through 1859 is derived from the ESNH Minute Book.

Relative isolation and difficulties of transportation probably hampered the growth of the ESNH more than that of the ANSP and the BSNH, but it was in the realm of financial support that the ESNH suffered more than its sister societies. Although both of the northern associations experienced financial difficulties in their early years, they eventually received large donations from wealthy benefactors. The ESNH never had such good fortune, however, and had to depend mainly upon membership dues and the sale of its publications for income. With a limited membership, revenue from dues was always very small, and the Society was never able to sell many copies of its *Proceedings* and *Journal*. Moreover, it did not succeed in getting its *Proceedings* into print until long after meetings had been held. By 1859 Gibbes and John McCrady had persuaded the Society to publish a journal, but the effort came on the heels of increasing sectional hostility, and only three numbers of the *Journal* ever found their way into print. The Society had managed in 1859 to get the South Carolina legislature to allocate $500 for support of its activities. Most of this appropriation was funneled into the publication of the *Journal*, a very costly venture, yet one that stood a very good chance of bringing notice to the Society. Thus, through its *Proceedings* and its *Journal*, the ESNH disseminated many of the papers presented by its members. Although most of those papers were devoted to descriptions of botanical and zoological specimens, they nevertheless represented contributions to scientific knowledge.[12]

During its formative years the Society tried hard to attract national and international attention by electing several prominent scientists to corresponding membership, but its efforts were not nearly as successful as those of the ANSP and the BSNH. Indeed, the Society's records indicate that many of those chosen never bothered to respond to the invitation. Of fifty-one corresponding members elected during the first four years, for example, only twenty-eight accepted. Thereafter the Society extended fewer invitations. A special category of honorary membership was never used, thanks to the efforts of Holmes, who thwarted the attempt of John McCrady to invite fifteen eminent scientists to accept the honor. Piqued over some action taken by the Society during his absence from the city, Holmes, who seems to

12. ESNH Minute Book, February 14, 1866, October 1, 1867, and July 9, 1868; Baillière Bros. to Lewis R. Gibbes, October 1, 1867, and October 21, 1867, in the Gibbes Papers, Library of Congress; John McCrady to Edmund Ravenel, January 7, 1858, in E. Ravenel Letters, Charleston Museum Library. See also A. Hunter Dupree, "The National Pattern of American Learned Societies, 1769–1863," in Oleson and Brown (eds.), *The Pursuit of Knowledge*, 24–29.

have viewed the Society as something of a personal possession, managed to table McCrady's motion. It was never submitted again. The BSNH, on the other hand, used the category to good advantage, electing thirty-two renowned scientists, mostly from abroad, to honorary membership during its first decade of existence.[13]

Gibbes and his fellow members of the ESNH also failed to recognize the benefits of publicizing the association's activities. In fact, the Society evolved into something like an exclusive private club. Although Gibbes managed to build attendance to an average of ten at each meeting, which compares favorably with the BSNH during its early years, he and the Society did not provide for popular lectures by reputable scientists, and many Charlestonians were totally unaware of the existence of this professional association.[14] In one way at least, this choice made sense: the ESNH was intended to promote professionalism by encouraging rigorous scientific observation and research, fostering scrutiny of papers presented before the Society, and disseminating through its publications the critical studies offered by its members. In another way, the decision to exclude popularization of scientific knowledge from its activities was injurious to the association's wider interests. Why should the public take any interest in the doings of a private club of scientists whose discussions centered around esoteric matters? Other matters of concern, such as improvements in agriculture and domestic economy, were more important to the public than abstract research.

This is not to suggest that the Society engaged in useless discussions and the presentation of meaningless papers. On the contrary, the small handful of devoted members took their task seriously. But, from 1853 to 1867, when the name was changed to the Elliott Society of Science and Arts, only ten persons presented papers before the Society. In all, forty-one papers were read during this period, the great majority by Gibbes and McCrady. The former read nine papers and the latter, fourteen. Gibbes' papers covered a total of approximately fifty-three pages, all published in the *Proceedings* except for a separate pamphlet on the accentuation of scientific names, which won the praise of his

13. ESNH Minute Book; *Constitution and By-Laws of the ESNH*, containing "List of Members," 1857; BSNH, "List of Members," 1840–1841.
14. A series of fifty-eight articles on the museum appeared in the Charleston *Courier* between March 13 and October 23, 1858, but the ESNH was hardly noticed. On October 21, 1882, a Charleston citizen, who had some acquaintance with science, wrote to the *News and Courier*, expressing the belief that the city had never had "a natural history society."

colleagues but was viewed by his northern peers as a pedantic exercise. Those of the marine invertebrate specialist McCrady, who is undoubtedly one of the most underrated of all the Charleston naturalists, covered well over 200 pages in both the *Proceedings* and the *Journal*, and they would have covered more had not many of them been lost when Columbia was burned in 1865—before the *Proceedings* of the meetings in 1859–1861 could be published. Holmes read three short papers before he quit the Society in 1857 in a fit of petulance. Other papers presented included four each by the nationally recognized conchologist Edmund Ravenel and the able but relatively unknown botanist William Wragg Smith; two by William H. Ford, including a lengthy monograph on the chemistry of human blood; and one brief report each by Henry William Ravenel, Francis P. Porcher, and A. M. Forster.

Corresponding member William Sharswood of Philadelphia presented two brief papers on chemistry. He was the only "outsider" who did so, indicating that, unlike the BSNH and the ANSP, the Society attracted little more than local attention. The overwhelming majority of the papers dealt with zoological and botanical topics. But, despite the aim and the name of the Society, other topics were allowed, which perhaps indicates a lack of enough papers on natural history subjects. It also probably indicates that many of the members were really cultivators, not practitioners or researchers.[15] Obviously, the members of the Society viewed the dissemination of new scientific knowledge through publication of their studies as an important objective of their association, and they endeavored repeatedly to foster an exchange of publications with other scientific societies, both at home and abroad. No doubt, they also did so for personal enhancement, but that was not a peculiar trait of southerners. What is more significant, perhaps, is that they sought to publish and exchange publications in order to show that the South was no backwater of scientific achievement.

As an association of natural historians, the Society was concerned with the classification of species. In an age before photography and illustrated field guides, naturalists depended heavily upon viewing specimens to assist them in identifying species. Though in part the collection and preservation of specimens represented a fad of the era, the advancement of knowledge in botany, zoology, chemistry, mineralogy, and paleontology depended upon the development of well-organized and carefully arranged cabinets of specimens. Moreover, pictures in books could never take the place of specimens on display in

15. *Proceedings of the ESNH,* I (1857); ESNH Minute Book.

museums of natural history. Such collections required a permanent place for storage and display, and both the ANSP and the BSNH succeeded fairly early on in establishing permanent cabinets and museums. The ESNH, on the other hand, maintained only one principal cabinet. Many of its specimens had to be placed in the Charleston Museum for display. In large measure, this arrangement was due to the development of the Charleston Museum as a branch of the College of Charleston. Since the ESNH held most of its meetings at the college, was centered mainly around Gibbes, and lacked sufficient funds, members of the Society soon came to accept their dependence upon the college and the museum for assistance in displaying their collections. They endeavored to set their collections apart and to maintain a special identity for them, but their arrangement with the museum ultimately worked against the independent development of the Society. By 1857, the Society was already having difficulty gaining access to its collections in the museum, run by Holmes, and finally had to petition the college trustees for clarification of the museum's rules. Gibbes was able to bring his influence to bear, and the matter was finally settled to the benefit of the Society.[16] Yet the relationship between the Society and the museum always remained tenuous and ill-defined, and the museum remained dominant as the place for display of specimens.

After December 15, 1860, the Society temporarily suspended meetings. Since average attendance had already fallen to four or five, the Society could not carry on during the war. By February 1866, however, Gibbes had managed to revive the association. The few faithful members carried on with their scientific discussions and endeavored to find ways to increase attendance and membership. Despite difficulties resulting from lack of funds and reduced membership, the ESNH managed to remain fairly active until 1869, but the effort was clearly a losing cause. In 1867 the association had changed its name to the Elliott Society of Science and Arts in an attempt to attract more members. Although this brought a minor surge of new life to the Society, the effect was temporary. In the face of declining interest, the loss of several members during the war, and the departure from the city of some of the older Charleston naturalists, the Society's prospects were practically hopeless. Moreover, when McCrady left in 1873 to take a post

16. ESNH Minute Book; ESNH "Memorial" to the President and Board of Trustees of the College of Charleston [1857], in the Lewis R. Gibbes Scrapbook, Special Collections Division, College of Charleston; College of Charleston Trustees Minute Book, August 31, 1868–January 25, 1869, Special Collections Division, College of Charleston.

with Agassiz at Harvard University, the Society lost one of its most active and able members. Gibbes and a handful of stalwarts tried vainly to carry on, and eventually managed to publish additional *Proceedings*, which attracted virtually no attention. The number of meetings dwindled drastically, and from 1875 to 1885 the Society held none at all, although Gibbes continued to request scientific reports and monographs for the association's library. Gibbes managed to revive the Society in 1885, but he relinquished the presidency late in 1889. The Society ceased to meet after June 1891.[17]

The Elliott Society of Natural History never equaled its Boston or Philadelphia counterparts in size, financial stability, or total productivity during the antebellum years, but then it had a much later start and lacked both the financial and the human resources necessary to sustain it at the same level. Moreover, it gained neither the preeminence nor the respect among its own people or in the eyes of the scientific world that would assure its longevity and leadership in the promotion of scientific inquiry. Far removed from the center of ESNH activities, professors of science in southeastern colleges could not find the Society very helpful, and they had to carry the burden for the advancement of science on their own shoulders, cut off as most of them chose to be from scientific associations in the rest of the nation. The ability of the ESNH to survive the ravages of the Civil War and to take up where it had left off in 1861 was insufficient to the task. Nevertheless, the Society had served a useful purpose by bringing together a small but talented and dedicated group of scientists who were not only geographically isolated from their peers in the North and from their peers in the region but also, by virtue of their culture and by volition of their will, from the seedbed of scientific growth. The accomplishments of the Society were indeed notable and indicate that scientific work in the Old South could easily equal that in the North. Conditions prevented the ESNH from achieving its potential, however, and, the effects of the Civil War aside, the fate of the ESNH would in all likelihood have been the same as that of the ANSP and the BSNH in later years when their status declined. The scientific enterprise was simply becoming too vast

---

17. *Proceedings of the Elliott Society,* II (1891), 259; ESNH Minute Book, June 11, 1885, July 9, 1885, and November 25, 1886. Between March 1859 and July 1868, sixteen of the relatively active members of the Society died. From June 9, 1870, to October 26, 1875, the Society held only two meetings. It met again on November 5, 1875, and thereafter not until January 22, 1885. An attempt was made to revive the Society in 1900–1901. On the effects of the Civil War upon scientific activity in the South, see Robert V. Bruce, *The Launching of Modern American Science, 1846–1876* (New York, 1987), esp. 271–344.

and too specialized to sustain local societies as major bodies for the advancement of science. Still, the ESNH demonstrated for a time, however brief, that scientific activity could flourish respectably where common interests were shared.

In many ways the history of the New Orleans Academy of Sciences parallels that of the ESNH. Founded in the same year as the ESNH, the Academy also depended during its formative period primarily upon the leadership of one man, namely, John Leonard Riddell. In addition, its regular membership was confined to a single city; its average attendance at meetings was small, although larger than that of the ESNH; it had similar financial difficulties and problems with publications; and it likewise had to disband during the Civil War. Yet, in other ways, the NOAS differed from its sister association in Charleston. Unlike the ESNH, the NOAS did not restrict its primary interests to natural history. In fact, the New Orleans group specified that "its sole object shall be the advancement of Science, properly so called, in all its various departments." Moreover, the NOAS constitution stated that the Academy could "establish Lectureships, in the various sciences," though it did not often take advantage of this provision. Like the ESNH, the Academy sought to be selective in accepting candidates to regular fellowship. Originally, the NOAS constitution stipulated that "no person shall be eligible to membership until he shall have given proof of his devotion to Science by the production of a paper on some scientific subject." Within a year after its founding, however, the Academy added the provision that membership was open also to persons who "by some act of genuine liberality" advanced the Academy's interests. This revision apparently stemmed from the reality that no more than a small handful of eligible members would qualify under the original provision. In fact, as with the ESNH, the vast majority of potential members were really cultivators or practitioners of science, not researchers.[18]

18. Records of the Transactions of the New-Orleans Academy of Sciences, Instituted April 25, 1853, I (a manuscript ledger containing the minutes of all except the executive proceedings from the first through the seventh and final preliminary sessions, March 21 to April 25, 1853, and the regular sessions, May 2, 1853 to December 11, 1854; continued in a second untitled manuscript ledger for the period 1854–1857; each hereinafter cited respectively as NOAS Records of Transactions, 1853–1854, and NOAS Records of Transactions, 1854–1857). Early executive-session minutes are recorded in an untitled manuscript ledger for the period June 6, 1853 to March 31, 1856 (hereinafter cited as NOAS Registrar's Minute Book). On the original membership provision, see the entry for October 19, 1853, NOAS Records of Transactions, 1853–1854. See also "Constitution and By-Laws of the New Orleans Academy of Sciences," 1854. All items are in the NOAS Papers, Special Collections Division, Tulane University.

The NOAS constitution also provided for the election of honorary and corresponding members. During its first six years the Academy chose several prominent scientists as honorary members, six of whom accepted the invitation. In the eyes of NOAS members the names of Louis Agassiz, A. D. Bache, and Joseph Henry certainly added to the Academy's prestige. Likewise, the election of other able scientists from the nation and from abroad indicated that the Academy was well on its way to serious recognition prior to the Civil War. In 1859, the NOAS claimed ninety-five corresponding members. Yet, like its sister society in Charleston, the NOAS issued many invitations to potential corresponding members who never bothered to reply. Still, it was more successful than the ESNH in soliciting corresponding members, probably in part because of its broader scope. The ESNH was, of course, essentially interested in natural history and made no concerted effort until the postbellum years to extend its range to all areas of science. The NOAS included members from disciplines that are now called social sciences as well as from agriculture and other peripheral fields of study. By 1859, it had created twelve "scientific sections," and though these divisions rarely functioned, they nevertheless enhanced the notion that the NOAS was interested in all scientific pursuits.[19]

The NOAS was not as successful in increasing the size of its regular membership, however, and during the period from its founding to 1860, it managed to enlarge its roll of fellows to only seventy-one, which was eight less than the number of regular members in the ESNH. Given that the population of New Orleans was then over four times larger than Charleston's, it seems that the NOAS should have been comparably larger. The difference may have been due to its more exclusive process of electing fellows. In fact, the Academy's records of executive sessions indicate that many nominees were rejected, and in 1855 one of the faithful fellows complained that his peers were turning down every candidate he put forward. A few months earlier another fellow had already expressed the view that his colleagues were "too eager to add members" and that the Academy was presently large enough "to carry out its objects." Indeed, a few months later, the Academy voted to restrict the number of fellows to fifty. It appears that before the Civil War the NOAS, like the ESNH, refused as a general rule to admit those they deemed to be mere science buffs or hobbyists. Although later abandoned, this restriction helped to ensure that on the whole only the most rigorous scientific inquiry would prevail in the

19. "Constitution and By-Laws of the New Orleans Academy of Sciences, Together with a List of Fellows, Honorary and Corresponding Members," 1859; NOAS Records of Transactions, 1853–1854; NOAS Records of Transactions, 1854–1857.

presentation and publication of papers and thrive under the sanction of a formal association to which most of the accomplished scientists of the city belonged. But the limitation on membership probably also excluded many interested cultivators of science who could not only have profited from an association with their peers but also have broadened the Academy's base of support.[20]

A group of five New Orleans medical doctors interested in forming a professional society first met on the evening of March 21, 1853, to consider "the expediency of some kind of organization, with a view to mutual improvement in medical and natural sciences." Among them were Bennet Dowler, Noah B. Benedict, and Josiah S. Copes, all recognized men of scientific accomplishments. Agreeing upon the potential benefits of a scientific association as a means of sharing and criticizing research and as a source of encouragement to each other, the group decided to invite eight of their colleagues to the next meeting a week later. Not all attended, but the group pushed forward through six additional "preliminary meetings," and by April 25, they had prepared a constitution and a set of bylaws, to which twelve members subscribed. Josiah Hale, a graduate of Transylvania College and former student of the naturalist Constantine Rafinesque, as well as a successful physician and a noted botanist, was elected as the first president of the NOAS. The newly formed Academy held its first regular meeting on May 2, 1853. During the next few years it had an average of fifteen members present at its weekly meetings. Occasionally attendance rose to around twenty, and from time to time, especially during the hot summer months, it fell below the quorum of nine.[21]

A gross profile of the occupations of the members of the NOAS in 1853 and in 1859 reveals them to be closely similar to those of ESNH members. Medical doctors constituted 40 percent of the membership in the charter year, but by 1859 the ratio had dropped to 25 percent, somewhat less than that in the ESNH. The percentage of clergymen admitted to the NOAS declined from 12 percent during the founding year to 8 percent six years later. College professors associated with the NOAS always constituted a smaller number than in the ESNH, ranging from 9 percent in 1853 to 12 percent in 1859. But the percentage of members engaged in other pursuits was roughly the same as in Charleston: 39 percent of those enrolled in the year of the founding of the Academy and 55 percent of those listed as fellows in 1859. The difference in the makeup of the two societies was thus minimal. Signif-

20. NOAS Registrar's Minute Book, November 6, 1854, February 5, 1855, and October 6, 1855.
21. NOAS Records of Transactions, 1853–1854, and 1854–1857.

icant perhaps is the fact that medical doctors also played an important part in the founding of the NOAS, and, though the proportionate number of physician members of the Academy declined as it did in the ESNH, it is clear from the minutes of the NOAS meetings that they played a greater role in the subsequent work of the Academy than did their counterparts in the ESNH.

From 1853 to 1857, the reading of original papers and formal reports before the Academy was the exception rather than the rule. Existing records for the period indicate that NOAS members were less active in this respect than were members of the ESNH. Of twenty papers presented before the NOAS, six were in fields that can be broadly defined as social science; four in chemistry; three in medicine; two in agriculture; one each in physics, astronomy, and geology; and two on technological subjects. One of the papers was presented by a corresponding member, all others by a total of eleven fellows, five of whom each read two papers and two of whom each presented three papers. Two of the three antebellum presidents of the Academy, E. H. Barton and J. L. Riddell, each read one paper before the society. In November, 1857, Dr. Noah B. Benedict, among the most faithful in attendance and longtime recording secretary of the Academy, noted the paucity of formal papers and urged upon his fellow members "the desirability of a regular series of papers to be read before the Academy, at the regular weekly meetings." Such, he maintained, "would be in accordance with the very purpose of this organization." Benedict likewise encouraged the Academy to invite guests to hear these papers. The result was remarkably good, if only temporary. On November 30, 1857, some twenty-two fellows turned out, as did "about one hundred and fifty persons—ladies and gentlemen." In part, the splendid showing was due to effective solicitation by Academy members, the topic of the paper, and the willingness of the NOAS to allow women to attend the special meeting. The paper was presented by Samuel A. Cartwright, an articulate writer, if not a good scientist. Titled "On the Ethnological Peculiarities of Prognathous or Negro Race," the paper expounded Cartwright's theory of the innate inferiority of Negro intelligence.[22] It did not, however, typify the papers presented at NOAS meetings, though it does perhaps reveal that Academy members were keenly attuned to received southern views on race.

22. *Ibid.*; Johnson, *Scientific Interests*, 161–69; John Duffy, *The Rudolph Matas History of Medicine in Louisiana* (2 vols.; Baton Rouge, 1958, 1962), II, *passim*; Joseph Ewan, "Josiah Hale, M.D., Louisiana Botanist, Rafinesque's Pupil," *Journal of the Society for the Bibliography of Natural History*, VIII (1977), 235–43; James O. Breeden, "States-Rights Medicine in the Old South," *Bulletin of the New York Academy of Medicine*, LII (1976), 348–72.

While the number of papers presented before the Academy was limited, the amount and the range of discussion at the meetings were not. Indeed, the faithful fellows freely discussed many subjects, most of which dealt with scientific matters. Typically a member made an observation before the group, and from that point others proceeded to comment upon it. In some cases, the initiator had prepared some informal remarks, and in others, he apparently spoke as the spirit moved him. As might be expected, the topic of yellow fever and other epidemics often served as the focus of discussion. Among other topics included were animal behavior, the power of serpent charmers, the principles of psychology, ocean waves, the Gulf Stream, physiology and medicine, meteorology, animal embalmment, chemical properties, and, especially, historical geology. While uninformed opinion and speculation occasionally characterized the discussions, a remarkably critical attitude generally prevailed. On the occasion of a discussion of "animal behavior," for example, J. S. Copes noted that "natural science as well as medicine is injured by hasty presumption and ignorance, to say nothing of downright arrogance and quackery." Yet when the discussion turned to the question of the antiquity of certain fossils, Copes argued against the hypothesis. J. L. Riddell complained that he "perceived in Dr. Copes . . . an apprehensiveness lest the facts of Geology might be found to conflict with the statements of the Bible" and then reminded his colleague that the goal of the Academy was simply to search for "truth as the most precious of all things."[23] Tolerant and basically open-minded, despite their predisposition to reconcile scientific propositions with the Scriptures, Academy members generally displayed a genuine spirit of inquiry, even if they did so from a Baconian frame of reference.

The NOAS, like the ESNH, sought to emulate the older northern scientific societies, most especially the ANSP. In 1855, for example, Benedict reported on his recent visit to the Philadelphia academy, and after giving a glowing account of ANSP accomplishments, he said that the NOAS had "cause only for gratulation and encouragement" as it moved from its infancy toward maturity. Noble as was Benedict's optimism, it represented a somewhat unrealistic view, given the difference in the size of the populations of New Orleans and Philadelphia. Yet it did reflect the belief of enthusiastic NOAS members that they could not only promote scientific pursuits but also demonstrate the viability of inquiry in their own city and region. Their pride was not purely parochial, however. Indeed, the extant minutes do not suggest any overweening notion of a peculiar southern flavor in the Academy's

23. NOAS Records of Transactions, 1853–1854.

70

scientific discussions. In fact, in 1857, Benedict announced his pleasure over the spread of "scientific pursuits" in "our country." Moreover, NOAS members expressed their delight in the formation of the Chicago Academy of Science (CAS) in that same year. A letter from the CAS contained the "very gratifying information" that it was "the offspring of the New Orleans Academy . . . projected solely in consequence of the visit, two years ago, of one of its founders, to the New Orleans Academy, and that it is very closely modelled after the pattern of our own Academy." Shortly thereafter, Benedict, recently returned from the AAAS meeting in Montreal and subsequent visits with CAS members and New York scientists, reported that he was generously received by his northern cohorts.[24]

From its beginning, the NOAS recognized the importance of developing museum collections, exchanging specimens, securing scientific works for its library, and publishing its papers and proceedings. It never succeeded as well as its sister society in Charleston, nor did it even come close to rivaling the scientific societies in Boston and Philadelphia—though, of course, both of the latter had a big jump on the NOAS, and neither of them was seriously affected by the Civil War. If the NOAS received as many donations of specimens as did the ESNH, the records do not indicate such. This probably resulted from the fact that the NOAS generally showed less interest in natural history than did the ESNH. Yet, the NOAS was certainly aware of a need to build a good museum, and it did purchase some specimens at its own expense. It also received many donations from individuals. But, unlike their counterparts in Charleston, NOAS fellows did little to collect specimens from their own region, a point that especially bothered Benedict. "It is peculiarly mortifying," he said, "to be unable to exhibit in our collection a single specimen of those objects of prime interest to strangers which are indiginous [sic] with us." Thereafter, the Academy strove to rectify the problem, although its fellows never did much to collect specimens locally. By 1857, however, Benedict could report that donations were "pouring in upon the Academy, from every quarter of the globe."[25] Still, in comparison with the ESNH, the ANSP, and the BSNH, the NOAS devoted relatively little attention to the development of its museum.

The NOAS was typically more interested in such matters as sanitation, levee construction, an artesian well, and a geological survey of the state. Certainly, problems with epidemics, flooding, drainage, and a pure water supply loomed large in the city, and the NOAS actively

24. NOAS Records of Transactions, 1854–1857.
25. Ibid.

supported efforts to remedy these problems. No doubt, the influence of physicians in the Academy and the peculiar problems associated with the terrain of the city resulted in the unusual emphasis upon matters of medical import. Members of the Academy strongly urged the boring of an artesian well in New Orleans, and they followed its progress closely. However, they were apparently more interested in the geological information it yielded than in its potential as a source of pure water. In fact, their interest in geology led them to press the state legislature for a geological survey of Louisiana.[26]

In 1855, the Academy petitioned the legislature to authorize a geological survey of the state and offered to draft a detailed plan at a cost of $500, which would be borne by the Academy. Other matters commanded the attention of Louisiana legislators, however, and the petition came to nought. The hopes of the NOAS did not die, and two years later the Academy drafted a bill for a state geological survey and sent it to the legislature. However, the chairman of the legislative committee on internal improvements replied that the request had arrived too late for consideration in the current session but added his hope that the next legislature would "be composed of men of different stuff from this." Unfortunately for Louisiana, the next legislature was not composed of men of different stuff, and Louisiana did not conduct a geological survey until 1871. The NOAS, then, had not been very effective as a lobbying agent in spite of the effectiveness of its argument for a state geological survey.[27]

Shortly after its founding, the NOAS arranged for publication of its transactions, and by October, 1854, the first volume of the NOAS *Proceedings*, covering the period from May, 1853, to March, 1854, was in print. In keeping with NOAS activities for the period, the bulk of the *Proceedings* consisted of the record of discussions, business, donations, and a few original papers. Of seven papers presented during the period, six were published, comprising a total of seventeen pages. Three of the papers dealt with chemical analyses, while one each consisted of comments on specimens of Indian pottery, Roman coinage, and a plan for underground privy drainage in New Orleans. Thus

26. NOAS Records of Transactions, 1853–1854 and 1854–1857; Letter of Transmittal, February 14, 1855, and Copy of Report of the Academy of Sciences on a Protection Levee (with map attached), in NOAS Papers, Special Collections Division, Tulane University; *Report of the Special Committee of the New Orleans Academy of Sciences, Appointed December 7, 1858, to Investigate and Report, at as Early a Day as Practicable, Upon the Subject of a Geological and Scientific Survey of the State of Louisiana* (New Orleans, 1858).

27. NOAS Records of Transactions, 1854–1857, March 5 and March 12, 1855, and February 2, March 16, and March 23, 1857.

72

lacking much substance, the *Proceedings* was not especially impressive. But NOAS members took great pride in their accomplishment and vowed to continue with the publication of their transactions.[28] Their hopes were never realized, however, for the Academy lacked sufficient income to carry out one of its major goals. In 1855 the NOAS asked the state legislature for "an annual appropriation, for a limited time, for a sum of money which would suffice to print the *Proceedings*." The request fell on deaf ears. Eventually, Benedict suggested that the Academy should appeal to the public for subscriptions to a second volume of proceedings. "Southern pride and the municipal spirit of our Citizens would," he insisted, "induce a spontaneous offering of the sum necessary" to publish the Academy's transactions. The Academy approved the recommendation, but its appeal brought in only a small amount of money. Unlike the ESNH, then, the NOAS managed to publish very little.[29]

In the case of each society, publishing its own papers was important, for there were very few opportunities to publish scientific works in the South. Occasionally, a brief, popularized scientific piece was printed in the pages of *De Bow's Review* or in other southern, mostly literary, journals, or in local newspapers. At least some southern scientists suspected that northern scientific journals were not receptive to their papers, and though the evidence belies that charge in general, it was nonetheless true that southern scientists had limited opportunities to publish their works, especially when their subjects dealt with local scientific studies. Aside from that, as sectional rivalry increased, so did the desire of southern scientists to produce publications at home. This point was forcefully stressed by ESNH member John McCrady in 1856 in an address calling for the development of journals in the land of "a peculiar people" who must stop looking toward "Europe and . . . the hostile Northern States." Lewis Gibbes, who before 1853 had published several worthy papers in northern-based journals, apparently came to share this view. He virtually ceased thereafter to submit papers other than to the ESNH *Proceedings*, except for three articles sent in 1859 and 1860 to the *Mathematical Monthly*, published by J. D. Runkle, who wrote to Gibbes that he received few "contributions from your part of the country."[30] Although no evidence has been uncovered to show that members of the NOAS held the same views as McCrady and

28. NOAS Records of Transactions, 1853–1854, and 1854–1857; *Proceedings of the New Orleans Academy of Sciences*, I (March 1, 1854).

29. NOAS Records of Transactions, 1854–1857, December 24, 1855.

30. McCrady, "A System of Independent Research"; J. D. Runkle to L. R. Gibbes, March 2 and November 2, 1859, in the Lewis R. Gibbes Papers, Library of Congress.

Gibbes, it seems safe to guess that they too desired to publish their scientific works at home.

The role of John Leonard Riddell in leading the NOAS was comparable to that of Gibbes in the ESNH. Born in Ohio in 1807, Riddell studied under the noted geologist and naturalist Amos Eaton at the Rensselaer Institute in New York and eventually took a degree in medicine. Extremely able and well read but irascible and somewhat arrogant, Riddell was a man of broad learning who could speak knowledgeably on many scientific topics. He was especially well informed in medicine, microscopy, chemistry, geology, and botany. A freethinker, he did not hesitate to voice his views on religious topics. In 1836 he accepted an appointment as a professor of chemistry in the Medical College of Louisiana and eventually earned a deserved reputation for his botanical and microscopic studies, the latter of which he improved by his development of the binocular microscope. Soon after the NOAS was established, Riddell became a fellow. He was elected a vice-president in 1854. One year later he was chosen to serve as president and was reelected every year thereafter until his death in 1865. By his sheer breadth of scientific knowledge, his wide range of investigations, and his strong personality, Riddell tended to overpower most of his colleagues in the Academy. As the records of NOAS proceedings seem to indicate, he took greater delight in his own projects and in playing the role of critic than he did in promoting the general welfare of the Academy. Certainly his criticisms often helped to deflate loose speculations; his interests in such matters as the artesian well and a state geological survey helped to promote scientific interests; and his efforts to develop specialization of scientific inquiries aided the Academy in achieving a reasonable degree of professionalization. But unlike ESNH leader Lewis Gibbes, Riddell did not set an example by presenting original papers before the Academy, nor did he articulate any clear goals for the organization. Still, he kept NOAS affairs going well until the Civil War forced a general suspension of meetings from 1861 to 1866.[31] The NOAS experienced a resurgence in membership and activity from 1885 to 1890, and, despite ups and downs thereafter, it was still active at the time of its centennial celebration.

Certainly, a review of the origins and development of the ESNH and the NOAS reveals that many able scientists in the Old South were not

31. Karlem Riess, "John Leonard Riddell, Scientist-Inventor, Melter and Refiner of the New Orleans Mint, 1839–1848, Postmaster of New Orleans, 1859–1862," *Tulane Studies in Geology and Paleontology*, XIII (1977); Karlem Riess, "The New Orleans Academy of Sciences: Its First Hundred Years (1853–1953)," *Scientific Monthly*, LXXVII (1953), 255–59.

only genuinely interested in the advancement of science but also keenly aware of the importance of forming close ties with their peers in promoting professionalization of their endeavors. Although both of these southern scientific societies got a late start, they made impressive strides toward elevating the status of science, enhancing a sense of professionalism, and developing the unity of efforts necessary to advance scientific interests, including a sharing of information and criticism of ideas and explanations. Unquestionably, their endeavors received a devastating setback from the Civil War, but even before the war began both the ESNH and the NOAS were unable to advance their activities as fully as their founders desired.

The NOAS and especially the ESNH were handicapped by limiting conditions and circumstances, among which were the size of the populations from which they could draw their members, the relative isolation of their activities from the mainstream of American scientific life, their somewhat narrow scope of interests, their views on professionalism, and their philosophy of inquiry. In comparison with major northern cities where scientific activity flourished, neither New Orleans nor, particularly, Charleston contained populations large enough to support an expansion of membership that would ensure sustained growth and renewed vitality. This condition was made worse in both instances by a reluctance to elicit the support of the cultivators of science and to publicize effectively the activities of the societies among the local populace. The situation constituted a dilemma, however, for on the one hand to take such steps would have lowered standards and therefore hampered the development of professionalization, while on the other, not taking them created a barrier between the organizations and their potential patrons.

Had the societies created a special category of membership for professionals and had they enlarged the geographic range from which regular members could be drawn, they might have increased the sizes of their organizations. Many able scientists were, after all, scattered throughout the region. It is true, of course, that such members would have been unable to attend meetings regularly, but both they and the respective societies could have benefited from a greater mutual exchange. At the very least, the NOAS and the ESNH could have followed the lead of the ANSP and the BSNH by promoting public lectures on scientific topics. The single effort by the NOAS in 1857 to appeal to the public with a popular lecture demonstrated that the Academy could attract wider interest in scientific affairs, at least when the topic dealt with a popular subject like the "Ethnological Peculiarities of . . . [the] Negro Race." Less sensational but nonetheless

75

thoughtful lectures on scientific topics could almost certainly have drawn a sizable number of local citizens, but the NOAS did not view such as a purpose for its existence. Neither did the ESNH, which declined even to make such an attempt during the antebellum period.

Unlike the ANSP and the BSNH, neither southern scientific society benefited substantially from private financial contributions, and though in the antebellum years the ESNH received some state funds, it, like the NOAS, had insufficient income to reach fully its goal of publishing scientific proceedings and papers. This situation deterred both organizations, but especially the NOAS, from their missions of exchanging scientific materials, and, particularly, from establishing widespread reputations as accomplished scientific associations. Yet it was not financial difficulty alone that accounted for the failure of either group to achieve national recognition. Despite their commendable efforts to promote science in the South, both societies did so from a somewhat narrow point of view. Certainly, the NOAS recognized the importance of all the sciences, but it also declined to identify itself as a body devoted solely to the physical and natural sciences. By including peripheral areas of interest under the same umbrella with science, the Academy probably stretched itself too thin. This arrangement reflected an older universalist philosophy that promoted the advantages of a general learned society, but the NOAS was created during an era when scientific specialization was becoming the order of the day. On the other hand, the ESNH generally restricted its interests to natural history. These interests really represented the old-style natural history, however, and thus tended to stress the pursuit of specimen collection and classification. Only one member of the ESNH, John McCrady, persistently sought to go beyond taxonomic work into comparative analysis. Indeed, his studies of the life cycles of marine Hydrozoa were forward-looking, but they were the exception, not the rule. In addition, the ESNH tended to place too much value on such pedantic matters as the accentuation of scientific terms.[32] This, in part, stemmed from its excessive dependence upon the leadership of one man, a situation that also characterized the development of the NOAS, which too relied primarily upon a single individual.

32. ESNH Minute Book. On McCrady's studies, see *Proceedings of the ESNH*, I (1857), and *Proceedings of the Elliott Society*, II (1891). A sketch of McCrady is given in *Cyclopedia of Eminent and Representative Men of the Carolinas of the Nineteenth Century*, I, 158–62; the bulk of his extant papers are in the private possession of Mrs. Edith McCrady, Sewanee, Tennessee, and Dr. Edward McCrady, Greensboro, North Carolina. See also Lester D. Stephens, "John McCrady, Pioneering Embryologist in the Old South" (Paper delivered at the annual meeting of the American branch of the Society for the History of Natural History, October 29, 1987, Raleigh).

In general, both the NOAS and the ESNH were guided by a Baconian philosophy of scientific methodology. As noted by George H. Daniels, Baconianism meant different things to different people. To some it was synonymous with "empiricism," or the direct observation of phenomena from which facts could be derived that could ultimately lead to generalizations when a sufficient number accumulated. Inquiry by observation and induction was thus the only proper approach to the development of valid scientific knowledge. A second meaning followed from the first, namely that because direct observation was so important, hypothesizing was dangerous to the gathering of facts. In other words, to guess at the probable outcome of an investigation was to run the risk of obscuring the facts that would emanate from careful observation free of preconceived views. Finally, to others Baconianism signified that the goal of scientific inquiry was to identify and classify natural phenomena. In brief, the scientists who subscribed to this view saw their task as no more and no less than taxonomy. Ultimately, the Baconian method, as Herbert Hovenkamp notes, became "the only one a Christian could use" and really served less as a tool than as a "symbol . . . to show that one was on guard against rationalism, deism, speculative science, or anything else that might approach infidelity." Thus compatible with the American frame of mind, Baconianism "reigned" in the United States until the mid-nineteenth century. Yet it did not go untested, and by the 1830s it had begun to come under fire. Significantly in the context of scientific activity in the Old South and among the members of the ESNH and the NOAS, however, the Baconian ideal was never brought into serious question. For the most part, then, antebellum southern scientists continued to believe that taxonomy was the chief aim of inquiry, for, after all, each natural phenomenon was but a manifestation of God in nature.[33]

Throughout the antebellum period religion continued to play a significant role in the work of the southern naturalists. Although not unimportant to other scientists of the age, it had a pronounced place in the minds of the members of both the ESNH and the NOAS, even if it was not often the focus of discussions at their meetings. The question of the relation of science to religion did enter into some of the discussions conducted at NOAS meetings, but religion was rarely discussed

---

33. Daniels, *American Science*, 63–162; Herbert Hovenkamp, *Science and Religion in America, 1800–1860* (Philadelphia, 1978). On the trend toward scientific specialization and professionalization, see Kohlstedt, *The Formation of the American Scientific Community*, and Howard S. Miller, *Dollars for Research: Science and Its Patrons in Nineteenth-Century America* (Seattle, 1970), 3–23.

at ESNH gatherings. Yet, the correspondence of Gibbes indicates that he and his colleagues firmly believed that scientific inquiry was primarily intended to reveal God at work in nature. It would be incorrect, however, to say that either society placed any limitations upon the scientific subjects it chose to pursue. Indeed, despite occasional questions about the right to discuss any topic lest it invade the realm of Providence, the members of both organizations displayed a commendable spirit of free inquiry.

Perhaps members of the societies were limited in their inquiries because of fixed cultural views, on race, for example. Certainly, they were limited to an extent by provincial loyalties. The harsh comments of ESNH member John McCrady in the late 1850s indicate clearly that anti-North feelings were indeed strong among at least some of the scientists. However, neither society recorded in its minutes any formal discussion of the growing rift between North and South. In their meetings the scientists continued right up until the outbreak of hostilities to go about the business of their societies. To be sure, each organization definitely took pride in its southern origins, and each, particularly the ESNH, tended more and more to isolate itself from the AAAS, thereby diminishing fruitful contact with the largest scientific association in the nation. Some individuals, such as Francis S. Holmes and Edmund Ravenel, did continue right up to the last days before the Civil War to correspond with scientific friends above the Mason-Dixon Line, and both Gibbes and Ravenel published papers in northern scientific journals at the peak of political animosity. When the crunch came, however, the southern scientists proved themselves to be southern patriots, and they readily pushed aside their scientific interests for their cultural and political loyalties. They had wanted it both ways, but it could not be. For them and for their scientific societies, the result was catastrophic.

Nevertheless, before the war, both the ESNH and the NOAS contributed effectively to the professionalization of science in the Old South, and for that reason alone, if for no other, they had a positive, if short-lived, effect upon the intellectual development of the region. While the antebellum southern colleges bore the burden of educating young men in science, the southern scientific societies added impetus to the promotion of scientific activity. Their effect was limited, of course, but it was nonetheless important. As their impact was retarded, so was a part of the region's cultural development.

CHAPTER 4

SCIENCE ON THE PLANTATION

William K. Scarborough

The association between science and agriculture was tenuous at best until about the fourth decade of the nineteenth century. The natural sciences of chemistry, biology, and botany, still in their infancy, could not yet offer applications for such pressing agricultural concerns as restoring soil fertility, breeding improved strains of plants and livestock, or eradicating diseases and insect pests. Geology, soon to become useful in determining soil-fertilizer relationships, did not emerge as a recognized profession until the 1830s. Indeed, the word *scientist* did not even enter the English vocabulary until that decade.[1]

In the absence of any meaningful assistance from the scientific community, southern planters, in company with their counterparts in the free states, began as early as the 1780s to conduct systematic experiments and to communicate their findings through newly organized agricultural societies and available print media.[2] As a consequence of such empirical investigations, undertaken by increasing numbers of planters in subsequent years, the foundations were laid for much of modern agricultural science. A notable case in point is the science of plant breeding, which, as John Hebron Moore has so convincingly demonstrated, originated in the efforts of early nineteenth-

1. Percy W. Bidwell and John I. Falconer, *History of Agriculture in the Northern United States, 1620–1860* (1925; rpr. Clifton, N.J., 1973), 255; James X. Corgan, "Early American Geological Surveys and Gerard Troost's Field Assistants, 1831–1836," in James X. Corgan (ed.), *The Geological Sciences in the Antebellum South* (University, Ala., 1982), 40–41.

2. Bidwell and Falconer, *History of Northern Agriculture*, 184, 186; Lewis C. Gray, *History of Agriculture in the Southern United States to 1860* (2 vols.; 1933; rpr. Gloucester, Mass., 1958), II, 612, 779.

century Mississippi planters to develop a strain of cotton better suited to their particular environment.[3]

Although ignorant of the most elementary principles of the science of botany, planters in southwestern Mississippi succeeded between 1810 and 1830 in crossing strains of cotton indigenous to the diverse locales of Siam, Mexico, and the West Indies to produce a new variety, the so-called "Mexican cotton," which "became the standard breed of ante-bellum American cotton and parent of most of the modern American strains as well." Initially, this hybridization was effected accidentally through the natural processes of cross-pollination and evolution. However, in the early 1830s Dr. Rush Nutt and other planters near Rodney, Mississippi, inaugurated a primitive method of seed selection that yielded an improved variety known as "Petit Gulf cotton." Superior to its predecessors in yield, quality of fiber, resistance to disease, adaptability to various soils, and ease of picking, this strain was first sold commercially in 1833 and soon captured the bulk of the southern market.[4] In later years other Mississippi cotton planters, most notably Richard Abbey and Henry W. Vick, used somewhat more sophisticated breeding techniques to improve the Petit Gulf strain. Vick's "Hundred Seed" cotton, the product of some ten years of experimentation, ultimately earned the reputation of being "the very best Mexican, or Petit Gulf" cotton in the state.[5]

Although planters continued to render notable service to southern agriculture through such trial-and-error methods, in the quarter century preceding the Civil War the growing professionalization of science finally engendered the first significant efforts to apply science directly to agriculture. Of particular note were advances in chemistry and geology that promoted chemical analysis of soils and suggested means for rejuvenating exhausted lands and increasing productivity. Earlier writings of European scientists, of which Sir Humphry Davy's *Elements of Agricultural Chemistry* (1803) was perhaps the most important, had attracted the attention of some progressive southern planters. But it was the seminal work of the German scientist Justus von Liebig that most profoundly affected American agriculture.[6]

3. I am grateful to Professor John Hebron Moore for calling my attention to the important contributions of antebellum Mississippi cotton breeders in his commentary on the original version of this paper, which was presented at the first "Barnard-Millington Symposium on Southern Science and Medicine" in March, 1982.

4. John Hebron Moore, *Agriculture in Ante-Bellum Mississippi* (New York, 1958), 28–35.

5. *Ibid.*, 147–54; *De Bow's Review*, X (1851), 568.

6. Paul Wallace Gates, *The Farmer's Age: Agriculture, 1815–1860* (New York, 1960), 295; Bidwell and Falconer, *History of Northern Agriculture*, 319.

First published in this country in 1841, Liebig's *Chemistry in Its Application to Agriculture and Physiology* was an immediate sensation. By explaining the relationship between soil composition and plant nutrition, Liebig elucidated more clearly than any before him the fundamental principles underlying soil fertilization. In essence, he explained that plant growth depends upon minerals in the soil and that these minerals—chiefly lime, potash, sulphur, and phosphorous—must be restored by artificial means as they become depleted for the soil to remain productive. Liebig's work won immediate acclaim from such southern agricultural reformers as John S. Skinner and Edmund Ruffin. Addressing the Louisiana Agricultural and Mechanics' Association in 1845, Louisiana sugar planter Pierre Rost likened Liebig's contributions to agriculture to those of Lavoisier in chemistry. And the following year, in an oration before the same body, James D. B. De Bow asserted, somewhat optimistically, that "the profound investigations of Liebig in the vegetable world have already created a revolution."[7]

The scientific theories of Liebig and other European scholars were disseminated widely in the United States during the last two decades of the antebellum period, largely through agricultural journals. These periodicals, which first appeared in the second and third decades of the nineteenth century, mushroomed after 1830, though most were short-lived and had a limited circulation. Their purpose, as enunciated in the inaugural issue of John Skinner's pioneering journal the *American Farmer*, was "to collect information from every source, on every branch of husbandry, thus to enable the reader to study the various systems which experience has proved to be the best, under given circumstances."[8]

At least a hundred such journals were established at one time or another in the South before 1860, but only a few lasted for any appreciable length of time. Among the most notable of these were Skinner's *American Farmer* (1819–1834), Edmund Ruffin's *Farmers' Register* (1833–1842), the *Southern Agriculturist* (1826–1846) of Charleston, the *Southern Planter* (1841–) of Richmond, the *Southern Cultivator* (1843–1935) of Augusta, and the *American Cotton Planter* (1853–1861) of Montgomery. In addition, many daily and weekly newspapers featured articles on agricultural topics, as did periodicals of broader scope, such as *De Bow's Review*, published in New Orleans. These publications thus in-

---

7. Bidwell and Falconer, *History of Northern Agriculture*, 319; Gates, *Farmer's Age*, 317, 345; *De Bow's Review*, IV (1847), 427, 443.

8. Quoted in Bidwell and Falconer, *History of Northern Agriculture*, 316.

creased their subscribers' awareness of the benefits to be derived by applying science to agriculture.[9]

Some of the articles that appeared in *De Bow's Review* during the late 1840s reflected the new enthusiasm for science. Although this celebrated journal was oriented more toward the commercial than the agricultural interests of the South, one of its stated goals was to disseminate information relating to "the soil and its capacities for improved growth and cultivation, the variety and tests of soils, their relative value and productiveness, their yield in the most and least favorable circumstances, their best sites and locations."[10]

From the journal's inception, *De Bow's* correspondents extolled the virtues of scientific agriculture. Arguing that a knowledge of plant physiology and soil chemistry was essential to success in agriculture, one writer asserted that many errors committed in farming could be avoided "if the planter would consent to unite a larger portion of scientific information with his practical skill." Another contributor, William P. Hart, reporting on an analysis of soils in Brazoria County, Texas, that he had conducted using the procedures established by Sir Humphry Davy, reminded readers that chemical analysis was particularly important in determining the mode and amount of fertilization. Yet another, lauding the work of Hart, opined that in recent years "chemistry has become the handmaid of agriculture" by lessening the cost of labor and increasing production. These sentiments were echoed by Judah P. Benjamin, one of the most progressive sugar planters in Louisiana. After recounting the benefits that the beet-sugar industry of France had reaped by applying scientific principles, he urged his fellow Louisiana planters to become acquainted "with at least those general elementary principles of Chemistry, of which our sugar-houses show us the application on a large scale."[11]

Benjamin was a frequent contributor to *De Bow's*, which, because of its location, catered particularly to the sugar interests. Sugar was unique among southern staples in that the boiling of cane juice constituted a manufacturing process, and it therefore stood to benefit more from the proliferation of scientific knowledge in the mid-nineteenth century than did any other commercial crop produced in the slave states. Accordingly, during the initial years of his editorship,

9. Gray, *History of Southern Agriculture*, II, 788; Gates, *Farmer's Age*, 341–42; Bidwell and Falconer, *History of Northern Agriculture*, 320.

10. *De Bow's Review*, I (1846), 5.

11. *De Bow's Review*, III (1847), 302, 557; *De Bow's Review*, IV (1847), 319; *De Bow's Review*, V (1848), 44–49.

De Bow published "a great variety of papers" touching upon every facet of the sugar industry by "the best informed and accurate sources, at home or abroad."[12]

In a particularly notable article published in the fall of 1846, Benjamin presented in elaborate detail the fruits of his studies "on the cultivation and manufacture of sugar in this State." Demonstrating a remarkable familiarity with international scientific literature—citing, among others, the works of Davy, Benjamin Silliman, the eminent German chemist Hochstetter, and the French chemist Peligot—Benjamin reviewed the chemical constitution of cane as established by organic analysis and argued that the practice of plowing in trash improved fertility by adding carbon and inorganic bases to the soil. Turning next to the manufacturing process, the author discussed the relative merits of the open-kettle and vacuum-pan methods of boiling cane juice and alluded to "the researches and experiments of eminent chemists, who have devoted their time and labor to this subject."[13] In a piece published two years later, Benjamin described and explained the principles underlying "Soleil's Saccharometer." This instrument, invented in Paris in 1846 on the basis of "discoveries in optics made by modern science," measured the quantity of crystallizable sugar in saccharine solutions and was thus of obvious utility to sugar planters.[14]

Unfortunately, support for the new scientific agriculture was far from unanimous among southern agricultural proprietors or, for that matter, among their northern counterparts. Farmers have traditionally been conservative, and those in nineteenth-century America were no exception. Stung by various crazes, such as the silkworm mania of the 1830s, and by exaggerated claims for new methods of cultivation or new varieties of seeds and livestock, many farmers grew wary of the agricultural press.[15] Such distrust was expressed vividly in the *Southern Planter* shortly after the American edition of Liebig's celebrated work was published. In marked contrast to the praise lavished upon the German scientist by such reform-minded observers as Rost and De Bow, this writer declared:

> Mr. Justus Liebig is no doubt a very clever gentleman and a most profound chemist, but in our opinion he knows about as much of agriculture as the horse that ploughs the ground, and there is not an old man that stands

12. *De Bow's Review,* IX (1850), 109.
13. *De Bow's Review,* II (1846), 322, 327–28, 341, 343.
14. *De Bow's Review,* V (1848), 357.
15. Gates, *Farmer's Age,* 296; Gray, *History of Southern Agriculture,* II, 789.

between the stilts of a plough in Virginia, that cannot tell him of facts totally at variance with his finest spun theories. The same thing is true pretty much of the balance of the agricultural philosophers; they are smart men, and in the multiplicity of their guesses they may strike right, but we hardly esteem their works, with one or two exceptions, worth the notice of the practical farmer.[16]

In vain, the reformers railed against the enemies of so-called book farming. Declaring flatly that "farmers are opposed to innovation," a disillusioned Richard Abbey charged that "there is almost an organized opposition to change or reform in any particular." Another Mississippian, expressing agreement with Napoleon's assertion that "the world was governed by epithets," lamented that "the name of theorist, or book-farmer, has deterred many from improving their minds, and their condition of life." Even the usually optimistic De Bow, in the lead article of the December, 1847, issue of his review, deplored what he perceived as the tendency of the South "to prosecute agriculture with little regard to system, economy, or the dictates of liberal science."[17]

Of course, opposition to agricultural experimentation and innovation was not confined solely to the South. American farmers in general were more conservative in this respect than their counterparts in Europe. Perhaps the most obvious explanation lies in the abundance of fertile and salubrious land available in most parts of the United States. Quite simply, American farmers failed to adopt progressive agricultural methods because they had no motive to do so. As Lewis Gray has remarked, "broadly speaking, interest in fertilization or in scientific field systems did not develop anywhere so long as fresh fertile land was locally available." De Bow repeatedly offered the same explanation.[18]

Despite regional similarities reflected in such factors as the ready availability of fertile land and the crazes and puffs propagated by the agricultural press, the South was apparently less receptive than the North to scientific agricultural practices. Although quantification of this type is hazardous at best, a comparison of the number of agricultural societies, periodicals, and state-aided surveys in each region reveals a significant sectional differential. For example, in the late 1850s more than 900 local and state agricultural societies existed in the

16. Quoted in Gray, History of Southern Agriculture, II, 789.

17. De Bow's Review, III (1847), 4; De Bow's Review, V (1848), 365; De Bow's Review, IV (1847), 419.

18. Gray, History of Southern Agriculture, II, 806; Moore, Agriculture in Mississippi, 41; De Bow's Review, IV (1847), 419, 443; De Bow's Review, IX (1850), 382.

United States, of which no more than 165 were located in the South.[19] Similarly, on the eve of the Civil War there were approximately 25 farm journals in the free states with an estimated circulation of 250,000, while the slave states had but 6 to 8 such papers with a circulation of 35,000.[20] Finally, of the 24 state agricultural societies and boards of agriculture organized in the 1840s and 1850s, only a fourth were below the Mason-Dixon Line.[21] Southern spokesmen such as De Bow recognized these manifest disparities and tried valiantly to stimulate their countrymen to greater activity. In an article promoting the fifth anniversary meeting of the Louisiana Agricultural and Mechanics' Association, the indefatigable editor praised the quantity and quality of agricultural societies, fairs, and journals in Massachusetts and New York and called for the establishment of local societies in every parish in Louisiana.[22] Such pleas, however, were largely unheeded.

Why did the South languish behind the rest of the nation in adopting a more scientific approach to agriculture? Slavery, of course, was the most obvious factor differentiating the two sections, and it has been fashionable to attribute most of the ills of the South to that benighted institution. Thus, in assessing the general intellectual atmosphere in the South during the late antebellum period, Clement Eaton termed the southern mind "essentially unscientific" and attributed this condition, in large measure, to the "inhibiting influence of slavery." Recently, this view has been challenged by Ronald and Janet Numbers, who contend that the South's relative backwardness in promoting science "resulted more from demographic and environmental factors than from slavery-related mental attributes."[23]

The Numberses are correct, but only up to a point. Clearly, slavery per se did not stifle the spirit of intellectual inquiry or the application of scientific principles, for it was the planters—particularly the large slaveholders—who were most inclined to adopt scientific agricultural practices.[24] Yet slavery did have important side effects that were inimical to a broader application of science to agriculture by the southern population as a whole. Chief among these were the impediments the

19. Bidwell and Falconer, *History of Northern Agriculture*, 318; Gates, *Farmer's Age*, 314.

20. Gates, *Farmer's Age*, 343. For slightly different figures, see Gray, *History of Southern Agriculture*, II, 788.

21. Bidwell and Falconer, *History of Northern Agriculture*, 318.

22. *De Bow's Review*, IV (1847), 419–21, 445.

23. Clement Eaton, *The Mind of the Old South* (Baton Rouge, 1964), 156; Ronald L. Numbers and Janet S. Numbers, "Science in the Old South: A Reappraisal," *Journal of Southern History*, XLVIII (1982), 184.

24. Gates, *Farmer's Age*, 138.

slave system placed upon white immigration; the growth of industry; and the development of transportation facilities, urban centers, and schools. In short, slavery saddled the region with an overwhelmingly rural agricultural economy.[25]

The lack of urbanization and the absence of adequate educational facilities were especially critical, for both significantly affected the ability to communicate scientific ideas to a broad spectrum of the agricultural population. Considering that only twenty-two towns, five of them in Virginia, had a population of ten thousand or more in 1860, it is little wonder that the slave states had so few agricultural societies and journals. Yet these agencies were essential to the dissemination of scientific information.

Even if urban growth in the South had been sufficient to support the publication of additional agricultural periodicals, there would have been no market for them. As it was, editors of southern journals were so strapped financially by the lack of popular support that they had to borrow much of their material from more affluent northern and English magazines.[26] The paucity of potential readers for such journals is primarily attributable to the woeful state of education in the South. Not until the 1840s did anything approaching a public school system emerge, and the illiteracy rate remained more than twice as high as that of the Northeast until the end of the antebellum period.[27] Southern leaders recognized these deficiencies and labored diligently to correct them, but progress was slow. As late as 1856, Philip St. George Cocke, in his presidential address to the Farmers' Assembly of the Virginia State Agricultural Society, called attention to the deplorable state of education in the South and delivered a fervent plea for both public school and agricultural education. Noting, perhaps with some exaggeration, that 70,000 adult white Virginians could neither read nor write, Cocke charged that the small landholders, overseers, and managers who constituted 95 percent of southern agriculturists were "universally and utterly ignorant of every abstract principle of physical or natural science."[28]

In the face of such realities, it was the planters who assumed the

25. Eugene D. Genovese, "The Significance of the Slave Plantation for Southern Economic Development," *Journal of Southern History*, XXVIII (1962), 422–23, 437; Gray, *History of Southern Agriculture*, II, 940–42.

26. Gates, *Farmer's Age*, 347.

27. Numbers and Numbers, "Science in the Old South," 177–79.

28. *De Bow's Review*, XXII (1857), 499, 501. For a similar plea by the governor of Georgia, see *ibid.*, 665–66.

burden of applying scientific practices to southern agriculture. Only they had sufficient leisure, education, and familiarity with the literature to make science the true handmaid of agriculture. Consequently, it was this group that organized agricultural societies, supported fairs, and instituted systematic efforts to improve soils, crops, and livestock. It was to them that the contents of southern farm journals were directed.[29] And many were equal to the challenge.

In the following pages I hope to demonstrate that a significant relationship existed between science and the plantation in the Old South and that members of the planter elite were not only receptive to new ideas from the realm of science, but made notable contributions to the development of scientific agriculture. To facilitate this analysis, I shall divide antebellum planters into three categories. The first group, the "planter-scientists," includes those persons who, by training and experience, were scientists as well as planters. Their scientific achievements were not necessarily related directly to agriculture, though they tended to focus their attention on those branches most congenial to the rural, agricultural society in which they resided (e.g., geology, soil chemistry, botany, conchology). A second group of planters, whom I shall call "amateur scientists," had no scientific training and little or no professional experience outside of agriculture. However, though they were concerned primarily with the application of science to farming, they had other scientific interests as well. The third, and by far the largest category, the "scientific agriculturists," comprises those who applied scientific knowledge and methodology exclusively to the solution of agricultural problems. The northern agricultural reformer Solon Robinson called them "improving planters." Whatever one chooses to call them, they were a large group and had a profound impact upon the agricultural economy of the Old South. Admittedly, these divisions are fragile and, in some cases, perhaps arbitrary. However, this system of classification will, I hope, prove useful in the discussion that follows.[30]

Two of the most distinguished early planter-scientists were William Dunbar of Mississippi and Stephen Elliott of South Carolina. The son of a Scottish earl, educated in Glasgow and London, Dunbar came to America shortly before the Revolution and eventually established his residence on a plantation near Natchez. There he applied his scientific knowledge to agriculture and soon prospered sufficiently to indulge his paramount interest in scientific investigation. Particularly fasci-

29. Gates, *Farmer's Age*, 138, 342, 347; Moore, *Agriculture in Mississippi*, 85.
30. See Eaton, *Mind of the Old South*, 154–56, for a somewhat similar classification of southern scientists.

nated by astronomy, he erected his own observatory and in 1799 made the first significant meteorological observations in the Mississippi Valley. Regarded as the "foremost scientist of the Southwest," Dunbar corresponded extensively with Thomas Jefferson and other noted intellectuals of his generation. As a member of the renowned American Philosophical Society, he contributed papers to the *Transactions* of the Society on such diverse subjects as Indian sign language, fossil bones, and plant and animal life in his area.[31]

No less impressive was the career of Stephen Elliott, one of the most versatile intellects of the early nineteenth-century South. A graduate of Yale, Elliott was active in politics, banking, agriculture, the literary and creative arts, and the natural sciences. To name but a few of his distinctions, he was the first president of the State Bank of South Carolina, a founder and president until his death in 1830 of the Literary and Philosophical Society of South Carolina, president of the Charleston Library Society, a founder of the Medical College of South Carolina and its first professor of botany and natural history, the founder with Hugh Swinton Legaré of the *Southern Review,* to which he frequently contributed essays, and author of the two-volume *Sketch of the Botany of South Carolina and Georgia.* He collected and prepared material for the latter during an extended residence on his Beaufort District plantation before moving to Charleston in 1812. Eloquent testimony to Elliott's success in the dual role of planter-scientist is afforded by the fact that the Elliott Society of Natural History, organized in Charleston in 1853, was named in his honor and that his immediate descendants owned nearly five hundred slaves on the eve of the Civil War.[32]

After 1830 three members of the Ravenel family of South Carolina successfully combined planting careers with noteworthy achievements in various scientific fields. Edmund Ravenel, a pioneer American conchologist, received a medical degree from the University of Pennsylvania in 1819 and served for more than a decade as professor of chemistry in the Medical College of South Carolina. Resigning his position in 1835, he purchased a Cooper River plantation with more than a hundred slaves and by the 1850s had expanded his holdings to more than 7,500 acres. Yet Ravenel retained an active interest in scien-

31. *Dictionary of American Biography,* V, 507–508; Thomas Cary Johnson, Jr., *Scientific Interests in the Old South* (New York, 1936), 175.

31. *Dictionary of American Biography,* V, 507–508; Thomas Cary Johnson, Jr., *Scientific Interests in the Old South* (New York, 1936), 175.

32. *DAB,* VI, 99; Johnson, *Scientific Interests,* 63, 128, 149; Eaton, *Mind of the Old South,* 155; MS census returns, 1860, in National Archives, Washington, D.C. (Schedule 2, Slave Inhabitants), Beaufort and Colleton districts, S.C.. Those listed include William Elliott, 256 slaves; Stephen Elliott, Sr., 190; Stephen Elliott, Jr., 49.

tific matters: he published an important work on the marine shells of South Carolina in 1848 and contributed several articles to the Elliott Society of Natural History, of which he was a vice-president.[33] Edmund's nephew, St. Julien Ravenel, was a noted physician and agricultural chemist. After studying medicine at the Charleston Medical College and pursuing additional studies in Philadelphia and Paris, he soon turned his talents to agriculture. In 1857 he established on his Cooper River plantation a "perpetual kiln" for converting marl into lime, the first lime works in the state. Earlier, he had proposed the artesian well system inaugurated by the city of Charleston in the late 1850s. During the Civil War, St. Julien Ravenel administered the Confederate laboratory in Columbia that manufactured most of the medical supplies for southern troops. After the demise of the Confederacy, he returned to the task of trying to revitalize the soils of the South Carolina low country and developed processes for producing both ammoniated and phosphate fertilizers.[34]

Perhaps the most distinguished member of this Huguenot family was Henry William Ravenel. Born on a Charleston District plantation, he graduated from South Carolina College in 1832. His father, himself a former physician, dissuaded him from pursuing a career in medicine and, instead, provided him with a plantation and slaves. After embracing the life of a low-country planter, young Ravenel developed an avid interest in cryptogamic botany, the study of fungi, lichens, moss, and algae. This interest led to the publication in the 1850s of his five-volume work *Fungi Caroliniani Exsiccati*. After the war, he collaborated with the celebrated English botanist M. C. Cooke in publishing a second series entitled *Fungi Americani Exsiccati*. Together, these monumental contributions established Ravenel as the preeminent American authority on fungi and precipitated an extensive correspondence with botanists all over the world. In 1883 he was elected to membership in the Royal Zoological and Botanical Society of Vienna, and a decade later the British Museum purchased the cryptogamic portion of his famous herbarium.[35]

For reasons not immediately apparent, planters of Huguenot descent seem to have been particularly attracted to the world of science. In addition to the Ravenels, two of the most distinguished scientists in the Old South, Joseph and John LeConte, were of Huguenot ex-

33. *DAB*, XV, 394–95; Johnson, *Scientific Interests*, 136, 141, 149.

34. *DAB*, XV, 397; William K. Scarborough (ed.), *The Diary of Edmund Ruffin* (3 vols.; Baton Rouge, 1972–1989), I, 564; Johnson, *Scientific Interests*, 136, 146.

35. *DAB*, XV, 396; Johnson, *Scientific Interests*, 135, 143.

traction. Although both were professional scientists, they retained substantial land and slave holdings along the Georgia rice coast until after the Civil War.[36] Yet another Huguenot planter-scientist was John Wesley Monette of Washington, Mississippi. In contrast to the LeConte brothers, Monette did not inherit a plantation but acquired one late in life as he, like other professionals, succumbed to the temptation of the agrarian ideal that pervaded the antebellum South. A native of Staunton, Virginia, Monette grew up in Ohio and studied medicine at Transylvania University before settling in the Natchez area. While still a young man, he wrote a notable, but unpublished, essay in which he anticipated some of Darwin's ideas on natural selection. His study of yellow fever epidemics in Mississippi led him to suggest the quarantine as a preventive measure in combating that dreaded scourge. But his primary interest was natural history and his magnum opus a monumental study of the history and geography of the Mississippi Valley. Shortly before his death in 1851, Monette, his scientific curiosity presumably satiated, established his residence on a cotton plantation in northern Louisiana, where in 1850 he owned seventy-seven slaves.[37]

Although he lacked the formal professional training of planter-scientists like the Ravenels and LeContes, James Hamilton Couper of Georgia was destined to attain distinction not only as one of the foremost scientific planters of the Old South, but as an amateur natural scientist of extended reputation. His interest in science came quite naturally, for one of his uncles held the chair of practical astronomy at the University of Glasgow until his death in 1836, and another was a noted surgeon in the same city. Couper, like many others of his class, received a first-rate education in northern preparatory schools before matriculating at Yale, from which he graduated in 1814. Returning to Georgia, he was soon entrusted with the management of the vast Hopeton plantation, a tract of some two thousand acres owned in partnership by his father, John Couper, and James Hamilton and situated on the Altamaha River in Glynn County. As the years passed,

36. The entire LeConte family owned nearly two hundred slaves in Liberty County, Georgia, in 1850, and a decade later, Joseph and John together owned more than one hundred (MS census returns, 1850 and 1860, in National Archives, Washington, D.C. [Schedule 2, Slave Inhabitants], Liberty County, Ga.). For a recent study of the younger of the LeConte brothers, see Lester D. Stephens, *Joseph LeConte: Gentle Prophet of Evolution* (Baton Rouge, 1982).

37. *DAB*, XIII, 85; Johnson, *Scientific Interests*, 195–96; Eaton, *Mind of the Old South*, 152; MS census returns, 1850, in National Archives, Washington, D.C. (Schedule 2, Slave Inhabitants), Madison Parish, La.

Couper purchased a half-interest in Hopeton, inherited a plantation on St. Simon's Island, and acquired other properties in his own right. At the peak of his planting career in the mid-1850s, Couper was directing the labor of nearly fifteen hundred slaves on four plantations in the fertile Altamaha delta.[38]

From the outset, Couper conducted his agricultural operations on the basis of scientific research and experimentation. Shortly after assuming the management of Hopeton, Couper journeyed to the Netherlands to study firsthand that country's method of water control preparatory to establishing an elaborate system of dikes and drainage for his own rice fields. For a decade and a half, he experimented successively with sea island cotton, sugarcane, and rice before finally settling upon the latter as the principal staple at Hopeton. An entire volume of Couper's surviving plantation record books is devoted exclusively to copious notes on various aspects of sugar and rice culture as well as notes on other crops grown on his agricultural units. But he did not confine his propensity for experimentation to commercial crops. A strong advocate of diversification, he experimented at one time or another with such exotic products as oranges, date palms, and olives, achieving his greatest success with the latter. He was the first to use Bermuda grass to forestall erosion on the embankments surrounding rice fields. Couper also pioneered in the extraction of oil from cotton seed and operated two crushing mills, one in Natchez and the other in Mobile, for a brief period in the 1830s before a series of unpropitious circumstances caused the venture to end in failure.[39]

In company with other progressive planters, Couper sought to devise methods of preserving the fertility of his lands and rendering them more productive. To this end, he advocated deep plowing and the application of such natural fertilizers as cane leaves and rice straw in combination with animal manures. He also fell prey to the guano craze that swept across the South during the last decade of the antebellum period. But Couper was most innovative in the practice of crop rotation. Convinced that "rotation was nature's great fertilizer," he developed a highly sophisticated land-use pattern for Hopeton. Underlying his scheme of rotation, which comprised a sixteen-year cycle for highlands and a nine-year cycle for tidal swamplands, was a con-

38. James E. Bagwell, "James Hamilton Couper, Georgia Rice Planter" (Ph.D. dissertation, University of Southern Mississippi, 1978), 25, 41, 106, 231–32; *DAB*, IV, 468.

39. Bagwell, "James Hamilton Couper," 171, 107–108, 202–204, 68, 77; James Hamilton Couper Plantation Records, in the Southern Historical Collection, University of North Carolina, Chapel Hill, vols. 3, 4; *DAB*, IV, 468.

viction that plants could be divided into two basic categories: the broad-leaf or leguminous type, which had an ameliorative effect on the soil, and the narrow-leaf or culmiferous type, which had a debilitating effect. By skillfully alternating crops on the various fields of his plantation, Couper found that he was able to sustain high crop yields over an extended period of time.[40]

Although Couper was one of the greatest of the rice barons and one of the largest slaveholders in America, he found time to indulge a variety of scientific interests that were quite distinct from his business operations. Characterized by one authority as a true Renaissance man, Couper made significant contributions in the fields of geology, conchology, herpetology, paleontology, ornithology, and botany. Noted particularly for his knowledge of the geology of coastal Georgia, he presented a paper on that subject in 1845 to the Geological Society of London, of which he was a corresponding member. He corresponded with and entertained at Hopeton such notable figures as William Cooper, a prominent New York naturalist, and Sir Charles Lyell, perhaps the most celebrated British scientist to visit the United States before the Civil War. A member of the Academy of Natural Sciences in Philadelphia, Couper donated a number of valuable fossil specimens to that institution, and in 1861 he presented a collection of several thousand items to the Museum of Natural History in Charleston.[41]

Couper received his greatest plaudits from the scientific community when, in the course of superintending construction of the Brunswick canal in the late 1830s, he unearthed the remains of a number of prehistoric animals, of which the most important was a gigantic sloth known as the Megatherium. There had been earlier discoveries of this animal in both Spain and Georgia, but relics from those excavations had been only fragmentary. Now an entire skeleton was available for study. Couper hastened to present his findings in a paper read before the Academy of Natural Sciences of Philadelphia in the autumn of 1842. Four years later, a Savannah planter, William B. Hodgson, incorporated Couper's geological observations in his *Memoir on the Megatherium and Other Extinct Gigantic Quadrupeds of the Coast of Georgia, with Observations on Its Geologic Features.*[42] Hodgson, who had acquired the famous Retreat plantation in Jefferson County through his marriage to the daughter of Alexander Telfair and who by 1860 was the largest

40. Bagwell, "James Hamilton Couper," 211–27.

41. *Ibid.*, ix, 269, 271, 280–82; Johnson, *Scientific Interests*, 98–99, 149.

42. Bagwell, "James Hamilton Couper," 276–77; Johnson, *Scientific Interests*, 64–65, 98.

slaveowner in the state, was yet another member of the planter elite who displayed more than a passing interest in science.[43]

Although he did not match Couper in either the size of his agricultural holdings or the diversity of his scientific interests, Benjamin L. C. Wailes of Mississippi was also an amateur scientist of considerable reputation. Like Couper, Wailes manifested an interest in scientific agricultural practices, serving as president of the short-lived Jefferson College Agricultural Society in the early 1840s and experimenting with a variety of vegetables and fruits on his farm near Washington, Mississippi. He was also one of the leading sheep breeders in the Natchez area. Like his Georgia counterpart, however, Wailes exhibited a scientific curiosity that transcended the immediate needs of his planting enterprise. He too accumulated a large collection of rocks, fossils, flora, and fauna from his region and eventually donated them to appropriate depositories within the state. He maintained contact with such noted contemporary scientific figures as John J. Audubon, Louis Agassiz, and Benjamin Silliman. Most important of all, while serving as assistant professor of agricultural and geological sciences at the University of Mississippi, he conducted the first agricultural and geological survey of the state and published his report in 1854.[44]

Despite the undoubted contributions of those planters who were also professional scientists and those, like Couper and Wailes, who merely pursued scientific interests as an avocation, the most persistent link between science and the plantation was formed by the large body of southern agriculturists who applied scientific knowledge and methodology specifically and exclusively to agricultural concerns. As Clement Eaton has remarked, a "surprising number" of antebellum planters "closely observed nature, read agricultural publications, and experimented with new crops."[45] Anyone conversant with the contents of extant plantation record books can affirm the validity of that assertion. Whether science is defined simply as "knowledge obtained by study and practice" or, more specifically, as "a branch of study concerned with observation and classification of facts, especially with the establishment of verifiable general laws," the planters more than met the

43. Hodgson ranked third among the large slaveholders of Georgia in 1850, when he had 450; ten years later, his holdings had increased to nearly 600 (MS census returns, 1850 and 1860, in National Archives, Washington, D.C. [Schedule 2, Slave Inhabitants], Burke, Chatham, Jefferson counties, Ga.).

44. Charles S. Sydnor, *A Gentleman of the Old Natchez Region: Benjamin L. C. Wailes* (Durham, 1938), 152–53, 160, 83, 183; *DAB*, XXIV, 315–16.

45. Eaton, *Mind of the Old South,* 155.

test.[46] Their meticulous notations in plantation journals relating to meteorological phenomena, agricultural experiments, crop yields, characteristics of the labor force, and the like afford abundant evidence of their use of scientific procedures. As noted at the outset of this chapter, science was not the precise and highly structured discipline in the nineteenth century that it is today. One did not have to earn an advanced degree or use the facilities of a sophisticated laboratory to apply the techniques encompassed within the general definition of science.

One fact that emerges from a perusal of both the business records of the planters and the agricultural press of the late antebellum period is the emphasis upon system and order in plantation operations. Many proprietors prepared a written set of regulations for the governance of their properties. They maintained precise logs of the amount of cotton picked by every hand during each day of the harvest season. They carefully noted in their plantation journals the daily activities of each segment of the work force. And they recorded in detail the results of the experiments in which they were continually engaged. Typical is the journal of Francis Terry Leak, who operated a moderate-sized plantation in northeastern Mississippi. His plantation diary, covering 1839–1862, contains numerous speculations on how to increase crop yields, frequent references to agricultural experiments, meticulous observations on the progress of various crops, and even suggestions of mechanical devices that would benefit the cotton planter.[47]

The success of scientific experiments on the plantation necessarily depended upon the cooperation of such subordinate functionaries as the overseer. Unfortunately, the members of that unlettered and largely unmotivated class did not perceive this to be one of their primary functions—or so their employers claimed. "It would seem as if my blundering Overseers would forever put it out of my power to ascertain facts from the accuracy of experiments," complained an exasperated George Washington in 1794. A half-century later, the South Carolina planter-politician James Henry Hammond discharged one of his overseers "because he would not weigh measure & attend properly to the details of my affairs—experiments particularly." Another South Carolina proprietor charged that overseers "uniformly set themselves against any improvement that is attempted, and in most cases will lose their places rather than permit any important experiment to succeed

46. *Webster's New Collegiate Dictionary* (Springfield, Mass., 1949), 757.
47. Francis Terry Leak Diary, in the Southern Historical Collection, University of North Carolina, Chapel Hill, vols. 2, 3, 5.

which they can thwart."[48] Despite such annoying opposition, progressive planters continued to apply scientific principles to their business operations in the hope of improving both the quality and quantity of their crops and livestock. Whether they employed the sophisticated methodology of Edmund Ruffin, who conducted nineteen separate experiments over more than fifteen years on his James River farm to ascertain the effect of marling, or the haphazard methods of Charles Whitmore, who frequently neglected to record the results of his various experiments, southern planters were well aware of the benefits to be derived from the application of science to agriculture.[49]

It was the agricultural reform movement of the 1830s and 1840s, however, that especially promoted a more scientific approach to agriculture in the Old South. Plagued by widespread soil exhaustion, the product of nearly two centuries of tobacco culture, the upper South was in the throes of a severe economic depression by the end of the second decade of the nineteenth century when a number of reform advocates made their appearance. The first significant reformer was John Taylor of Caroline, who in 1813 published his pioneering work *Arator*. In that book Taylor championed such innovative practices as subsoil plowing, a four-field system of crop rotation, prolonged fallowing of exhausted soils, and the use of vegetable materials for manure. Unfortunately, Taylor's efforts had little immediate effect, but others soon assumed the mantle of leadership and brought to fruition the agricultural renaissance he had initiated. Chief among these were John Skinner of Maryland, founder of the *American Farmer*, the first important agricultural periodical in America, and Edmund Ruffin, editor of the *Farmers' Register* and chief proponent of the gospel of marl.[50]

The movement thus spawned in the upper South in the 1820s spread to the Southwest twenty years later as the once-prosperous cotton kingdom fell victim to the Panic of 1837 and plummeting cotton

48. George Washington to William Pearce, November 23, 1794, in Moncure Daniel Conway (ed.), *George Washington and Mount Vernon, Long Island Historical Society Memoirs*, IV (1889), 130; James Henry Hammond to Edmund Ruffin, August 7, 1845, Edmund Ruffin Papers, Virginia Historical Society, Richmond; *American Agriculturist*, IV (1845), 319. See also William K. Scarborough, *The Overseer: Plantation Management in the Old South* (Baton Rouge, 1966), 107; *Southern Cultivator*, II (1844), 170.

49. Edmund Ruffin, *An Essay on Calcareous Manures*, ed. J. Carlyle Sitterson (Cambridge, Mass., 1961), 83–119; Mack Swearingen, "Thirty Years of a Mississippi Plantation: Charles Whitmore of 'Montpelier,'" *Journal of Southern History*, I (1935), 203–205.

50. Clement Eaton, *The Growth of Southern Civilization, 1790–1860* (New York, 1961), 178–80.

prices. In desperation, agricultural leaders from the South Atlantic states assembled in a series of so-called planters' conventions to discuss various alternatives for raising the price of cotton. But these efforts proved abortive, and once again an impressive array of reformers came forward to plot a course toward renewed prosperity. Men like Martin W. Philips and John C. Jenkins of Mississippi, David Dickson and William J. Eve of Georgia—all of them planters—began to urge southern farmers to diversify their crops and to employ more intensive methods of farming. Agricultural journals were established to propagate the theories of the maturing sciences, and progressive agriculturists organized societies on both county and state levels to facilitate the exchange of new ideas and to exhibit quality livestock and farm produce at annual fairs.

After some prodding, state agencies also began to participate in the campaign to rejuvenate the southern agricultural economy. If farmers were to improve the productive capacity of their lands, they would first have to know something about their chemical content. Consequently, a number of states commissioned agricultural and geological surveys. At the invitation of Governor Hammond, himself a progressive planter, Edmund Ruffin conducted such a survey in South Carolina in 1843. During the following decade, four other southern states followed suit. In like spirit, Maryland, Virginia, North Carolina, Alabama, and Mississippi had, by 1851, appointed official agricultural chemists whose chief tasks were to analyze the soils in their respective states and communicate their findings to agriculturists.[51] Some states established agricultural bureaus to assist in the organization of local societies and to facilitate the collection and dissemination of information on all aspects of farming. Among the specific objectives of the Mississippi Bureau, created in 1857, was the establishment of "a Chemical Labratory [sic] and a Mineral Cabinet, where soils, manures, minerals and waters may be analyzed, and their constituents, in quantity and in quality, demonstrated to exact figures."[52]

An interest also developed, rather belatedly, in agricultural education. One of its chief proponents was Philip St. George Cocke, who was one of the largest slaveowners in the South and had extensive holdings in both Virginia and Mississippi. In 1856, while serving as president of the Virginia State Agricultural Society, Cocke called for a dual system of agricultural education that would consist of a depart-

51. Gray, *History of Southern Agriculture*, II, 790.
52. Moore, *Agriculture in Mississippi*, 200–203; *De Bow's Review*, XXIII (1857), 639.

ment of agriculture with three professorships at the University of Virginia and, for those in the lower stratum of society, an agricultural institute having a less demanding and more practical curriculum. Estimating the total cost of his proposed package at $200,000, half of which would be subscribed by the farmers themselves, he offered to initiate the plan by donating $20,000 to the society for the first of the professorships. But when Cocke insisted on naming the initial incumbent, the offer was rejected and the money diverted, instead, to establish a school of agriculture at the Virginia Military Institute.[53] Shortly before this controversy erupted in Virginia, chairs of agricultural chemistry had been established at the state universities in both North Carolina and Georgia.[54]

Among those who had opposed the Cocke donation was Edmund Ruffin, without doubt the premier scientific agriculturist of the Old South. Unfortunately, his notoriety as a political extremist has clouded public awareness of his extraordinary agricultural contributions—so much so that his latest biographer makes only brief mention of the latter.[55] Others, however, have been more appreciative. Former president John Tyler hung Ruffin's portrait over his fireplace next to that of Daniel Webster, thereby honoring, as he said, the one as "the first among American statesmen, & the other [as] the first of American Agriculturists," and praised his fellow Virginian for having contributed "more good to the country than all our political great men put together." More recently, he has been hailed by one authority as "the father of soil chemistry in America" and by another as "the most influential leader of Southern agriculture and one of the greatest agricultural figures America has produced."[56] Such praise seems well merited.

The son of a prosperous James River planter, Ruffin attended the College of William and Mary, served briefly in the War of 1812, and then commenced farming at Coggin's Point in Prince George County. His agricultural debut, however, proved to be anything but auspicious. Plagued by the impoverished soils for which his compatriot

---

53. *De Bow's Review*, XXII (1857), 502–504; *Ruffin Diary*, I, 12–13, 117, 173. In 1860 Cocke owned more than 650 slaves in the two states of Virginia and Mississippi (compiled by author from MS census returns, 1860, in National Archives, Washington, D.C. [Schedule 2, Slave Inhabitants], Brunswick and Powhatan counties, Va.; Lowndes and Yazoo counties, Miss.).

54. Gray, *History of Southern Agriculture*, II, 792.

55. Betty L. Mitchell, *Edmund Ruffin: A Biography* (Bloomington, Ind., 1981).

56. *Ruffin Diary*, I, 123, 619; Avery O. Craven, *Edmund Ruffin, Southerner: A Study in Secession* (1932; rpr. Baton Rouge, 1966), 60; Gray, *History of Southern Agriculture*, II, 780.

John Taylor had proposed remedies, he followed the advice propounded in *Arator* but to no avail. The application of vegetable manures had but little effect in increasing the productivity of his exhausted lands. Just as he was about to abandon his farm in despair and seek greener pastures in the West, a chance reading of Davy's *Elements of Agricultural Chemistry* suggested a possible solution to his problem. Was it possible that organic acids had rendered his soil immune to the beneficent effects of putrescent manures? If so, perhaps this acidity could be neutralized by the application of marl, a shell-like deposit consisting primarily of clay mixed with calcium carbonate, which was abundantly available in eastern Virginia. Eagerly Ruffin commenced marling operations on his Coggin's Point property in 1818, and that autumn he presented to his county agricultural society the first of his many provocative and enlightening papers on agricultural topics. Three years later, John Skinner published a revised version of that paper entitled "On the Composition of Soils and their Improvement by Calcareous Manures" in the *American Farmer*.[57]

Though without scientific training, Ruffin conducted over the next decade an elaborate series of experiments designed to test the validity of his new theory. First, he perused the pages of European works on soil chemistry. Next, he took soil samples and, with scientific precision, measured the proportion of calcareous earth in each by means of a pneumatic apparatus first proposed by Davy. With the knowledge thus acquired, he then applied to carefully measured experimental plots on his Coggin's Point farm various quantities of either marl alone or marl in combination with organic manures and meticulously recorded the results of each trial. These carefully structured experiments confirmed "in almost every particular the chemical powers" Ruffin had attributed theoretically to calcareous manures. In no instance had the increase of the first marled crop of grain planted on "worn acid soil" been less than 50 percent above the previous crop, and frequently the increased yield had been as great as 100 percent. Buoyed by this dramatic confirmation of his theories, the enthusiastic young gentleman farmer hastened to spread the glad tidings to other farmers in his region and, indeed, throughout the South.[58]

During the course of his experiments at Coggin's Point, Ruffin had

---

57. Scarborough's introduction to *Ruffin Diary*, I, xviii; Craven, *Edmund Ruffin*, 54–56; Sitterson's introduction to Ruffin, *Essay on Calcareous Manures*, xii–xiv; Gray, *History of Southern Agriculture*, II, 780–81; Johnson, *Scientific Interests*, 180–81.

58. Ruffin, *Essay on Calcareous Manures*, 40–42, 125–27; Gray, *History of Southern Agriculture*, II, 781.

gradually expanded his original seven-page article prepared for Skinner into a book of nearly 250 pages, which he published in 1832 under the title *An Essay on Calcareous Manures*. This work, later hailed by a Department of Agriculture expert as "probably the most thorough piece of work on a special agricultural subject ever published in English," established Ruffin's reputation as a scientific agriculturist and attracted such favorable notice that four subsequent editions were published during the next twenty years.[59] In essence, Ruffin argued that naturally poor soils differed from once-fertile soils exhausted by excessive cultivation in their capacity for enrichment from putrescent manures, and that the capacity for improvement of any soil depended upon its natural fertility. The exhausted soils of eastern Virginia, he further contended, were suffering from excessive vegetable acidity and a deficiency of calcareous earth. The application of marl was merely the indispensable first step toward restoring the productive capacity of these lands. It did so by maximizing the fertilizing effect of vegetable and animal manures, by neutralizing acids in the soil, and by improving the texture and absorbency of the soil. Or, as Ruffin explained more succinctly, calcareous earth "destroys the worst foe of productiveness, and uses to the greatest advantage the fertilizing powers of other manures."[60] In his conception of soil fertility as a dynamic condition, subject to change as a consequence of organic action, Ruffin was, as Avery Craven has observed, "a half-century or more ahead of his time."[61]

During the decade that followed the publication of his famous *Essay*, Ruffin gradually withdrew from the active management of his farm and turned his attention to other activities. From 1833 to 1842 he was engaged chiefly with the publication of his distinguished agricultural journal, the *Farmers' Register*, which has been described by one scholar as "the most important single force in producing the agricultural revolution that transformed the agriculture of the upper south from its moribund state in the 1820's to its prosperous condition in the 1850's." When his editorial tirades against the evils of wildcat banking caused this publication to fail in December, 1842, he embarked immediately upon his agricultural survey of South Carolina. Upon his return to Virginia the following year, Ruffin, having previously relinquished

59. Sitterson's introduction to Ruffin, *Essay on Calcareous Manures*, xvi; Craven, *Edmund Ruffin*, 56.

60. Ruffin, *Essay on Calcareous Manures*, 21–22, 73–75.

61. Sitterson's introduction to Ruffin, *Essay on Calcareous Manures*, xv; Craven, *Edmund Ruffin*, 58, 60.

control of his James River place to his eldest son, purchased a new plantation of some one thousand acres along the banks of the Pamunkey River northeast of Richmond. During the next decade he transformed this property, appropriately named Marlbourne, into a model estate. He constructed an elaborate system of covered drains, applied large quantities of marl, and by these and other means increased dramatically the productivity of his land. Once again, the veteran farmer had proved that his theories could be effectively translated into practice.[62]

Having demonstrated beyond question his capability as an agricultural entrepreneur, Ruffin retired from the active direction of his farming operations in the mid-1850s and devoted his attention increasingly to political affairs. Still, until the war itself became the all-absorbing topic in his mind, he found time to indulge his interest in agriculture and to render additional services to the field that had claimed the bulk of his energy for more than forty years. In the course of his extensive journeys through the South, the ever-inquisitive Ruffin took copious notes on the various soil formations and types of vegetation he encountered. He continued the practice he had begun many years before at Coggin's Point of testing various soils with muriatic acid to determine their calcareous content. These observations furnished the basis for a number of valuable articles on such topics as the swamplands of eastern North Carolina, the canebrake lands of Alabama, and the "peculiarities of the soils of Florida."[63] He also continued his efforts to promote agricultural reforms in his native state. Thus, when the Virginia State Agricultural Society was organized in 1852, Ruffin accepted the presidency and remained one of its most active leaders for the balance of the decade.

Although Ruffin, like others of his class, was primarily concerned with agriculture and politics, he had other intellectual interests as well. Among these was a natural curiosity about scientific phenomena quite apart from his pragmatic interest in soil chemistry. Like Couper and Wailes, he developed an extensive collection of fossil shells, many of

62. Sitterson's introduction to Ruffin, *Essay on Calcareous Manures*, xix; Scarborough's introduction to *Ruffin Diary*, I, xviii–xx. For a recent interpretation that emphasizes personal and economic, rather than political, factors in the downfall of the *Farmers' Register*, see W. M. Mathew, "Edmund Ruffin and the Demise of the *Farmers' Register*," *Virginia Magazine of History and Biography*, XCIV (1986), 3–24.

63. *Ruffin Diary*, I, 192–93, 518–19, 536; Johnson, *Scientific Interests*, 181. See, for example, Edmund Ruffin, "Agricultural Features of Virginia and North Carolina," *De Bow's Review*, XXII (1857), 462–79; *De Bow's Review*, XXIII (1857), 1–20.

which came from various European sites and were sent to him by Sir Charles Lyell. He was intimately acquainted with a number of the most prominent members of the southern scientific community, most notably Matthew F. Maury, whom he visited frequently; Michael Tuomey, whom he personally recommended for the position of geological surveyor of South Carolina and, subsequently, as the first professor of agricultural chemistry in the University of Alabama; and, above all, the Reverend John Bachman, the renowned Charleston naturalist and Lutheran minister. Ruffin's scientific interests ranged from geology to ethnology. Though utterly without training in the former, he complained that some of his practical observations had been "stolen without being acknowledged" by the celebrated William B. Rogers. He read "everything I have met with" on the subject of ethnology but found "more amusement than reliable information" because virtually all authorities seemed bent on proving one or the other of the antithetical doctrines of the unity or diversity of the origin of man.[64] Thus, Ruffin, like Couper, was something of a Renaissance man.

Despite his other scientific interests, however, Ruffin made his most notable contribution in his application of science to agriculture. In a moment of self-reflection shortly after he entered his seventieth year, he assessed his agricultural labors in these terms: "As an agriculturist, I have made discoveries, & have introduced in Virginia improvements of the most important value—which have already added many millions to the intrinsic value of this region, & have enabled thousands of individual farmers to triple & quadruple the productive value of their property." If his own generation did not appreciate his efforts—and he complained bitterly that it did not—he was content to await vindication from future generations. For the most part, the latter have responded favorably to his appeal, at least with respect to his agricultural achievements.[65]

Next to Ruffin, probably the most significant advocate and practitioner of scientific agriculture in the Old South was Dr. Martin W. Philips. A native of South Carolina, Philips abandoned the practice of medicine while still a young man and in 1831 moved to Hinds County, Mississippi. Five years later, he established his residence at Log Hall, a small cotton plantation on the Big Black River midway between Jackson

64. *Ruffin Diary*, II, 472; *Ruffin Diary*, I, 55, 42; *Ruffin Diary*, III, January 10, 1864.

65. *Ruffin Diary*, II, 545–46, 549. For a provocative new study of Ruffin and the relationship between slavery and agricultural reform, see William M. Mathew, *Edmund Ruffin and the Crisis of Slavery in the Old South: The Failure of Agricultural Reform* (Athens, Ga., 1988).

and Vicksburg. There he proceeded to put his progressive theories into practice and soon developed a model estate.[66]

Sharply critical of then-current agricultural practices in the cotton states, Philips emphasized the need for greater production of subsistence crops and livestock to reduce operating expenses, but, at the same time, he advocated improved techniques to increase cotton yields. For more than a quarter-century he promoted the ideal of self-sufficiency with his own investigations and experiments and through countless articles in the agricultural press. He developed and tested farm implements, conducted extensive experiments in cotton hybridization and corn cultivation, imported quality livestock into central Mississippi, helped to organize local and state agricultural societies, and, in partnership with two relatives, founded in 1857 the only farm-implement factory in the state. But Philips' influence was not confined to Mississippi. He communicated his views and findings to agricultural journals throughout the nation. It would be difficult to quarrel with John Hebron Moore's assertion that Philips "was the most prolific American agricultural writer of the ante-bellum period."[67]

At the same time, Log Hall became an example of the economic diversification preached by its proprietor. As one visitor put it, Dr. Philips "practices what he professes." Cotton and corn were the basic crops, but Philips also planted substantial amounts of oats, sweet potatoes, and millet, and he experimented with rice, tobacco, and Chinese sugarcane. In addition, he raised a varied assortment of vegetables and fruits, procuring seeds and trees from plant breeders and nurserymen throughout the country. Included in the magnificent fruit orchards at Log Hall, which reputedly contained more than 2,000 trees, were 150 varieties of peaches and numerous kinds of apples, pears, plums, apricots, cherries, figs, and grapes. Philips also raised and bred substantial numbers of quality livestock, achieving his greatest success with Black Berkshire hogs. Constantly augmenting his herds with thoroughbred animals purchased from such leading breeders as Richard Peters of Georgia, Mark Cockrill of Tennessee, and James H. Hammond of South Carolina, Philips developed a stock in-

66. Gray, *History of Southern Agriculture*, II, 781; Gates, *Farmer's Age*, 145; Moore, *Agriculture in Mississippi*, 97.

67. Moore, *Agriculture in Mississippi*, 85, 97–98, 158–59, 189–91, 198; Gray, *History of Southern Agriculture*, II, 782; Franklin L. Riley (ed.), "Diary of a Mississippi Planter, January 1, 1840 to April, 1863," *Publications of the Mississippi Historical Society*, X (1909), 305–481.

ventory that included Durham and Ayrshire cattle, Bakewell and Merino sheep, Berkshire and Essex hogs, and Cashmere goats.[68]

It would be difficult to imagine a more clear-cut example of the application of the scientific method to agriculture than that afforded by the career of Martin W. Philips. Theory, experimentation, observation, interpretation, and dissemination of results—these are the quintessential elements of scientific inquiry, and all were reflected in Philips' approach to agricultural problems. In contrast with Couper and Ruffin, however, the Mississippi planter apparently never manifested much interest in scientific fields extraneous to agriculture. After the war, in which his plantation suffered irremediable losses, he remained dedicated to the improvement of agrarian pursuits, first as a nurseryman, later as editor of the *Southern Farmer* in Memphis, and finally as the first head of the department of agriculture at the University of Mississippi.[69]

The career of yet another Mississippian, John Carmichael Jenkins, will suffice as a final illustration of that remarkable group that I have chosen to call scientific agriculturists. Born in Lancaster, Pennsylvania, Jenkins graduated from Dickinson College, took a medical degree from the University of Pennsylvania in 1833, and shortly thereafter moved to Wilkinson County, Mississippi, to assist an uncle with his medical practice. Following the death of his uncle four years later, Jenkins embarked upon a planting career, married the daughter of William Dunbar, and in 1840 shifted his residence to Elgin plantation in Adams County. In the ensuing years Jenkins achieved great success as a cotton planter, ultimately operating four plantations with a combined slave force of nearly four hundred. When he inherited his uncle's properties in 1837, they were encumbered by a debt of more than $150,000. However, during the next seven years, in the midst of a depression, he produced nearly seven hundred bales of cotton annually, which yielded an average gross income of $23,600 per year. As a consequence, Jenkins was able to retire his debt completely by the mid-1840s. He went on during the next decade to accumulate an estate valued at nearly $200,000 before he and his wife met their untimely deaths in a yellow fever epidemic.[70]

68. *Southern Cultivator,* XVI (1858), 177; Riley (ed.), "Diary of a Mississippi Planter"; Gates, *Farmer's Age,* 260.

69. Riley (ed.), "Diary of a Mississippi Planter," 308.

70. Albert G. Seal, "John Carmichael Jenkins: Scientific Planter of the Natchez District," *Journal of Mississippi History,* I (1939), 14–16, 27; Plantation Diary of John Carmichael

Much of Jenkins's success can be attributed to his superb managerial ability and his progressive methods of agriculture. Though not a propagandist like Ruffin or Philips, he was constantly experimenting—with different varieties of seed cotton, with various types of fertilizer, and, above all, with fruit culture. He converted his home plantation of Elgin into a veritable agricultural experiment station. Termed by one authority a "ranking pioneer in Southern horticulture," Jenkins maintained meticulous records of the experiments conducted in his elaborately planned orchard, which was carefully divided into large sections, each confined to a particular fruit, and subsections for individual varieties in which each tree and row were numbered. The orchard at Elgin reportedly contained more than a hundred varieties of apples and pears, and Jenkins himself developed and marketed at least eighteen new varieties of peaches.[71] Thus, although he made his fortune in cotton, the Natchez planter-physician responded enthusiastically to the call for economic diversification sounded by his fellow countryman Martin W. Philips and in the process rendered notable service in the field of southern horticulture.

What, then, may we conclude about the relationship between science and the plantation and, more generally, that between science and agriculture in the Old South? As early as the 1780s such progressive-minded planters as George Washington and Thomas Jefferson began to undertake formal experiments designed to increase the productiveness of their increasingly exhausted lands. Although conversant with similar experimentation being conducted in England and in the North, they received little guidance from the still undeveloped sciences.[72] Operating largely by trial-and-error methods, southern planters in the early nineteenth century made important discoveries (e.g., in plant breeding) that laid the foundations for many of the achievements associated with modern agricultural science.

The agricultural reform movement of the late antebellum period, however, provided the main impetus for a more scientific approach to agricultural problems. Coinciding with important advances in the emerging sciences of biology, geology, and chemistry, the movement spawned a number of agricultural journals that disseminated the theo-

---

Jenkins, January 11, 1845, John C. Jenkins and Family Papers, Louisiana State University Department of Archives, Baton Rouge; MS census returns, 1860, in National Archives, Washington, D.C. (Schedule 2, Slave Inhabitants), Wilkinson County, Miss.

71. Seal, "John Carmichael Jenkins," 16–25.

72. Gray, History of Southern Agriculture, II, 612, 779.

ries of such scientists as Liebig, along with the practical findings of progressive planters. Taking their cue from the private sector, states soon began to render assistance in various ways. They sponsored agricultural and geological surveys, appointed official agricultural chemists, established state agricultural bureaus and societies, and funded agricultural professorships in state institutions of higher learning. As a consequence of these endeavors, both public and private, the 1850s became the most prosperous decade in southern agriculture during the entire antebellum period.

Although a few planters, like the Ravenels of South Carolina, successfully combined planting careers with notable professional achievements in the sciences, most were dissuaded by the agrarian, country-gentleman ideal from embarking upon careers as professional scientists. That cult, which emphasized the preeminent position in southern society of agriculture and politics, not only diverted some bright young men from potential careers in science but also influenced the direction taken by science in the region. As the Numberses have remarked, southern scientists tended to focus their attention primarily on "the biological and geological sciences"—those most closely related to the agrarian orientation of the section— "rather than on the physical sciences and mathematics." The emphasis on agricultural subjects in state geological surveys, observed another historian, "bore witness to the fact that geology was widely regarded as the handmaid of agriculture rather than as a distinct science."[73] Still, science had a profound impact even upon those who subscribed fully to the agrarian ideal that permeated the slave South. It is worthy of note that many of the so-called scientific planters discussed in the preceding pages received their first exposure to science in the course of preparing for their initial vocations as medical doctors. Perhaps that training made them particularly receptive to the scientific approach when they later concentrated their attention on agricultural pursuits.

Whatever the reason, many members of the southern planter elite clearly embraced with enthusiasm new theories propagated by the scientific community, put them into practice on their own estates, and labored assiduously to persuade the lesser planters and yeoman farmers to emulate their example. However, they met with only limited success in the latter endeavor. Their failure was not a result of the

73. Numbers and Numbers, "Science in the Old South," 184; Charles S. Sydnor, *The Development of Southern Sectionalism, 1819–1848* (Baton Rouge, 1948), 265.

intellectual rigidity associated with the hardening proslavery orthodoxy of the late antebellum period, as some have alleged;[74] rather, it
was a consequence of certain residual effects engendered by the peculiar institution. Chief among these was a predominantly rural society
that discouraged formation of those agencies necessary to communicate scientific information to the general population and a seriously
defective system of public education. As Lewis Gray has observed,
agricultural periodicals did not flourish in a region populated largely
by Negro slaves and "illiterate poor whites occupying non-commer-
cial farms."[75] Thus, despite the many impressive accomplishments of
the large slaveholders, southern agriculturists as a whole did not take
full advantage of the opportunities afforded them by the advances in
scientific knowledge in the mid-nineteenth century.

74. Eaton, *Mind of the Old South*, 137, 156–57.
75. Gray, *History of Southern Agriculture*, II, 788–89.

CHAPTER 5

SLAVERY AND TECHNOLOGY IN THE ANTEBELLUM SOUTHERN IRON INDUSTRY: THE CASE OF BUFFALO FORGE

Charles B. Dew

A nyone attempting to discuss the relationship between science and industry in the Old South has to face the fact that such industrialization as occurred in the region prior to the Civil War was almost totally unaffected by early nineteenth-century scientific knowledge and inquiry. The primary industrial activities of the antebellum South—textile manufacturing; coal mining; lumbering; the production of naval stores; shipbuilding; iron manufacturing; and the processing of southern-grown cotton, tobacco, sugar, hemp, rice, corn, and wheat—were based largely on the technology of the earlier phases of the Industrial Revolution. Thus to assess the place of science in the industrial life of the Old South, we must turn rather quickly to the technologies employed in southern manufacturing. The Old South seems to afford a striking illustration of a point made by Thomas C. Cochran: "In early industrialization what may be called the workbench skills and imagination were more important than scientific knowledge or the kinds of intellectual skills required in the twentieth century."[1] This chapter will focus on the technology and "workbench skills" used in the manufacture of iron in the antebellum South. Iron-making was one of the most significant elements in the industrial life of the pre–Civil War (and wartime) South. Even more important, the process by which iron ore was converted into finished goods reflected the close relationship between the technology used in much of southern iron manufacturing and the South's most peculiar form of industrial labor, slavery.

1. Thomas C. Cochran, *Frontiers of Change: Early Industrialism in America* (New York, 1981), 54.

In the summer of 1862, William Weaver, one of the leading iron-masters in the Valley of Virginia, received what can only be described as a plea from the president of an important Richmond manufacturing establishment. "We have been brought pretty near the point that un-less we can very soon get some Iron we must close our Works," wrote William S. Triplett of the Old Dominion Iron and Nail Works. This would be a serious blow to the Confederate war effort, he went on, because the government depended on his mill for a number of critically needed items. "I therefore write to you in perfect frankness to say we have no Iron, or next to none, and to enquire at what price you will send us, or make for us, . . . 200 Tons Iron," Triplett told Weaver. "We will pay a high price to get it, but hope you will be as moderate as you can."[2]

William Weaver had devoted most of his eighty-two years to trying to make money in the Virginia iron trade, and the chance virtually to name his own price for two hundred tons of pig iron must have been tempting to him. But even that generous prospect would not induce him to put his Etna Furnace in Botetourt County, Virginia, back into blast. "I have no metal for sale, nor am I making any, having closed my furnace last Christmas," Weaver replied. "My reason for relinquishing the furnace business was, that Richmond was always a bad market and we could not compete with northern iron, as it always had a preference over our mountain iron and I had become tired of supplying an article at a loss," he continued. "The present price would pay well," Weaver readily agreed, "but when the blockade is opened where will the profit be?"[3]

Weaver's refusal to resume the manufacture of pig iron, even in the face of the unprecedented wartime demand, was a forceful reminder of the declining fortunes of the Virginia iron industry during the late antebellum years. A committee report to a miners and manufacturers convention assembled in Richmond in 1850 had told much the same tale as Weaver's letter. "Virginia has an unlimited supply of the finest ores, easily accessible for use and transportation, with the greatest abundance of coal, wood and limestone for their manufacture," wrote the members of the "Committee to enquire into and report on the condition of the Coal and Iron Trades." And yet, despite her abundant raw materials, the manufacture of iron in Virginia had "shrunk to an inconsiderable amount," and the industry was "in danger of utter

2. William S. Triplett to William Weaver, August 21, 1862, in William Weaver Papers, Duke University Library, Durham.
3. Weaver to Triplett, August 25, 1862, in Buffalo Forge Letterbooks, Weaver-Brady Collection, University of Virginia Library, Charlottesville.

ruin," the report concluded. In 1850, the year of this bleak forecast, twenty-nine Virginia blast furnaces employing 1,129 workers produced 22,163 tons of pig iron. Ten years later, sixteen Virginia blast furnaces employed only 529 men, and production had fallen to only 11,396 tons. During that same decade, the manufacture of pig iron in Pennsylvania rose from an 1850 level of 285,702 tons to 580,049 tons in 1860.[4]

Virginia's iron men, and the merchants who sold their products, were well aware of the sad plight of their industry in the years leading up to the Civil War. "In reference to Iron Masters, we have to say, if they continue to go out of the market in this next 12 months in proportion to the past year say three a year, we shall have none to begin 1860 with, as three more will include you," Weaver's Lynchburg merchants wrote him in January 1859. The problem, quite simply, was that Virginia's producers of pig and wrought iron were being squeezed out of their own market by low-cost northern and British iron. "I cannot sell [pig] metal at less than $26 per ton," Weaver complained in June 1859, and he insisted that even at that price he was taking a loss on his pig. "Sales cannot be made now at either 25 or 26$," his Richmond commission merchants informed him in August, and the next month they told him bluntly that "metal cannot be sold at anything like your prices." During this same period, Joseph R. Anderson of Richmond's sprawling Tredegar Iron Works was buying pig iron in thousand-ton lots in Philadelphia and Baltimore for $19 to $21 per ton. No wonder Anderson warned his brother Francis, who owned Glenwood Furnace in Rockbridge County, Virginia, to think about his future operations. "If I were in your place I would during the present year carefully investigate the question whether it is [in] your interest to continue the Iron Business," Anderson cautioned in July 1857. Although Joseph had an "abundance of good ore" on property he owned in an adjoining county, he refused even to consider the possibility of erecting a blast furnace on his land. "It seems to be worthy of inquiry whether you cannot make more money with less outlay and trouble by making other uses of your valuable land and timber," Joseph advised his brother.[5]

4. Richmond *Whig*, December 17, 1850; Charles B. Dew, *Ironmaker to the Confederacy: Joseph R. Anderson and the Tredegar Iron Works* (New Haven, 1966), 32.

5. Lee Rocke & Co. to Weaver, January 8, 1859, Weaver to F. B. Deane, Jr., & Son, June 22, 1859, and Shields & Somerville to Weaver, August 3 and September 3, 1859, all in Weaver-Brady Collection, Charlottesville; Dew, *Ironmaker to the Confederacy*, 33; J. R. Anderson to F. T. Anderson, July 12, 1857, in Anderson Family Papers, University of Virginia Library, Charlottesville.

The same depressing picture faced Weaver and other Virginia iron-masters when they attempted to sell their wrought iron, generally referred to in the iron trade as "merchant bar," on the Richmond or Lynchburg markets. Weaver's Buffalo Forge, located some nine miles southeast of Lexington in Rockbridge County, Virginia, produced a high-quality bar iron much prized by local blacksmiths and implement makers, but he asked $90 per ton for his metal in the late 1850s. Common English wrought iron could be had in Richmond for as little as $65 per ton in 1860, and the best English bar sold there for $75 per ton, prices even J. R. Anderson's local Tredegar rolling mills could not match. Northern-produced wrought iron, like that made in England, also undersold the Virginia-manufactured bar iron in the Virginians' own market.[6]

On the eve of the Civil War, the figures for wrought iron production in Virginia were as dismal as those for pig iron. In 1860, Virginia's sixteen forges, located mostly beyond the Blue Ridge Mountains in the Valley and employing only 154 hands, produced a total of 1,709 tons of merchant bar; the Tredegar Iron Works rolled 6,000 tons of bar in Richmond. That same year, Pennsylvania's eighty-seven mills and forges, employing 10,177 workers, manufactured 112,276 tons of bar iron and 133,577 tons of railroad iron. Not a single ton of railroad iron was produced in the Old Dominion during 1860.[7]

A close student of iron manufacturing in antebellum Virginia concluded that the basic structure of the industry just before the Civil War was little different than it had been in the early decades of the eighteenth century. "Individual iron plantations . . . formed the backbone of the iron industry in Virginia," writes S. Sydney Bradford, "and at them the basic product, pig iron, was manufactured for the whole of the period from 1716 to 1861." And just as the eighteenth-century iron plantation survived into the industrial age of mid-nineteenth-century America, so too did the primitive iron-making technology of an earlier era. The basic techniques of operating both blast furnaces and forges remained "largely unchanged," Bradford notes. "While British and Northern ironmasters lowered costs through adopting improved processes of manufacture" in the first half of the nineteenth century, "Virginia's iron makers paid such changes little heed." As a consequence,

6. William D. Couch & Co. to Weaver, February 9, 1859, and McCorkle & Co. to Weaver, February 22, 1859, both in Weaver Papers; McCorkle & Co. to Weaver, January 15, 21, 1859, both in Weaver-Brady Collection, Charlottesville; Dew, *Ironmaker to the Confederacy*, 30.
7. Dew, *Ironmaker to the Confederacy*, 88.

"by 1861, Virginia's iron industry was moribund," Bradford concludes, "with its most successful days a thing of the past."[8]

Anyone who has studied the iron industry of antebellum Virginia can attest to the accuracy of Bradford's description, which could be applied to the entire region.[9] The blast furnaces that dotted upland areas of the South during the Civil War were little different in form or technology from those that had existed in the days of the American Revolution. And the mountain forges that produced horseshoe iron for the Army of Northern Virginia or the Army of Tennessee were refining pigs and hammering out bars in almost exactly the same manner as their predecessors had done for the Continental forces fighting the war for independence some eighty-five years before.

Why was this so? Why had technological innovation largely bypassed the South's iron industry? The answers are complex and include a variety of factors. Certainly one major reason for the backwardness of southern iron manufacturing was an accident of nature: anthracite coal, the fuel that helped transform the northern iron industry in the 1830s and 1840s, was mined only in eastern Pennsylvania in the decades prior to the Civil War and was not available to southern ironmasters.[10] As a result, ironworks in the South continued to rely almost exclusively on charcoal, a very expensive fuel to produce, and southern iron carried the burden of this expense into the marketplace wherever it was sold.

Other important technological advances, however, could have increased the production of pig and wrought iron in the South and substantially reduced the cost of that iron. The hot-blast technique, for example, first introduced in England in 1828, was a marked improve-

8. Samuel Sydney Bradford, "The Ante-Bellum Charcoal Iron Industry of Virginia" (Ph.D. dissertation, Columbia University, 1958), 184–85.

9. See Dew, *Ironmaker to the Confederacy*, 32–34, 87; Lester J. Cappon, "Trend of the Southern Iron Industry Under the Plantation System," *Journal of Economic and Business History*, II (1930), 353–81, and "Iron-Making—A Forgotten Industry of North Carolina," *North Carolina Historical Review*, IX (1932), 331–48; Ernest M. Lander, Jr., "The Iron Industry in Ante-Bellum South Carolina," *Journal of Southern History*, XX (1954), 337–55; Frank E. Vandiver, "The Shelby Iron Works in the Civil War: A Study of a Confederate Industry," *Alabama Review*, I (1948), 12–26, 111–27, 203–17; Kathleen Bruce, *Virginia Iron Manufacture in the Slave Era* (New York, 1930); and Ethel M. Armes, *The Story of Coal and Iron in Alabama* (Birmingham, 1910).

10. Alfred D. Chandler, Jr., "Anthracite Coal and the Beginnings of the Industrial Revolution in the United States," *Business History Review*, XLVI (1972), 141–81; Frederick Moore Binder, *Coal Age Empire: Pennsylvania Coal and Its Utilization to 1860* (Harrisburg, Pa., 1974), 41–84.

ment over existing blast-furnace technology and could easily have been adapted to charcoal-fired southern stacks. The process basically involved heating the blast of air that was sent into the furnace to help bring the mixture of iron ore, fuel, and limestone to the proper temperature. As Peter Temin notes:

> This innovation could be attached to any existing blast furnace. In its simplest form, it was just a set of pipes over a fire in which the blast was heated on its way to the furnace. A more economical version, because it did not use any extra fuel, was to place the pipes through which the blast passed at the top of the blast furnace where they could be heated by the combustion of the waste gases from the furnace itself. It was in this form . . . that the innovation was generally adopted in America.[11]

The conversion of a New Jersey furnace to hot blast in 1834 marked the beginnings of this new process in America, and it spread rapidly across the North. A standard treatise on iron manufacturing, published in 1854, stated that a charcoal-fired blast furnace equipped with hot blast could "save twenty per cent of fuel, and augment the product fifty per cent." This new technology was almost totally ignored in the South.[12]

The production of wrought iron in the southern states reflected the same general pattern as the production of pig iron: a lack of concern for technological change. The use of the puddling furnace and the rolling mill to manufacture wrought iron—greatly improved techniques that swept across the northern iron industry in the three decades prior to the Civil War—accounted for most of the tremendous upsurge in the production of bar and railroad iron in Pennsylvania and other states in the North during the 1850s. In the eleven states that formed the Confederacy in 1861, there were exactly six modern rolling mills: two at the Tredegar Iron Works in Richmond, the Gate City rolling mill at Atlanta, the small Etowah rolling mill near Cartersville in northern Georgia, the Shelby rolling mill in Alabama, and the Cumberland rolling mill near Fort Donelson, Tennessee. The typical southern facility for producing wrought iron in 1860 was exactly what it had been one hundred years before—a charcoal-fired forge, where workers used refinery hammers to purify the iron and chaffery hammers to pound it into merchant bars.[13]

11. Peter Temin, *Iron and Steel in Nineteenth-Century America: An Economic Inquiry* (Cambridge, Mass., 1964), 58–59.
12. Frederick Overman, *The Manufacture of Iron* (3rd ed.; Philadelphia, 1854), 442; see also the entries for individual blast furnaces in J. P. Lesley, *The Iron Manufacturer's Guide to the Furnaces, Forges and Rolling Mills of the United States* (New York, 1859), 63–83.
13. Temin, *Iron and Steel in Nineteenth-Century America*, 100–101; Dew, *Ironmaker to the Confederacy*, 87; Lesley, *Iron Manufacturer's Guide*, 178–216, 244–46, 259.

The largely stagnant state of the iron industry in Virginia and throughout the antebellum South can be explained in a variety of ways. Capital for new industrial plants—modern hot-blast furnaces and large-capacity rolling mills, for example—was not easy to come by in the slave South. As Fred Bateman and Thomas Weiss point out, "planters and slaveholders, the chief potential source of capital within the South, failed to participate adequately in the development of manufacturing." Bateman and Weiss are undoubtedly correct when they conclude that "it seemed to take more evidence and more time to convince southerners to enter the murky waters of the American Industrial Revolution."[14]

But what about those men who did take the plunge, those southern ironmasters who invested substantial amounts of capital in blast furnaces and forges in the early nineteenth century and then, almost to a man, sat back and watched the technological innovations of the 1830s and 1840s pass them by? How do we explain their failure to use state-of-the-art industrial technology? The answer, it seems, lies at least partly in the nature of their labor force.

The career of William Weaver of Buffalo Forge, Rockbridge County, Virginia, provides an excellent example of my central thesis: that slave labor, once it was trained and functioning in the traditional ways of making iron, exerted a powerful, conservative influence on the technology of the southern iron industry. Slave workers predominated wherever iron was made in the Old South, and they had a great deal to say about the technology used and the methods employed in the manufacture of iron. No record better illustrates this than that of William Weaver's ironworks in the Valley of Virginia.

William Weaver apparently had all of the attributes of a hard-driving nineteenth-century American entrepreneur. He was, first of all, a Yankee, born in 1781 on a farm at Flourtown, Pennsylvania, not far from Philadelphia. His parents, pious, industrious, sober-minded folk, were German Dunkers, and young William learned the benefits of hard work and the value of a dollar at an early age. As he grew into manhood, he engaged in a variety of profitable enterprises in and around Philadelphia, including farming, merchandising, milling, marble-quarrying, textile manufacturing, and, during the War of 1812, blockade-running. Another one of his wartime ventures was his chance investment in the Virginia furnace and forge that later became the central focus of his life. Those ironworks, purchased in partnership

14. Fred Bateman and Thomas Weiss, *A Deplorable Scarcity: The Failure of Industrialization in the Slave Economy* (Chapel Hill, 1981), 127, 163.

with a Pennsylvania ironmaster named Thomas Mayburry in 1814, also provided his principal livelihood after he moved permanently to the Valley in 1823. From that time on, Buffalo Forge, his home base in Rockbridge County, and Etna Furnace, in neighboring Botetourt County, occupied most of his time and energy. In the late 1820s, Weaver also developed a third property called Bath Iron Works, a furnace and forge complex in northern Rockbridge County, to expand his production of both pig and bar iron.[15]

Weaver realized very quickly that he would have to rely heavily on slave labor if he were to make his Virginia investments pay off. "A very limited view of things" in the Valley convinced him that "no reliance could be placed in the free White laborers who are employed about Iron Works in this country," he wrote later. Free laborers were "generally very poor" workmen, in Weaver's view, and, even worse, in "moments of the greatest pressure and necessity, the proprietor must either make them advances which they will never repay, or they leave his service to the ruin of his business." Weaver clearly believed that in addition to being relatively unskilled, undependable, and prone to extortion, white ironworkers were also liable to be "idle half their time drunk," as Thomas Mayburry told Weaver in 1817, or, to use Weaver's phrase, off "on a Frolic" when most needed.[16] Excessive consumption of alcohol was a perpetual problem at almost all ironworks, North and South, where free labor was employed, and the use of slaves would help remedy that problem. When the manager of an extensive iron plantation in Botetourt County was asked whether he preferred white or black labor, he answered in words Weaver himself might have chosen: "I would rather have slaves," he said, "they are less trouble."[17]

15. "Weaver Family: Memo and Historical Notes," in Weaver-Brady Papers in the possession of T. T. Brady, Richmond; Donald F. Durnbaugh (ed.), *The Brethren in Colonial America* (Elgin, Ill., 1967), 214, 219, 244; deposition of William Weaver, December 10, 1840, Case Papers, *Alexander v. Irvine's Administrator,* Superior Court of Chancery Records, Rockbridge County Court House, Lexington, Va. (hereinafter cited as Case Papers, *Alexander v. Irvine's Administrator*); bill of complaint of *William Weaver v. Thomas Mayburry,* November 19, 1825, Case Papers, *Weaver v. Mayburry,* Superior Court of Chancery Records, Augusta County Court House, Staunton, Va. (hereinafter cited as Case Papers, *Weaver v. Mayburry*).

16. Bill of complaint, *Weaver v. Mayburry,* November 19, 1825, and Thomas Mayburry to William Weaver, August 16, 1817, both in Case Papers, *Weaver v. Mayburry;* William Weaver to John Doyle, January 7, 1828, Case Papers, *Doyle v. Weaver,* Superior Court of Chancery Records, Rockbridge County Court House, Lexington, Va. (hereinafter cited as Case Papers, *Doyle v. Weaver*).

17. Deposition of James T. Martin, May 23, 1826, Case Papers, *Weaver v. Mayburry.* See also Joseph F. Walker, *Hopewell Village: A Social and Economic History of an Iron-Making Community* (Philadelphia, 1966), 266, 381; Bradford, "Ante-Bellum Charcoal Iron Indus-

Weaver bought his first slaves in 1815. In October of that year he paid $3,200 for eleven slaves, divided into two quite distinct groups. The first parcel consisted of a valuable ironworker named Tooler, his wife Rebecca, and their four sons: Bill, seventeen; Robert, seven; Tooler, Jr., four; and Joe, two. The second group contained no males at all. It consisted of a woman named Mary and her four daughters: Sally, thirteen; Amey, ten; Louisa, six; and Georgianna, two. The ages given for Rebecca's and Mary's children on the bill of sale were all approximations, a frequent occurrence in transactions of this sort.[18]

The acquisition of these slaves provided a modest start toward the solution of Weaver's labor needs, but it was essentially a long-range remedy. Tooler and his oldest son, Bill, could go to work at once, but it would be years before Robert, young Tooler, and Joe could enter the labor force. They were, nevertheless, all boys, so there was a strong possibility that they would become productive furnace or forge hands. Such was not the case with Mary and her four girls, however. They might all eventually serve as cooks, house servants, or farm hands, but it was highly unlikely that they would ever be called upon to perform the heavy work required around a forge or blast furnace. In fact, just about the only iron-making job that ever used female labor was leaf-raking at the charcoal pits. In obtaining Mary and her daughters, Weaver appears to have been looking toward his future labor needs in a far different way than he was with the acquisition of Tooler and his family. Mary, in short, seems to have been a "breeding woman" in Weaver's eyes, to use a description Weaver later employed to describe a somewhat similar situation.[19] And Sally, Amey, Louisa, and Georgianna might play the same role as they grew up and took husbands.

If, as seems most likely, Weaver bought Mary and her children looking toward the natural increase of his slave force, then he knew exactly what he was doing. The purchase of Tooler and his wife and children and Mary and her four girls turned out to be one of the most significant acquisitions Weaver made during his long career as a Virginia ironmaster. In a life filled with many successful deals, Weaver probably looked back upon his first venture into the slave market as a stroke of the greatest good fortune.

It was not his last foray into the slave trade by any means. After he

<hr />

try," 90–92; Arthur Cecil Bining, *Pennsylvania Iron Manufacture in the Eighteenth Century* (2nd ed.; Harrisburg, Pa., 1973), 29–30.

18. Charles B. Dew, "Sam Williams, Forgeman: The Life of an Industrial Slave in the Old South," in James M. McPherson and J. Morgan Kousser (eds.), *Race, Region, and Reconstruction: Essays in Honor of C. Vann Woodward* (New York, 1982), 201–202.

19. *Ibid.*, 202.

moved permanently to Virginia in 1823, he steadily increased his force of slave workers until he had freed himself from any dependence on free labor at Buffalo Forge. "I bought a Forgeman for which I have to pay 300 D in Cash . . . and 2 tons castings," Weaver reported with obvious satisfaction in October 1827. "I should not have bot [sic] him at this time when money is much wanted but I have been endeavoring to purchase him ever since I have been in the Country," he went on. The slave was "the only one I know of—for sale—and such a negro in reality, will be worth two common hands," he added. Even more important, "I shall now have 6 Forgemen of my own," Weaver wrote; "I need hardly say it is all important particularly in this country." By buying the men he needed for a full forge crew in the 1820s, and by training his own younger slaves as they came of age in the 1830s and 1840s, Weaver was able to operate Buffalo Forge almost exclusively with slave labor from the late 1820s until his death in 1863. His heirs continued this practice until emancipation came to the Valley in the spring of 1865.[20]

Forge work demanded a combination of skill, brawn, and good judgment. The process began with the master refiner and his underhand working bars of pig iron in specially constructed charcoal fires until the iron turned into a ball of glowing, pasty metal. The refiner would then sling this semimolten mass of iron onto his anvil, where it was pounded and shaped under the rhythmic blows of a huge, water-powered hammer. Through successive reheatings and poundings, the refiner and his helper removed enough of the impurities in the pig iron to work it into a bloom, or anchony, as it was more often called in the Virginia iron country.[21]

Weaver described a typical anchony produced at Buffalo Forge as a piece of malleable iron of arbitrary size, "sometimes probably six inches square with a blade of iron about the length of my cane" (Weaver's cane, which still hangs inside the front door of his imposing house at Buffalo Forge, is thirty-two inches long); "one end of the blade has what is called the *tail end*, which contains iron enough generally to make a shovel mould," he added, and "the weight is also arbitrary, ranging from 80 to 150 lbs." Producing high-quality anchonies was not

20. William Weaver to John Doyle, October 12, 1827, Case Papers, *Doyle* v. *Weaver.* See also Buffalo Forge Negro Books, 1830–40, 1839–41, 1844–50, 1850–58, Buffalo Forge Iron Book, 1831–62, and Daniel C. E. Brady, Home Journal, 1858–60, all in Weaver-Brady Collection, Charlottesville; and Daniel C. E. Brady, Home Journal, 1860–65, McCormick Collection, State Historical Society of Wisconsin, Madison.

21. Bining, *Pennsylvania Iron Manufacture,* 72–73.

easy. The critical point in the refining process was knowing exactly when the pig iron heating in the special refinery fire had reached just the right temperature and consistency for pounding and shaping under the refiner's hammer. Bringing the pig iron "to nature," as this process was called, was the most difficult forge skill to learn, and it could only be acquired by many months of apprenticeship to a master refiner.[22]

Refining anchonies was the most important and difficult part of the forge operation, but it was only the first stage of the manufacturing process. The last step came when a second group of ironworkers, the hammermen, reheated the anchonies and worked them at another forge called a "chaffery." The hammermen drew wrought iron bars of various standardized sizes, shapes, lengths, and weights—merchant bars—which would be shipped to market and sold. Blacksmiths would then take these bars, heat them once more, and work them into a host of things needed for farm or home use—nails, tools, agricultural implements, horseshoes, and so forth.[23]

In order to discipline and motivate his forge crew, William Weaver, like almost all southern iron men, used a combination of coercion and reward. Surviving records show little evidence of the whip being used at Weaver's ironworks, but the threat of brutal punishment was always there. Even more intimidating was the possibility of sale. Slaves who tried to run away or who carried their resistance beyond Weaver's level of toleration could be placed in the hands of slave traders and sold. Yet force clearly had its limits, particularly when highly demanding industrial jobs were involved. No ironmaster would want to part with a trained slave ironworker, as Weaver's delight over acquiring his sixth forgeman in the fall of 1827 suggests. Buying a replacement might be difficult, if not impossible, and trying to hire skilled slave forge workers on a temporary basis was both uncertain and expensive. And if an ironmaster decided to punish rather than sell a slave artisan, he would be running risks there as well. A whipping administered to a skilled slave could easily backfire and damage the master's interests. A slave forgeman with his muscles sore and his anger near the boiling point would not work well, and retaliation would be relatively simple to

22. Deposition of William Weaver, December 10, 1840, Case Papers, *Alexander* v. *Irvine's Administrator*; Bining, *Pennsylvania Iron Manufacture*, 72–73; deposition of John Doyle, February 7, 1840, Case Papers, *Weaver* v. *Jordan, Davis & Co.*, Superior Court of Chancery Records, Rockbridge County Court House, Lexington, Va. (hereinafter cited as Case Papers, *Weaver* v. *Jordan, Davis & Co.*).
23. Bining, *Pennsylvania Iron Manufacture*, 73–74.

carry out around ironworking installations. From the ironmaster's point of view, it was far better to have reasonably willing workers than surly, rebellious slaves who could do considerable damage to forge machinery or perhaps burn the place down; live charcoal was there to do the job. The "overwork" system was the means by which southern iron men tried to secure voluntary performance of the slaves' duties.[24]

Payment for extra work was, as far as I have been able to determine, a universal feature of the labor system at ironworks that employed slave artisans. Slaves had to turn out so many pounds of iron or cut so many cords of wood for charcoaling, all on a daily or weekly basis. They were paid, in either cash, goods, or sometimes time off from work, for anything they produced over the required amounts. The task for slave refiners at Buffalo Forge, and everywhere else in the Valley, was a ton and a half of anchonies per week. Hammermen in the Virginia iron district were each required to draw a "journey" of 560 pounds of bar iron a day. Choppers had to cut nine cords of wood per week.[25] All of these had been the customary quotas for years, and they did not change during the forty years Weaver lived at Buffalo Forge. They were in place when he arrived; they were there when he died; and he never, as far as we know, made any attempt to increase them. To have done so would have been a very risky venture, and Weaver undoubtedly knew it.

What I am trying to suggest is that the ironmaster's twin needs to discipline and motivate his slave workers required that a rather delicate balance be worked out between the demands of the master and the wishes of the slave. The word "delicate" is not often used in describing any aspect of the slave regime, and the chances for misunderstanding here are obviously legion. But it seems fair to say that southern ironworks employing skilled slave artisans developed a labor system that brought the requirements of both master and slave into some sort of harmony. Once that balance had been achieved, it tended to continue from one generation to the next. The system placed a

24. See Buffalo Forge Negro Books, 1830–40, 1839–41, 1844–50, 1850–58, Weaver-Brady Collection, Charlottesville. The best discussions of the overwork system are in Robert S. Starobin, *Industrial Slavery in the Old South* (New York, 1970), 99–103; and Ronald L. Lewis, *Coal, Iron, and Slaves: Industrial Slavery in Maryland and Virginia, 1715–1865* (Westport, Conn., 1979), 119–27. See also Charles B. Dew, "Disciplining Slave Ironworkers in the Antebellum South: Coercion, Conciliation, and Accommodation," *American Historical Review*, LXXIX (1974), 405–10.

25. Depositions of John Doyle, February 5, 1840, Anthony W. Templin, January 24, 1839, John Jordan, July 22, 1836, and Henry A. Lane, February 5, 1840, Case Papers, *Weaver v. Jordan, Davis & Co.*; Dew, "Disciplining Slave Ironworkers," 406.

premium on stability, on getting the work done in old, familiar ways. It afforded precious little incentive toward change and technological innovation. It was, in sum, profoundly conservative, so much so that even a man like William Weaver, Pennsylvania-born entrepreneur though he was, became enmeshed in that very un-Yankee-like way of running an ironworks.

Part of Weaver's problem lay in the fact that his slave forgemen trained their own slave apprentices, often on a father-and-son basis. Frequently the slaves, young and old, had family roots that went back to the beginning, or near beginning, of Weaver's involvement in Virginia iron-making. They were, in a sense, "family servants," and he seems to have felt an obligation toward them and a genuine concern for their welfare. As his age advanced and his health deteriorated, he began to worry about the fate of his slaves, a force that numbered close to seventy men, women, and children in the 1850s. "I am old, all but 75," Weaver wrote in 1855. "The great object with me is, that my servants shall remain where they are, and have humane masters," he continued. "This point is the only difficulty on my mind in relation to my Estate. Giving them their freedom, I am satisfied, would not benefit them as much as having good masters, and remain where they are," Weaver concluded, a point about which he undoubtedly failed to consult his slaves.[26] The makeup of his forge labor force in the late antebellum years illustrates the extent to which his ironworkers were, indeed, part of Weaver's own Virginia experience.

Weaver's master refiner on the eve of the Civil War was a slave named Sam Williams. He traced his ancestry back to the first slaves purchased by Weaver; his mother was one of Mary's four daughters, Sally, who had been thirteen years old when Weaver bought her in 1815. Sally had married a man named Sam Williams, a slave ironworker Weaver had subsequently acquired, and in 1820 they had a baby boy. They named him Sam, after his father, and Sam Williams, Jr., had entered Weaver's forge as a refiner's apprentice at the age of eighteen. He learned the traditional art of refining pig iron into anchonies, became a master refiner, and in 1840 married a slave woman named Nancy Jefferson, whom Weaver also owned. They had four daughters, Betty, Caroline, Ann, and Lydia, all of whom were still alive at the beginning of the Civil War. Sam Williams had a lot to live and work for, and his overwork income was the highest earned by any slave at Buffalo Forge in the 1850s. His underhand at the refinery force was a

26. Weaver to Daniel C. E. Brady, August 27, 1855, Weaver Papers.

young slave named Henry Towles, who appears to have been related to Sam Williams, although the exact nature of the relationship remains obscure.[27]

The chaffery forgemen, like Sam Williams, went back to Weaver's earliest years in Virginia. One hammerman in the 1850s was Tooler (the son of the slave of the same name), who had been purchased by Weaver in 1815 when he was four years old. He had spent virtually his entire life at Buffalo Forge and served his apprenticeship there. The other chaffery forgeman, Harry Hunt, Jr., born in 1832, was the son of a slave named Harry, or Hal, Hunt, who had been one of the "6 Forgemen" Weaver was so pleased to have acquired by the fall of 1827.[28] The Hunts were certainly among the oldest slave ironworking families in Virginia at the time of the Civil War.

Harry Hunt, Sr., had been trained as a refiner at the Oxford Iron Works in Campbell County, Virginia, near Lynchburg. He had been born at Oxford in 1788, and *his* father, referred to in the Oxford records simply as "Old Hunt," born in 1747, had been a limestone miner at Oxford Furnace. When Harry Hunt, Jr., entered Weaver's Buffalo Forge as an apprentice hammerman, he was at least the third generation of his family to work in the iron trade. He may even have been the fourth. Young Harry Hunt's great-grandmother, a woman named Belinda born in 1731, was also an Oxford slave, and it seems reasonable to suppose that her husband (whose name does not appear in the surviving Oxford manuscripts) was also an ironworker.[29] Be that as it may, the ancestors of Harry Hunt, Jr., went a lot farther back in the Virginia iron industry than William Weaver did.

All the Oxford slaves had once been the property of David Ross, one of the legendary southern ironmasters of the Revolutionary and post-Revolutionary era. When Ross died in 1817 and his estate was broken up, a number of his best slave artisans were sold to iron men across the Blue Ridge Mountains. William Weaver was one of the Valley ironmasters who had purchased several of Ross's Oxford-trained forge hands, and Weaver considered himself fortunate to have acquired them.[30]

27. Dew, "Sam Williams, Forgeman," 202–19, 227.

28. Buffalo Forge Iron Book, 1831–62, Buffalo Forge Negro Books, 1830–40, 1839–41, 1844–50, 1850–58, Weaver-Brady Collection, Charlottesville; "Names, births &c: of Negroes," in Weaver-Brady Papers, Richmond.

29. "List of Slaves at the Oxford Iron Works in Families and Their Employment, Taken 15 January 1811," William Bolling Papers, Duke University Library, Durham; Charles B. Dew, "David Ross and the Oxford Iron Works: A Study of Industrial Slavery in the Early Nineteenth-Century South," *William and Mary Quarterly,* 3rd ser., XXXI (1974), 189–224.

30. Dew, "David Ross and the Oxford Iron Works," 222–24.

This web of family and personal ties in some ways embraced the ironmaster as much as the slave. Weaver clearly tolerated some poor work habits from men like Tooler and Sam Williams and Harry Hunt, Jr., that he would never have permitted in white forge laborers. It had been the unsatisfactory performance of white workmen that had originally prompted Weaver to begin his efforts to acquire slave ironworkers back in 1815. The slave-labor system had its *own* problems and limitations, however. The longstanding tradition of a reasonable task for each worker, and the fact that the slaves themselves decided if they would exceed those tasks in order to earn overwork compensation, placed constraints on productivity and performance that ironmasters had little choice but to accept. If his Buffalo Forge slaves were doing reasonably well—turning out eighty to one hundred tons of high-quality bar iron per year and not causing Weaver undue worry, trouble, or concern—he seemed content to live with the situation. If Tooler, Harry Hunt, Jr., Sam Williams, or Henry Towles "loafed" for several days, or longer, but then made up the shortfall, or most of it, with a spurt of activity toward week's or month's end, Weaver accepted that, too. The alternative—to sell a slave like Tooler, whom Weaver had owned since he had been a boy of four, and try to replace him with another slave forgeman (if one could be found)—was a step Weaver was unwilling to take.

Tooler must, in fact, have pressed Weaver's patience close to the limit. We know when Tooler was working well, working poorly, or not working at all because Weaver's manager wrote it all down during the late antebellum and Civil War years. His manager was his nephew-in-law, a Pennsylvanian named Daniel C. E. Brady, who had come down with his wife and children in 1857 to help Weaver run Buffalo Forge. Brady's journal, a daily description of work, weather, and notable events at Buffalo Forge, tells us what almost every one of Weaver's slave workers was doing almost every day of his life from March 1858 to June 1865.[31] It is a truly remarkable and exceedingly valuable record, and it describes a pattern of industrial slave life and work that was decidedly preindustrial.

One three-week period, running from April 29 to May 18, 1861, illustrates the nature of the industrial work regimen often followed by Tooler and Harry Hunt, Jr. On Monday, April 29, Tooler and Harry "drew 2 Jours," Brady wrote, and they continued to make their task every day that week through Friday, May 3. On Saturday, May 4, they

31. Dew, "Sam Williams, Forgeman," 219–20; Brady, Home Journal, in Weaver-Brady Collection, Charlottesville; Brady, Home Journal, in McCormick Collection.

drew only one journey of 560 pounds of bar iron between them, but Saturday was usually a slow day at the forge and a single journey for the two forgemen had become, over the years, an acceptable output.

On Monday, May 6, however, Tooler and Harry Hunt, Jr., began a week's unauthorized leave from the chaffery forge. "Tooler loafing Harry Hunt sick or loafing," Brady recorded in his journal. He entered exactly the same notations the next day for the two men, but by Wednesday, May 8, he had made up his mind about Harry. "Harry Hunt sick," Brady put down, "Tooler loafing." The following day, Brady changed his mind. "Harry Hunt loafing," was now his assessment, and he failed to record Tooler's status that day. On Friday, May 10, Tooler was out with the field hands planting corn, a common shift from industrial to agricultural work for Weaver's forgemen when planting or harvesting chores were pressing. Brady probably felt fortunate in having Tooler at least doing some sort of productive labor. Harry Hunt went that day with a crew of four other slaves to haul logs to Buffalo Forge, so he was back on the job, after a fashion, as well. Tooler remained with the corn-planting gang on Saturday, May 11, while Harry helped the forge carpenter, a slave named Henry Mathews, saw the logs they had brought to Buffalo Forge the previous day. Sunday was, as usual, a day of rest for all hands. The records show no indication that Weaver or Brady tried to force Tooler and Harry Hunt, Jr., back to their forge, despite Brady's conviction that the two slaves were shirking their duties.

On Monday, May 13, Tooler and Harry were back at the chaffery forge as if nothing had happened. "Tooler and Harry drew 2 Jours," Brady noted, and they continued this pace through Thursday, May 16. On Friday, after they had drawn one journey, the iron band holding the base of their anvil broke, presumably by accident, and they were forced to stop for repairs. The following day they drew the usual Saturday quota of one journey before ending their week's labor.[32]

A number of things might be said about this chronicle of two slaves' industrial work, agricultural work, and nonwork, but the basic point here is that William Weaver probably saw in the performance of his forgemen little incentive to invest in new iron-making technology. What, indeed, would have happened if he had altered the forge fires by installing improved furnace designs, something he knew about, thought about doing, but failed to carry out at Buffalo Forge?[33] These

32. Brady, Home Journal, in McCormick Collection.
33. Abram W. Davis to Weaver, September 3, 1830, in Weaver Papers.

technological innovations would have made it easier for Tooler and Harry Hunt, Jr., to make their tasks, but what then? If they chose to rest at that point, or to minimize their overwork, Weaver would have accomplished little or nothing toward increasing the output of bar iron. If, in the wake of possible improvements, he had tried to increase their *task* from its traditional weight of 560 pounds, how would Tooler and Harry have reacted to that step? One suspects that Weaver would have received his answer to this question in fairly short order.

Sam Williams, the master refiner at Buffalo Forge and probably the hardest-working slave Weaver owned, and Henry Towles, his helper, also had clear ideas about when they had labored long enough and hard enough to earn some rest. Following a period of very hot weather in the summer of 1860 when they had worked in brutal temperatures approaching one hundred degrees, Sam Williams and Henry Towles moved to take some much-needed time off. Towles took the first break. On Wednesday, July 18, Brady noted "Henry Towles sick." Jim Garland, a slave who served as a swing hand between the agricultural workers and the forge crew, was brought in from the fields to relieve Towles, and he and Sam Williams put in a full day at the refinery forge. Towles failed to show up for work the next day, Thursday, July 19, and this time Brady suspected that something was up. "Henry Towles sick i.e. loafing," he recorded in his journal. Jim Garland remained in the forge serving as Sam Williams' underhand, and he stayed there Friday and Saturday as well; Henry Towles was out "loafing" both days.[34]

The next week it was Sam's turn. Towles returned to work on Monday, July 23. He was experienced enough to handle Sam's job, and Jim Garland stayed on to serve as his helper. Sam was now "loafing," in Brady's estimation, and Weaver's master refiner stayed off the job *four* full weeks; Brady regularly identified him as "loafing" each day. At the end of Sam's first week of rest, a week in which the heat in the Valley had been particularly oppressive, Tooler and Harry Hunt, Jr., decided they had had enough as well. On Saturday, July 28, they carried out an act of industrial sabotage: "Tooler and Harry drew a few pounds and then broke down to loaf." At noon, Brady gave up: "All hands had a 1/2 [day] holiday."[35] A point of diminishing returns had obviously been reached. Again, as in previous, and subsequent, cases of "loafing" or slack work, there is no evidence in Brady's journal that any of the forge

34. Brady, Home Journal, in Weaver-Brady Collection, Charlottesville; Dew, "Sam Williams, Forgeman," 221–22.
35. Dew, "Sam Williams, Forgeman," 222.

workers were punished or that efforts were taken to try to make them return to their jobs.

Evidence as to why something like technological innovation does *not* occur is admittedly difficult to come by, but the three-week record of Tooler and Harry Hunt, Jr., in the spring of 1861 and Sam Williams' four-week absence from his post in the summer of 1860 would seem to offer at least a hint as to why southern iron manufacturing failed to keep pace technologically with northern and British competition. Weaver could count on his slave forgemen to keep things more or less operating, and they made a superior, albeit expensive, bar when they were working. But clearly Weaver could not count on a sustained, regular pattern of work from his forge crew that would justify the expense of technological modifications. And if his slaves did not like whatever new techniques he introduced, there was no guarantee they would do as well in the future as they had in the past. Labor conditions at Buffalo Forge, in short, were not conducive to change and innovation. Much the same pattern prevailed, one suspects, at furnaces and forges throughout the slave South.

There are other hints in the history of Weaver's iron operations that help explain the technological retardation of the South's iron industry. Experienced white forgemen who had spent some time in the Valley were frequently called upon to testify in the lawsuits in which Weaver and other local ironmasters seemed to be perpetually engaged. The evidence they gave concerning the skills and performance of slave refiners and hammermen was not encouraging. One such witness, who had worked with Harry Hunt, Sr., at Buffalo Forge was asked: "Do you believe or not that negro refinery men make a ton of anchonies out of a ton and half of pig metal?" The white artisan replied: "I do not. They are not as good workmen and do not take as good care or as much pains as good white workmen."[36] This observer may not have been entirely unbiased, since he had worked for Weaver at Buffalo Forge from 1825 until the latter part of 1827; he may well have lost his job when Weaver completed his slave crew by acquiring his sixth forgeman in October 1827.

His was not the only testimony, however. A former business partner of Weaver's, an ironmaster named John Doyle, provided the fullest comparison of slave and free labor in Virginia in a deposition he gave in 1840. "I have no doubt but it costs more to refine a ton of iron with slave

36. Deposition of William Narcross, August 22, 1840, Case Papers, *Alexander* v. *Irvine's Administrator*.

labor than it does with white labor," Doyle assured the court; "the reason is that they, slaves, do not understand it and they waste more metal and coal than greatly to overbalance the difference in other respects." Doyle had been "forcibly struck with this difference" by watching a white refiner and Harry Hunt, Sr., work in the same forge. "I procured a workman, a free man, from the North who put up a refinery fire in which he made an anchony that would go 18 to the ton with about 12 bushels of coal," Doyle testified. The white refiner "remained there but a short time," and after he left, Harry Hunt, Sr., went to work at the same fire. Weaver's slave refiner "took from 20 to 25 bushels [of charcoal] to make the same quantity of iron," Doyle reported. When asked if Rockbridge County's forges compared favorably with those he had seen in Pennsylvania, Doyle replied simply, "No, there is all the difference imaginable."[37]

In his superb study of Rockdale, Anthony F. C. Wallace describes the qualities that characterized the young mechanics emerging in that Pennsylvania community in the 1830s:

> Despite the arduous nature of the work, the machinist's trade attracted in general an extremely intelligent group of young men. They were aware of the vast industrial expansion under way in the textile and transportation industries, and looked forward to educating themselves widely and generally in manual skills, technical, and even scientific knowledge as preparation for the administrative role of master mechanic or engineer, where the earnings could be substantial and the work constantly called for a creative intelligence.[38]

Compare that passage with the following words written by David Ross, the master of the Oxford Iron Works, the forge where Harry Hunt, Sr., learned to refine iron in the early years of the nineteenth century. "I dare say you are correct as to my Forgemen," Ross admitted to a friend in 1812; "they were as good workmen 20 years ago as they are now." This was clearly not because of any lack of innate ability or capacity to learn. Ross's bondsmen, like Weaver's forge crew, were highly skilled men who had mastered an exceedingly difficult and demanding trade. The problem, as was certainly the case with Weaver's ironworkers, was the institution of slavery itself. As Ross put it, his forge workers "have had no chance to improve—they have not

---

37. Deposition of John Doyle, February 7, 1840, Case Papers, *Weaver v. Jordan, Davis & Co.*

38. Anthony F. C. Wallace, *Rockdale: The Growth of an American Village in the Early Industrial Revolution* (New York, 1980), 150.

[had] an opportunity of travelling to see other works and the annual improvements [made there]." Ross summed up his assessment of the capabilities of his own forgemen with a comment that stands as an indictment of the entire industrial slave system: "My people in every branch," he wrote, "have remained as it were stationary."[39] For this reason, and doubtless many more, the ironworks of the Old South were, almost without exception, technologically primitive and hopelessly inadequate in 1861 to the needs of a nation at war. The slave ironworkers, perhaps, had unwittingly helped to pave the way for their own freedom.

39. David Ross to Robert Richardson, November 10, 1812, in David Ross Letterbook, Virginia Historical Society, Richmond. See also Dew, "David Ross and the Oxford Iron Works," 216; and Lewis, *Coal, Iron, and Slaves*, 190–91.

CHAPTER 6

SCIENCE AND THEOLOGY IN THE OLD SOUTH

E. Brooks Holifield

W hen John Holt Rice became in 1824 the first professor of theology
at the Presbyterian Seminary in Hampden-Sidney, Virginia, he
was officially charged with the task of raising up a generation of scientifically minded clergymen: "And also as the cavils and objections of
infidels have been more readily answered as *natural science* has been
enlarged, that branch of knowledge should form a part of that fund of
information, which every minister of the Gospel should possess." The
charge to Rice reflected a consensus among the educated clergy of
the Old South that scientific investigation of the created order revealed
the existence and nature of the Creator and that theologians who knew
something about natural science could "see God . . . mirrored in his
works." Few people in the South outside the ranks of the physicians
and scientists could have exhibited greater enthusiasm for natural science than did the southern clergy.[1]

The ministers believed, of course, that the discoveries of the scientists would confirm the dogmas of Christian tradition. Their enthusiasm for geology and astronomy should not be confused with un-
qualified support for all scientific investigation or a willingness to
tolerate scientists whose conclusions threatened orthodox certitudes.
But most of the clergy had no difficulty sustaining their confidence in
science because many of the scientists had no trouble sustaining their

1. In this paper I draw on the conclusions of my book *The Gentlemen Theologians:
American Theology in Southern Culture, 1795–1860* (Durham, 1978). Clement Read,
"Charge Delivered to John Rice," in John Rice, *An Inaugural Discourse, Delivered on the
First of January 1824* (Richmond, 1824), 33; James Henley Thornwell, "The Philosophy of
Religion," *Southern Presbyterian Review*, III (1849–50), 519.

enthusiasm for theology. The *American Journal of Science*, after all, had in 1818 declared it the task of the scientist to demonstrate "the supreme intelligence and harmony and beneficence of design in the Creator," and many prominent American scientists, northern and southern, were as interested in the theological implications of their work as in its practical applications. Despite occasional squabbles, most theologians and scientists viewed themselves as allies, and the positions of southern theologians were identical to those held by most northern theologians.[2]

To be orthodox in the early nineteenth century was to assume the unity of truth and hence to affirm a "natural theology" based on human reason (and scientific method) as the normal prolegomenon, proof, and corollary of scriptural revelation. And the clergymen of the Old South's cities and small towns saw themselves as apostles of the unity of truth. They were convinced, as one Methodist theologian wrote, that God had "never enjoined upon man the duty of faith, without first presenting before him a reasonable foundation for the same," and they tried to establish orthodoxy on that foundation. The great irony in their construction of orthodoxy, however, was that natural science often became for them an implicit theological authority. The methods and conclusions of the scientists became unacknowledged criteria for the formulation of theological truth.[3]

As early as the first century, the apostle Paul informed the Christian congregation in Rome that ever since the creation of the world God's eternal power and deity had been "clearly perceived in the things that have been made" (Rom. 1:20). By the second century the Christian Hellenistic apologists, trying to demonstrate the compatibility of faith and reason, inaugurated the tradition of "Christian evidences," which presupposed that religious truth-claims were subject to an extrinsic mode of verification, logically antecedent to the doctrines themselves. Subsequent theologians eventually combined those two ideas in the tradition of natural theology, which reached an apex in the thirteenth century when Thomas Aquinas tried to present Christian truth in such a way that pagan philosophy could be seen as preparatory to faith. Just as Thomas argued that grace did not destroy but rather perfected nature, so he also claimed that revealed theology presupposed, used, and perfected natural knowledge. Each of the five major traditions of

2. Howard Mumford Jones, "The Influence of European Ideas in Nineteenth-Century America," *American Literature*, VII (1935), 241–73; "Introductory Remarks," *American Journal of Science*, I (1818), 8; Theodore Dwight Bozeman, *Protestants in an Age of Science* (Chapel Hill, 1977), 39–43.

3. Thomas Ralston, *Elements of Divinity* (Nashville, 1871), 361.

Christian religious thought in the Old South—Catholic, Lutheran, Reformed, Anglican, and Wesleyan—reflected that long heritage of natural theology.

The Catholic pastors in the coastal cities and the border states were the products of a continental "textbook theology" that taught them to begin their theological reflection with the *praeambula fidei*, a set of natural, rationally demonstrable truths that served as the prelude for understanding and accepting the revealed articles of faith. The nineteenth-century Lutheran pastors, having discarded Luther's deep reservations about natural theology, followed the Protestant scholastic theologians of the seventeenth century who had returned to Thomistic theses established with Aristotelian metaphysics. They spoke therefore of revelation as being "above," but not opposed to, reason—a recovery of scholastic hierarchical imagery. The southern Reformed theologians, the heirs of Ulrich Zwingli and John Calvin, followed the lead of seventeenth-century Reformed scholastics who believed that reason could demonstrate the existence and attributes of God, serve as a competent judge of religious teachings, and prove the Christian Scripture to be authentic and divine. The Episcopal clergy looked for guidance to English theologians whose determination to prove the credibility of revelation amply justified the later judgment of Mark Pattison that "the title of Locke's treatise, *The Reasonableness of Christianity,* may be said to have been the solitary thesis of Christian theology in England for the great part of a century." And even the patriarch of Methodism, John Wesley, who had confronted the English Enlightenment by counterposing an internal "spiritual sense" against a fallen "natural reason," declined to proceed to irrationalist conclusions. Wesley had written treatises on "natural philosophy" and argued that anyone who departed from "genuine reason" departed from Christianity.[4]

In eighteenth- and nineteenth-century England, especially, "the ra-

---

4. Giovanni Perrone, *Kompendium der katholischen Dogmatik* (Landshut, Germany, 1852), 342; Avery Dulles, *A History of Apologetics* (London, 1971), 150–97; Raymond M. Bost, "The Reverend John Bachman and the Development of Southern Lutheranism" (Ph.D. dissertation, Yale University, 1963), 194; E. C. Mayse, "Robert Jefferson Breckinridge: American Presbyterian Controversialist" (Th.D. dissertation, Union Theological Seminary in Virginia, 1975), 503; George Howe, *A Discourse on Theological Education* (New York, 1844), 229; John A. Broadus, *Memoir of James Petigru Boyce* (Nashville, 1927), 268; *History of the Establishment and Organization of the Southern Baptist Theological Seminary, Greenville, South Carolina* (Greenville, S.C., 1860), 46; John Hunt, *Religious Thought in England* (3 vols.; London, 1870), I, 271; Mark Pattison, "Tendencies of Religious Thought in England, 1688–1750," in *Essays and Reviews* (London, 1861), 258; Albert Outler (ed.), *John Wesley* (New York, 1964), 393–96.

tionalizing method possessed itself absolutely of the whole field of theology," and that heritage of Christian rationalism indelibly colored the outlook of the educated clergy in the Old South. It ensured that the tradition of natural theology would permeate the religious assumptions of the region's educated classes. And no advocate of natural theology could have ignored natural science.[5]

Of course, not every preacher waited eagerly for field reports from the geologists. Most of them were probably indifferent to the intricacies of debate over the nebular hypothesis. In 1850 there were 26,842 clergymen in the United States; some 7,514 were active in the South. Three years later the Southern Aid Society reported that "one fifth of the preachers are regularly educated for their business," an estimate suggesting that around fifteen hundred southern ministers might by that time be numbered among the clergy whom John Holt Rice had earlier described as "men of some literary attainments." Between 1800 and 1860, probably fewer than one hundred of them wrote the books, articles, and reviews that dealt with the relationship of theology to science. To be sure, the ministerial interest in scientific matters extended beyond that narrow circle of clerical authors; the ordination requirements in some denominations encouraged, even compelled, a broader interest. But the clerical elite of "gentlemen theologians" who dominated the intellectual life of the southern churches established the terms for the alliance of religion and science.[6]

A brief glance at the careers of one hundred "elite" southern clergymen reveals something about the intellectual background and social setting of the alliance. All held positions of regional and not simply local leadership; all were active in organizations, institutes, and movements to "improve" the clergy educationally and culturally; and all labored for portions of their careers in towns and cities. Such a sample does not reveal much about the typical preacher in the rural South. It does afford a perspective on the gentlemen theologians who defined the relationship between religion and science.

5. Pattison, "Tendencies of Religious Thought," in *Essays and Reviews*, 259.

6. Ronald L. Numbers, *Creation by Natural Law: Laplace's Nebular Hypothesis in American Thought* (Seattle, 1977), 38, shows, however, that some southern Christians were quite interested in the theological implications of the nebular hypothesis. For the statistics, see J. D. B. De Bow, *Statistical View of the United States* (Washington, D.C., 1854), 126–27; *The Seventh Census of the United States: 1850* (Washington, D.C., 1853), lxvii. I included figures from thirteen states: Maryland, Virginia, North Carolina, South Carolina, Georgia, Florida, Alabama, Mississippi, Louisiana, Texas, Arkansas, Tennessee, and Kentucky. The report from the Southern Aid Society is cited in Frederick Law Olmsted, *A Journey in the Seaboard Slave States in the Years 1853–1854* (2 vols.; New York, 1904), II, 82.

Although by 1860 three fourths of southern churchgoers were Methodists and Baptists, thirty-seven of the hundred elite clergy were Presbyterians, twenty-three were Baptists, eighteen were Methodists, fourteen were Episcopalians, six were Roman Catholics, and two were Lutherans. Most were native southerners; only twenty-eight were Yankees; only eight, including four of the Catholics, were born in Europe. Seventy-three had some college training; nine more received classical educations in private academies; only eighteen were self-educated or instructed solely by private tutors. Thirty-two attended theological seminaries, thirteen at Princeton, and fourteen more received some formal postcollegiate theological training from older ministers. Thirty-three attended southern colleges; thirty studied in the North; four tried both regions; and six went to school in Europe. Probably the most pertinent common feature, though, was that all one hundred labored for at least a portion of their careers in towns and cities.[7]

My generalizations in this paper are based mainly on the writings and activities of thirty-five clergymen from the group of one hundred and of twenty additional clerical writers (fourteen Presbyterians, three Methodists, two Catholics, and one Episcopalian) who commented on natural science. Most of the additional writers could probably be included in the ranks of the elite clerical gentlemen, but I did not secure detailed biographical information about them. My conclusions, then, are drawn from the work of fifty-five clergymen, twelve anonymous articles in the theological journals, and a number of book reviews. Of the fifty-five clergymen, thirty-one were Presbyterians, ten Methodists, five Baptists, four Catholics, three Episcopalians, one Lutheran, and one Unitarian. The leadership of the Presbyterian clergy was clearly disproportional to their numbers in the region. By 1860, 30 percent of the town clergy in the South were Methodists, 16 percent were Episcopalians, 14 percent Catholics, and only 12 percent Presbyterians. Yet the Presbyterians constituted 37 percent of my elite group of a hundred and 56 percent of the clergy whom I found to comment on science and religion. Their views on the issues, though, were precisely the same as those of the urban clergy in the other denominations.[8]

7. Holifield, *Gentlemen Theologians*, 25–28.

8. The fifty-five clergymen were the following: (Presbyterians) John Adger, George Armstrong, George Baxter, J. R. Blake, R. J. Breckinridge, W. T. Brooks, Joseph Caldwell, Edwin Cater, Alonzo Church, R. L. Dabney, W. C. Dana, Benjamin Gildersleeve, Richard Gladney, William Graham, L. W. Green, George Howe, Philip Lindsley, James Lyon, W. D. Moore, B. M. Palmer, Thomas Peck, William Plumer, Clement Read, John Holt

It was natural that ministers recognized as having superior abilities would ascend to the urban pulpits. It comes as no surprise that they assumed the lead in clerical reflection on scientific matters. But it is also arguable that the expectations and institutions of urban society encouraged clerical attention to the natural sciences. Fledgling urban pastors were sometimes explicitly reminded that they were now preaching to "town folks," who prided themselves on their "intelligence." In the estimation of their journalists, publicists, and professional classes, the towns were seats of "learning," elegant and enlightened oases where people were inclined to "patronize literature and science." It became an anxious cliché among the town clergy that the cities had "more literary and scientific men" and that "the ministry must be in advance of the people, leaders intellectually and socially as well as spiritually."[9]

Equally important, the towns created institutions that stimulated conversations about the sciences: lyceums, library companies, debating clubs, and literary societies, ranging from Charleston's pretentious Literary and Philosophical Society to the small debating club formed by the "gentlemen" of Athens, Georgia, in an unfurnished room over the post office. It was in such urban institutions that the Lutheran pastor John Bachman presented an early formulation of his *Unity of the Human Race Examined on the Principles of Science* and the Presbyterian Thomas Smyth delivered the lectures that became his *Unity of the Human Race Proved to be the Doctrine of Scripture, Reason, and Science.* Such institutions compelled the Methodist Lovick Pierce to maintain a regimen of study in logic and "physics," lest he be embarrassed before his better-informed peers. In any case, the town clergy took the lead in the discussion of religion and science. The expectations about "reasonableness" that emerged among the urban middle classes encouraged

Rice, E. F. Rockwell, B. M. Smith, Thomas Smyth, James H. Thornwell, A. B. Van Zandt, J. N. Waddel, John Young; (Methodists) A. T. Bledsoe, A. B. Longstreet, D. W. Martindale, T. V. Moore, Robert Paine, W. N. Pendleton, Lovick Pierce, Thomas Ralston, Edward D. Sims, T. O. Summers; (Baptists) Basil Manley, Jonathan Maxcy, Jesse Mercer, James Taylor, Alva Woods; (Catholics) Andrew Cornette, John England, John Spalding, Augustin Verot; (Episcopalians) Jasper Adams, A. P. Bernard, James Madison; (Lutheran) John Bachman; and (Unitarian) Samuel Gilman.

9. John G. Jones, *A Complete History of Methodism as Connected with the Mississippi Conference of the Methodist Episcopal Church* (2 vols.; Nashville, 1908), II, 142; C. S. Deems (ed.), *Annals of Southern Methodism for 1857* (Nashville, 1858), unpaginated; George G. Smith, Smith Diary (30 vols.; Southern History Collection, University of North Carolina, Chapel Hill), I, 111; LeRoy J. Halsey (ed.), *The Works of Philip Lindsley* (3 vols.; Philadelphia, 1866), I, 258; C. S. Deems (ed.), *The Southern Methodist Pulpit*, IV (1851), 52; Holifield, *Gentlemen Theologians*, 9, 39.

the clergy to continue and refine the tradition of natural theology in "the age of Natural science."[10]

The theologians agreed that natural theology, properly understood, furnished a foundation for revelation. They therefore assembled all the traditional religious arguments for the existence of God based on the harmony of the natural order, the mutual adaptation of its parts, its complexity, and the necessity of a sufficient cause for its existence. The insights thus garnered constituted a "natural" knowledge of God, independent of a special biblical revelation. Those insights permitted the theologians to look up "through nature's works to nature's God."[11]

Confident about the trustworthiness of natural theology, the southern theologians maintained a careful and hopeful watch over the physical sciences, with every assurance that "natural philosophy" would provide the nineteenth century's distinctive prospectus on divine truth. They believed that science could assume "a direct and active agency in the support and exposition of the Christian system." Hence they claimed to welcome scientific advance: "Shall we attempt to stop the march of science?" asked the Presbyterian W. C. Dana. "As well think to dam the Nile with bulrushes."[12]

The clergy believed that modern science was the product of Jewish and Christian tradition. A. B. Van Zandt, a minister in Petersburg, Virginia, explained to a university audience in 1851 that natural science presupposed an unspoken faith in purpose and rationality in the cosmos: "The maxim that 'Jehovah has created nothing in vain,' we hold to have been the basis of all those minute investigations of the scientists." A writer for the *Methodist Quarterly Review* suggested further that biblical tradition had undergirded the emergence of an inductive scientific method. The biblical interest in particular historical works of God had engendered a habit of mind attuned to "patient inquiry into facts," which subsequently issued in "the scientific method of seeking truth" through induction and generalization. A "tendency to glorify the Deity in his works gave rise to a taste for natural observation." The Protestant

10. John Bachman, *The Unity of the Human Race Examined on the Principles of Science* (Charleston, S. C., 1850); Thomas Smyth, *The Unity of the Human Race Proved to be the Doctrine of Scripture, Reason, and Science*, in *The Complete Works of Rev. Thomas Smyth*, ed. J. W. Flynn (10 vols.; Columbia, S.C., 1909–12); George G. Smith, *The Life and Times of George Foster Pierce* (Sparta, Ga., 1888), 41; Richard Gladney, "Natural Science and Revealed Religion," *Southern Presbyterian Review*, XII (1859–60), 449; Holifield, *Gentlemen Theologians*, 36.

11. Ralston, *Elements of Divinity*, 12.

12. W. C. Dana, "A Reasonable Answer to the Sceptic," *Southern Presbyterian Review*, XI (1859), 391.

clergy liked to think that the sixteenth-century revolt against both Rome and Aristotle had crystallized the movement toward a modern scientific worldview. Luther, Calvin, and Francis Bacon had overseen "the actual birth of modern science." And if science was the offspring of the Christian West, there was every reason to believe that the child would honor and obey the parent. Natural science would be one more weapon in the apologetic armory of Christendom.[13]

The theologians therefore argued that scientific investigation, properly conducted, provided a vast and grand extension of the traditional argument that design and order in nature demonstrated the reality and trustworthiness of God. They admired inordinately "the remarkable Mr. Hugh Miller," a Scottish naturalist whose combination of piety and geological acumen found expression in a series of popular treatises: *Footprints of the Creator, Popular Geology,* and *The Testimony of the Rocks.* Miller tried not only to prove the compatibility of geology and the Old Testament, but also to show the orderliness of nature under a superintending providence. He found even a numerical order in the creation: vertebrates always had ten digits, mammals always had seven neck vertebrae, and the leaf appendages of plants exhibited similar mathematical patterns. Nature was filled with pattern and regularity and therefore with intelligence.[14]

The theological journals occasionally carried articles by ministers or pious amateur scientists that promised to reveal the presence of design in leaf appendages or coal formations, or the orderliness within bee cells. For the most part, though, they were content with brief references to the ideas of "the strong men of science" whose findings

13. A. B. Van Zandt, "The Necessity of a Revelation," in William H. Ruffner (ed.), *Lectures on the Evidences of Christianity Delivered at the University of Virginia During the Sessions of 1850–51* (New York, 1852), 52; "The Progress of Science and Its Connection with Scripture," *Quarterly Review of the Methodist Episcopal Church, South,* XI (1857), 49, 55, 57, 63 (journal hereinafter cited as *Methodist Quarterly Review*).

14. L. W. Green, "The Harmony of Revelation and Natural Science; With Especial Reference to Geology," in Ruffner (ed.), *Lectures on the Evidences,* 463–76; T. V. Moore, "God's Method of Saving the World," *Methodist Quarterly Review,* IX (1855), 76; C. C. Pinckney, *The Testimony of Science to the Truth of Revelation* (Charleston, S.C., 1854), 3–4; Ralston, *Elements of Divinity,* 171; T. V. Moore, "English Infidelity," *Methodist Quarterly Review,* VII (1852), 9; "An Address on the Sphere, Interest, and Importance of Geology," *Southern Presbyterian Review,* III (1849–50), 662; B. M. Smith, *The Testimony of Science to the Truth of the Bible* (Charlottesville, 1850); "The Progress of Science and Its Connection with Scripture," 46–48. See also D. W. Martindale, "Footprints of the Creator," *Methodist Quarterly Review,* V (1851), 508; and W. N. Pendleton, "The Chronology of Creation," *Methodist Quarterly Review,* X (1856), 162, 178.

were vindicating religious truth. To them scientific research simply extended the old seventeenth-century tradition of "physico-theology," in which a small army of English and German theologians had produced an array of books on Astro-, Pyro-, Hydro-, and Litho-theology, even on Insecto-, Phylo-, and Bronto-theology, all intended to display the glory, wonder, and purposefulness of the divine creation.[15]

The high point of that tradition was the publication in England in 1802 of William Paley's *Natural Theology*. Paley argued that nature, in its purposeful regularity, was similar to a watch, except that the contrivances of nature, the structural adaptations within organisms, and the adaptations of living beings to their environment were so numerous, subtle, and complex that anyone who believed in watchmakers should believe even more in an intelligent Creator of the natural order. In subsequent years the argument from design assumed increasingly complicated and even fanciful forms. The *Southern Presbyterian Review* published arguments during the 1850s that based the proof of God's existence on the intricate modifications of the chemical elements.[16]

It was easy for the clergy to overlook the flaws in the argument because so many leading scientists found it compelling. Yale's geological star, Benjamin Silliman, was also a Christian apologist. When he came South in 1846, he lectured on chemistry and geology in the First Presbyterian Church in New Orleans. The naturalist Edward Hitchcock of Amherst studied for the ministry and wrote *The Religion of Geology and Its Connected Sciences* (1851), which received enthusiastic reviews in the southern theological journals. Joseph LeConte combined scientific and theological interests at Oglethorpe College in Georgia, as did Matthew Fontaine Maury in Virginia. The naturalist James Woodrow even accepted a position on the faculty of Columbia Theological Seminary. Hence the Reverend Richard Gladney felt no hesitation in declaring in 1860 that the future belonged not to the older philosophers but to scientists like Alexander von Humboldt and Justus von Liebig, William Buckland and Sir Richard Owen, and America's

15. "The Progress of Science and Its Connection with Scripture," 44–73; "Outlines of a System of Geology," *Methodist Quarterly Review*, III (1849), 120–42; E. F. Rockwell, "The Alphabet of Natural Theology," *Southern Presbyterian Review*, X (1857), 411–36; Martindale, "Footprints of the Creator," 511; Karl Barth, *Die protestantische Theologie im 19. Jahrhundert* (2 vols.; Hamburg, 1960), I, 133.

16. William Paley, *Natural Theology*, in *The Works of William Paley* (7 vols.; London, 1825), V, 129–206; Rockwell, "The Alphabet of Natural Theology," 411–36.

own Louis Agassiz, who had begun to show the consistency between science and religion.[17]

The clergy pledged their allegiance, then, to what T. Dwight Bozeman has called a "doxological science"—a conviction that scientific investigation, at its best, was a mode of piety. They worried about scientific atheism and about a purely utilitarian notion of science, but they were confident that science was, in the words of the Charleston Unitarian Samuel Gilman, a pathway to "better acquaintance with the thoughts of God." It was, said the *Methodist Quarterly Review*, a means of "being admitted to the decisions of heaven's chancery." To the Presbyterian James Henley Thornwell, it was a form of worship: "Science, when it has conducted us to God, ceases to speculate and begins to adore. . . . [T]he climax of its inquiries is a sublime doxology."[18]

To become an amateur scientist, then, was to extend and enrich the ministerial calling. Some presbyteries and synods required that prospective clergy study and take examinations on scientific subjects. The theological journals urged ministers to pursue scientific studies. The *Columbian Star*, the leading Baptist newspaper in the upper South, carried on its masthead the picture of a star flanked by two words: "religion" and "science." John Holt Rice's *Virginia Evangelical and Literary Magazine*, founded in 1818, consistently promoted clerical attention to scientific matters and carried regular items of "scientific intelligence" as objects of general interest. The southern *Methodist Quarterly Review* (1846) printed frequent articles on science along with a regular section of "scientific miscellanies" reporting the discovery of iron grains in fossil wood in Sweden, or the results of a microscopic examination of the alluvial deposit of the Nile, or the identification of new planets. The *Southern Presbyterian Review* (1847) explored the theological implications of scientific labor throughout the later antebellum period. The journals regularly reviewed the growing body of scientific

17. Bozeman, *Protestants in an Age of Science*, 43. See the reviews in *Southern Presbyterian Review*, II (1848–49), 164–65; *Methodist Quarterly Review*, VIII (1854), 611; *Methodist Quarterly Review*, XIII (1859), 271; Gladney, "Natural Science and Revealed Religion," 445. Clark Albert Elliott, "The American Scientist, 1800–1863: His Origins, Career, and Interests" (Ph.D. dissertation, Case Western Reserve University, 1970), studied biographies of 503 antebellum scientists, northern and southern. The biographies provided religious information about 233 of them. Only three of those were described as "agnostic" or uninterested in religion (p. 98).

18. Bozeman, *Protestants in an Age of Science*, 71–100; Samuel Gilman, *Contributions to Religion* (Charleston, S.C., 1860), 65; "The Dignity and Importance of Mathematical Science," *Methodist Quarterly Review*, I (1847), 25–37; John Adger (ed.), *The Collected Writings of James Henley Thornwell* (3 vols.; Richmond, 1871), I, 64.

literature, as well as the apologetic treatises written to prove "the harmony between the system of nature and that of revelation, through the entire course of the sciences."[19]

The nascent church-sponsored colleges tried to develop courses in chemistry and natural philosophy, sometimes in geology and astronomy, and their science instructors—such men as the Methodists Landon Garland of Randolph-Macon and Alexander Means of Emory, the Presbyterian W. C. Kerr of Davidson, W. G. Simmons of the Baptists' Wake Forest, and Father Andrew Cornette of the Jesuit Spring Hill College in Alabama—had every expectation of demonstrating the harmony of religion and science. Jesse Mercer in Georgia explained the religious import of the curriculum at Mercer College. Each of the academic disciplines, he said, exhibited the truth of God: to study geography, chemistry, history, or philosophy was to study "the works of God, in creation, and providence, and grace." When Alabama Baptists proposed a new college in 1834, they said it would promote "the cause of science and religion"; when the Disciples of Christ in Kentucky built Bacon College in 1836, they felt themselves to be honoring the founder of "the inductive method of reasoning and the new science." Whatever their influence on the advance of scientific research, the denominational colleges registered the favorable imprimatur of the southern churches on the scientific enterprise.[20]

The evidence abounds of clerical interest in science among the gentlemen clergy. They joined the movement to enhance the scientific offerings at state colleges and universities, and at least thirteen, and probably more, of our group of one hundred clerical leaders taught natural science or mathematics in southern colleges. In quaintly diverse ways they sought to inform themselves about the natural sciences: the Baptist James Taylor of Richmond attended lectures on natural philosophy and chemistry at the University of Virginia; the Catholic Bishop Augustin Verot, who had taught courses on geology and zoology at St. Mary's College, made regular geological excursions; the Methodist Bishop Robert Paine, who had also taught a college geology

19. Bost, "The Reverend John Bachman," 194; Bozeman, *Protestants in an Age of Science*, 42; *Columbian Star*, February 22, 1822, p. 1; "Remarks on the Study of Natural Philosophy," *Virginia Evangelical and Literary Magazine*, I (1818), 261–64; "Biblical, Literary and Scientific Summary," *Methodist Quarterly Review*, VI (1852), 331–32, 652; "Review of Thomas Dick, *The Christian Philosopher*," *Methodist Quarterly Review*, XI (1857), 461.

20. Thomas Cary Johnson, Jr., *Scientific Interests in the Old South* (New York, 1936), 39–43; Albea Godbold, *The Church College in the Old South* (Durham, 1944), 144–45; Charles D. Mallary, *Memoirs of Elder Jesse Mercer* (New York, 1844), 178–83; Bozeman, *Protestants in an Age of Science*, 28; B. F. Riley, *History of the Baptists of Alabama* (Birmingham, 1895), 87.

class, led small groups in search of fossils in Alabama. Indeed, the scientific avocations of the clergy were sufficiently visible to elicit a complaint from the anticlerical president of South Carolina College, Thomas Cooper, who thought that it was "high time" to "resist the inter-meddling of the clergy and their devoted adherents in matters of science."[21]

Cooper's complaint is a reminder that the clergy were not prepared to support every conclusion of every scientist. They joined the effort to remove Cooper from his position at South Carolina College after his unconventional views about the mythical character of Genesis became known. In their own estimation, though, they were ready to support science as long as it did not presume to be metaphysics. "Science, in general and in particular," wrote the Methodist W. N. Pendleton of Lexington, Virginia, "is merely accurate knowledge, systematically deduced from established principles and observed facts, by the mind acting according to its inherent powers and appointed laws." It should not be restricted by religious authority, he said, but he also implied that it should not be treated as a religious authority. The problem was that the clergy tended to accuse the scientists of metaphysical pretension whenever their scientific conclusions seriously threatened established religious tradition.[22]

The threat came from three sources. The ministers worried, first, about materialism. They opposed any scientific conclusion that seemed to them to reduce judgment, reason, and will merely to matter and force. They worried also about "developmentalism," which the Methodist D. W. Martindale defined as the notion that complex organisms were "called into being from the action of chemistry upon gelatine and albumen, and then through the long lapse of ages successively developed into the fish, the reptile, the bird, the quadruped, and the man." Developmental assumptions, they thought, led

21. Holifield, *Gentlemen Theologians*, 6; R. H. Rivers, *The Life of Robert Paine* (Nashville, 1844), 31, 34, 49; George B. Taylor, *Life and Times of James B. Taylor* (Philadelphia, 1872), 133; Michael V. Gannon, *Rebel Bishop: The Life and Era of Augustin Verot* (Milwaukee, 1964), 6–7; Thomas Cooper, *The Connection Between Geology and the Pentateuch in a Letter to Prof. Silliman, from Thomas Cooper* (Columbia, S.C., 1837), 74. The science teachers were Jasper Adams, George Armstrong, John Bachman, George Baxter, A. T. Bledsoe, Joseph Caldwell, Alonzo Church, A. B. Longstreet, James Madison, Jonathan Maxcy, Robert Paine, Edward D. Sims, and Alva Woods.

22. W. N. Pendleton, "The Parentage of Mankind," *Methodist Quarterly Review*, IX (1855), 324.

inexorably to metaphysical materialism. And they worried, finally, about the scientific challenge to the historical accuracy of Scripture.[23]

As long as the scientists remained within the confines of true scientific method, the theologians argued, no one should have to worry about those problems. One reason they could be so sanguine was their conviction that Lord Bacon had imposed proper restraint on scientific speculation. Bozeman has documented the attraction of conservative Presbyterians to the Baconian method; theologians of almost every denomination shared that admiration for Bacon. To them the name "Bacon" suggested scrupulous adherence to "facts," careful induction, and modest generalization. Combining their Baconianism with Scottish Realist Philosophy, they concluded that the task of the scientist was simply to discern through painstaking observation the laws that governed the phenomenal world. Any speculation about ultimate causes or substances, then, became an instance of illicit metaphysics.[24]

The ministers were inclined to sniff metaphysical odors, though, any time that scientists began offering hypotheses about the origin of the earth or the development of species. The problem was Genesis. Adherents of the prevailing nineteenth-century conservative doctrine of Scripture could not entertain the thought that the account of creation in Genesis might be simply religious poetry. Hence they struggled mightily to reconcile Genesis and geology.

The issue could preoccupy even as learned a scholar as the South Carolina Lutheran pastor John Bachman, who once said that he felt a sense of clerical duty to investigate the sciences. By 1830 Bachman was collaborating with J. J. Audubon; he wrote the text of the celebrated *Viviparous Quadrupeds of North America,* a book that struck Agassiz as having no equal in America. In the South, Bachman became better known for defending the unity of the human race. Between 1847 and 1853 Agassiz delivered lectures at Charleston proposing a polygenetic account of human origins. During the same period a small group of

23. Martindale, "Footprints of the Creator," 507. See Bozeman, *Protestants in an Age of Science,* 101–31.

24. Bozeman, *Protestants in an Age of Science,* 3–31. See also, as examples, D. D. Buck, *Our Lord's Great Prophecy* (Nashville, 1857), 50; Benjamin Palmer, "Baconianism and the Bible," *Southern Presbyterian Review,* VII (1852), 226–53; Neal C. Gillespie, *The Collapse of Orthodoxy: The Intellectual Ordeal of George Frederick Holmes* (Charlottesville, 1972), 13; George H. Daniels, *American Science in the Age of Jackson* (New York, 1968), 63–85. Daniels suggests, however, that high-church Anglicans and Catholics disliked Bacon because they thought he subverted history and tradition.

southern naturalists advanced the same hypothesis, partly to demonstrate that whites and blacks were members of different species. Bachman believed that they subverted the biblical account of a single creation, so in 1853 he published his *Unity of the Human Race* to show that humankind constituted a single species with an infinite number of varieties. He resolved to make no appeal to Scripture, and he confined his argument largely to demonstrating the existence throughout nature of variation within species, but he also wrote as a conservative Christian intent on proving the congruence between "the book of nature" and the revealed "truths of heaven." He was engaged in an enterprise that occupied dozens of ministers who published articles on science and religion in the theological journals. And to many of them it seemed that their labors had succeeded. By 1850 it was possible to speak of a "theology of natural science" that was supposedly in perfect harmony with the Bible.[25]

In developing such a theology, however, the ministers began to permit their science to govern their reading of Scripture. The most revealing test case was the creation narrative in Genesis. The problem was time: while the biblical account, as interpreted in conservative circles, suggested that the creation of the earth had occurred six thousand years ago, the geologists spoke of immense changes over a vast, indefinite period of time. Efforts to reconcile the two positions were, if anything, ingenious, and two solutions commanded widespread ministerial assent. Encouraged by Benjamin Silliman at Yale and Hugh Miller in Scotland, some of the ministers argued that each of the seven "days" in the creation story was a geological period of indefinite length. Moses Stuart of Andover offered a telling criticism when he pointed out that the Hebrew word for "day" meant in its grammatical and historical context exactly what it seemed to mean: a twenty-four-hour day. Nevertheless, one southern Methodist claimed as late as 1857 that his fellow theologians "generally admitted" the theory of Miller and Silliman to be true.[26]

Other scientists and ministers solved the problem by positing an

25. Fletcher Green, *The Role of the Yankee in the Old South* (Athens, Ga., 1972), 102; Bachman, *Unity of the Human Race*, 9, 292; Green, "Harmony of Revelation and Natural Science," in Ruffner (ed.), *Lectures on the Evidences*, 463.

26. "Hugh Miller on the Testimony of the Rocks," *Methodist Quarterly Review*, XI (1957), 626. See also Martindale, "Footprints of the Creator," 502; Pendleton, "Chronology of Creation," 162, 178; "The Progress of Science and Its Connection with Scripture," 46; "The Testimony of Geology and Astronomy to the Truth of the Hebrew Records," *Southern Baptist Review and Eclectic*, I (1855), 723.

immense period between the time that Genesis called "the beginning" and the concluding six days of creation, which were understood as merely the final stage in the creation of the species. Between the phrase "in the beginning" and the account of the six days of creation, they assumed, millions of years might have passed. The theologian Thomas Ralston claimed that this was the theory "adopted generally by Christian geologists" and "most intelligent Christians of the present day." The geologists William Buckland and Adam Sedgwick were among its English proponents, and it also carried the imprimatur of Thomas Chalmers in Scotland, whose *Natural Theology* had enormous influence on southern Presbyterians. Hitchcock popularized the theory in his *Religion of Geology.*[27]

The southern pastors could therefore appeal to the scientists as guardians of scriptural truth, but as the condition of their guardianship the geologists demanded a subtle rationalizing of the text, which the ministers began to interpret in accordance with the latest findings of nineteenth-century science. Relatively modern notions of geological time became interpretive clues for understanding the "real" meaning of Genesis, which was hidden behind its merely apparent meaning. The ministers were prepared to accept the possibility, in short, that "science may not only cast light upon the scriptures, but correct many false readings of them." An astute critic, Moses Stuart, for example, could see precisely what was happening: the clergy were imposing a nineteenth-century worldview on ancient Jewish literature. Natural science was becoming an implicit norm for biblical interpretation.[28]

Some of the theologians even tried to remodel theology itself after the image of the natural sciences. Among Reformed theologians, especially, it became an article of faith, as Thornwell wrote, that "all sciences have as their basis indisputable facts arranged and classified according to the necessary laws of the mind," and that the biblical revelation furnished "facts" just as susceptible to scientific ordering as any other. The attempt to construct an "inductive" theology endured among ministers of several denominations throughout the antebellum period. The postwar fundamentalist movement drew on that tradition in its later struggles with theological liberalism.[29]

27. Ralston, *Elements of Divinity,* 73; "The Nebular Theory," *Methodist Quarterly Review,* II (1848), 508.

28. "The Nebular Theory," 508.

29. "Report of Thornwell's Inaugural Address," *Southern Presbyterian,* XI (October 24, 1857), 1; Robert J. Breckinridge, *The Knowledge of God, Subjectively Considered* (New York, 1859), xii.

By the 1850s the early enthusiasm for science had begun to show signs of strain. There had, of course, been some tension from the beginning, but the expanding range of scientific investigation, especially the increasing interest in developmental hypotheses after the 1844 publication in England of the *Vestiges of the Natural History of Creation*, seemed to trouble the clergy. By the 1850s the *Presbyterian Critic* was speaking of the alliance of scientists and theologians as "a very delicate point in the present posture of opinion." The journal's editor, Thomas Peck, announced that the clergy had been too sensitive for too long about the pretensions of science. "The gospel of science," added the *Methodist Quarterly Review* in 1859, "is, for man, an infinitely poor gospel after all."[30]

The evidence for a transition, though, is impressionistic and inconclusive. The University of Virginia offered some lectures during the 1850s "to counteract the tide of infidelity threatened by the new scientific investigations," but the lecturers were still highly optimistic about the complementary relationships between religion and science. In 1857 the Tombecbee Presbytery in Mississippi complained of insidious scientific attacks on religion and recommended that chairs be established in theological seminaries "to refute the objections of infidel naturalists." But that was only one side of the story: the chairs were also intended "to evince the harmony of science with the records of our faith," an intention bespeaking the familiar confidence in the alliance of religion and science.[31]

The Presbyterian proposal illustrated, more than anything else, the ambiguity of the alliance in the 1850s. Among the clergy who favored the proposal, some felt defensive about the sciences; others had every expectation of maintaining cordial relations between the disciplines. James Lyon of Columbus, Mississippi, led the drive. A graduate of Princeton Theological Seminary who had interrupted a series of urban pastorates to spend a period in Europe, Lyon hoped that the new chair would preclude the "indiscreet zeal" of ministers who were un-

---

30. Thomas E. Peck, *Miscellanies of the Rev. Thomas E. Peck* (2 vols.; Richmond, 1895), II, 293, 295; "Scientific Import of the First Chapter of Genesis," *Methodist Quarterly Review*, XIII (1859), 568.

31. Van Zandt, "The Necessity of a Revelation," in Ruffner (ed.), *Lectures on the Evidences*, 31–33; Robert J. Breckinridge, "The General Internal Evidence of Christianity," in Ruffner (ed.), *Lectures on the Evidences*, 330; Green, "Harmony of Revelation and Natural Science," in Ruffner (ed.), *Lectures on the Evidences*, 463–76; William Childs Robinson, *Columbia Theological Seminary and the Southern Presbyterian Church* (N.p., 1931), 168–77; John B. Adger, *My Life and Times* (Richmond, 1899), 423–25.

equipped to defend the faith. He was confident about the continued apologetic potential of the sciences, for he believed that the works of nature constituted "the first great revelation that God has made of himself," and that therefore the revelation in nature was fully as authoritative and inspired as the Bible itself. Scripture, he said, was simply a "supplement" to nature, made necessary by human sinfulness.[32]

Others were uneasy, and Robert Dabney of Union Seminary in Virginia spoke for them when he complained that the proposed chairs would have "a tendency towards naturalistic and anti-Christian opinions." But in 1859 a member of Lyon's congregation, Judge John Perkins, donated $50,000, and the denomination promptly called James Woodrow to the Perkins Professorship of Natural Science in Connection with Revealed Religion at the seminary in Columbia. Woodrow's inaugural address spoke of the "harmony" of science and Scripture, but almost immediately he shifted his language to refer to the absence of "contradiction" between them, and within three decades Woodrow was the defendant in a heresy trial occasioned by his acceptance of evolutionary theory.[33]

The Perkins Professorship symbolized the end of an era, and the debates attending its formation signaled the beginning of the breakdown of clerical optimism about the sciences. Indeed, the sad conclusion of the affair portended the anti-science temper of later southern conservative theology during the Darwinian era. Throughout the antebellum period the gentlemen theologians had found in the sciences the data for a natural theology that prepared the mind to receive the biblical revelation. The study of the natural world enabled the theologian, so it was thought, to discover natural truths that confirmed the revealed truth. The very effort assumed that "the theology of natural science" was "in perfect harmony with the theology of the Bible."[34]

32. James A. Lyon, "The New Theological Professorship—Natural Science in Connection with Revealed Religion," *Southern Presbyterian Review*, XII (1859), 188–89.

33. Adger, *Life and Times*, 423–25; Robinson, *Columbia Theological Seminary*, 168–77. Numbers, *Creation by Natural Law*, 161, notes, however, Woodrow's observation that in the 1880s several denominational colleges taught evolutionary theory.

34. Green, "Harmony of Revelation and Natural Science," in Ruffner (ed.), *Lectures on the Evidences*, 463.

PART II

MEDICINE IN THE OLD SOUTH

INTRODUCTION

U nlike science, which directly involved only a small percentage of antebellum southerners, medicine influenced the lives of virtually everyone in the Old South. Thus the chapters in this part offer a less elitist and more inclusive view of southern society before the Civil War than those of the previous section. They examine not only the lives of orthodox physicians, but those of sectarian and folk healers as well. They explore both the myths and the realities associated with the medical geography of the region, and they attempt to identify the prevailing diseases and the elements of the population most at risk. They investigate the ways in which antebellum southerners, both individually and collectively, responded to the presence and threat of disease. And, like the chapters on science in the Old South, they seek to identify the distinctive aspects of medical life in the South by comparing it with what is known about medical life in other regions, a method that surprisingly few American medical historians have used.[1]

Although allusions to medical conditions and practices have long been common in studies of the Old South, the first systematic discussion of the subject did not appear until 1930, when the medical historian Richard Harrison Shryock published a brief survey entitled "Med-

---

1. An outstanding exception is John Harley Warner, *The Therapeutic Perspective: Medical Practice, Knowledge, and Identity in America, 1820–1885* (Cambridge, Mass., 1986), which compares therapeutic practices in the Northeast, Midwest, and South. See also Warner, "A Southern Medical Reform: The Meaning of the Antebellum Argument for Southern Medical Education," *Bulletin of the History of Medicine*, LVII (1983), 364–81.

ical Practice in the Old South."[2] In this classic essay, which touches on virtually every topic presented in this section of the book, Shryock pointed to the pervasive influence of the southern environment and the institution of slavery on the medical conditions, practices, and politics of the region. He addressed such issues as southern medical distinctiveness, the care of slaves, the quality of medical education, the development of public health, and the popularity of irregular medicine. His work has deservedly served as the starting point for most subsequent historical investigations of antebellum southern medicine.

Until recently the most extended studies of medicine in the Old South have generally been found in state histories of medicine, such as Wyndham B. Blanton's on Virginia, Joseph I. Waring's on South Carolina, and John Duffy's on Louisiana.[3] Although some of the local histories are marred by a chauvinistic tone and a provincial outlook, they all contain information of value to present-day scholars.

With the emergence of trained medical historians in the past couple of decades, attention has shifted from descriptive state surveys to more analytical and specialized studies. The issue of southern medical distinctiveness, however, has remained a subject of perennial interest. This concern is reflected in such diverse works as John Duffy's and James O. Breeden's provocative essays on sectional medical politics and states-rights medicine;[4] Duffy's and JoAnn Carrigan's investigations of the impact of yellow fever; Albert E. Cowdrey's evocative portrayal of the southern environment; and William D. Postell's, Todd

2. Richard Harrison Shryock, "Medical Practice in the Old South," *South Atlantic Quarterly*, XXIX (1930), 160–78, reprinted in Shryock, *Medicine in America: Historical Essays* (Baltimore, 1966), 49–70. For another early survey, see Martha Carolyn Mitchell, "Health and the Medical Profession in the Lower South, 1845–1860," *Journal of Southern History*, X (1944), 424–46.

3. Wyndham B. Blanton, *Medicine in Virginia in the Nineteenth Century* (Richmond, 1933); Joseph I. Waring, *A History of Medicine in South Carolina, 1825–1900* (Columbia, S.C., 1967); John Duffy (ed.), *The Rudolph Matas History of Medicine in Louisiana* (2 vols.; Baton Rouge, 1958, 1962).

4. John Duffy, "Medical Practice in the Antebellum South," *Journal of Southern History*, XXV (1959), 53–72; Duffy, "A Note on Ante-Bellum Southern Nationalism and Medical Practice," *Journal of Southern History*, XXXIV (1968), 266–76; James O. Breeden, "States-Rights Medicine in the Old South," *Bulletin of the New York Academy of Medicine*, LII (1976), 348–72. See also Harold J. Abrahams, "Secession from Northern Medical Schools," *Transactions and Studies of the College of Physicians of Philadelphia*, 4th ser., XXXVI (1968), 29–45.

L. Savitt's, and Kenneth Kiple and Virginia H. King's monographs on slave-related health and medicine.[5]

Building on these works and their own research, participants in the second Barnard-Millington symposium once again addressed the problem of southern medical distinctiveness, but this time from a comparative perspective. Were the medical needs and medical practices of the Old South, they asked, really so different from those of other regions? The answer that emerges from the following essays is a qualified yes—qualified for the reasons John Harley Warner outlines in Chapters 9 and 10. Observing that "the southern argument for regional medical distinctiveness was in itself not at all distinctive," he shows that residents of all regions viewed their health conditions and medical needs as unique, even when their practices were not always distinctive. Southerners pushed their claims more vociferously and vocally, he asserts, because they believed they had more at stake— politically, socially, and economically, as well as medically.

Warner's work exemplifies the importance of looking at sectional issues in a national, even international, context and illustrates the value of a comparative approach. After reading Chapter 9, a historian examining antebellum medical journals, for example, would better understand why so many physicians carefully noted such details as a patient's sex, age, nativity, race, length of residence, and previous residence in their case histories, because, according to the prevailing theory, the appropriate therapy depended on a knowledge of these variables.

As the chapters in this section demonstrate, it is nearly impossible to write about medicine in the Old South without considering two distinctive elements: slavery and the southern environment. In fact, these two issues were often closely related. As K. David Patterson points out in Chapter 7, "Disease Environments of the Antebellum South," when

5. John Duffy, *Sword of Pestilence: The New Orleans Yellow Fever Epidemic of 1853* (Baton Rouge, 1966); JoAnn Carrigan, "Privilege, Prejudice, and the Strangers' Disease in Nineteenth Century New Orleans," *Journal of Southern History*, XXXVI (1970), 568–78; Albert E. Cowdrey, *This Land, This South: An Environmental History* (Lexington, Ky., 1983); William D. Postell, *The Health of Slaves on Southern Plantations* (Baton Rouge, 1951); Todd L. Savitt, *Medicine and Slavery: The Diseases and Health Care of Blacks in Antebellum Virginia* (Urbana, 1978); Kenneth F. Kiple and Virginia H. King, *Another Dimension to the Black Diaspora: Diet, Disease, and Racism* (Cambridge, England, 1981). See also John S. Haller, "The Negro and the Southern Physician: A Study of Medical and Racial Attitudes, 1800–1860," *Medical History*, XVI (1972), 238–53.

blacks brought such diseases as malaria, yellow fever, and hookworm with them from Africa, they helped to create "a modified West African disease environment" in parts of the South. Slavery also contributed to the creation of a distinctive disease environment, argues James H. Cassedy in Chapter 8, by promoting extensive land clearing, soil exhaustion, and rural settlement.

But slavery and the environment also acted independently on many aspects of southern life and health, affecting such areas as public health, domestic medical care, and folk practices. In Chapter 11, "Public Health in the Old South," Margaret Warner examines the ways in which the stubborn persistence of yellow fever, one of the transplanted African diseases that thrived in filthy environments, prompted much of the public-health effort in the antebellum South.[6] In Chapter 13 on domestic medicine, Elizabeth B. Keeney shows how the region's poor roads, inadequate medical care, distinctive plants, and large black population influenced the popularity and content of domestic medical guides.[7] In Chapters 14 and 15, respectively, Elliott J. Gorn and Todd L. Savitt focus specifically on the medical needs and remedies of southern blacks, whose physical and cultural characteristics were used by some white southerners, including physicians, as a justification for slavery.

Although the essays in this section contribute much to our understanding of medicine in the Old South, considerable work remains to be done. Little, for example, is known about antebellum southern hospitals, despite the presence of such prominent institutions as the Charity Hospital in New Orleans and the Roper Hospital in Charleston. Thus we still do not know if southern hospitals played the same social roles as those in the North, or even how many general hospitals southerners established. In Chapter 12, however, Samuel B. Thielman analyzes the structure and function of mental hospitals in the Old South.[8]

6. A useful earlier discussion of public health in the Old South appears in David R. Goldfield, "The Business of Health Planning: Disease Prevention in the Old South," *Journal of Southern History*, XLII (1976), 557–70. See also Henry E. Sigerist, "The Cost of Illness to the City of New Orleans in 1850," *Bulletin of the History of Medicine*, XV (1944), 498–507.

7. The most popular of the southern antebellum domestic manuals, *Gunn's Domestic Medicine*, has recently been reprinted with an introduction by Charles E. Rosenberg (Knoxville, Tenn., 1986).

8. On southern asylums, see also Norman Dain, *Disordered Minds: The First Century of Eastern State Hospital in Williamsburg, Virginia, 1766–1866* (Williamsburg, 1971); Gerald N. Grob, *Mental Institutions in America: Social Policy to 1875* (New York, 1973); Savitt, *Medicine and Slavery*, 247–80.

The place of medical societies and journals in the professional lives of southern physicians also deserves attention. It would be useful to know, for example, how popular they were, how they influenced medical practice, how they differed from those in other regions, and how they were used by the medically orthodox to combat the threat of irregular practitioners—another topic in search of a historian.[9] Besides the standard references to James Marion Sims's repairs of vesico-vaginal fistulae and Ephraim McDowell's pioneering ovariotomies, not much is known about medical research and experimentation in the Old South.[10] In fact, with the exceptions of Joseph Jones and Josiah Nott, the subjects of recent biographies, the lives of antebellum southern physicians, including such luminaries as Bennet Dowler, John L. Riddell, and Samuel Cartwright, remain largely a mystery.[11] Clearly, the agenda sketched by Richard Shryock over fifty years ago remains unfinished.

9. James O. Breeden provides one of the few discussions of sectarian medicine in the Old South in "Thomsonianism in Virginia," *Virginia Magazine of History and Biography,* LXXXII (1974), 150–80.

10. But see Todd L. Savitt, "The Use of Blacks for Medical Experimentation and Demonstration in the Old South," *Journal of Southern History,* XLVIII (1982), 331–48.

11. James O. Breeden, *Joseph Jones, M.D.: Scientist of the Old South* (Lexington, Ky., 1975); Reginald Horsman, *Josiah Nott of Mobile: Southerner, Physician, and Racial Theorist* (Baton Rouge, 1987).

CHAPTER 7

DISEASE ENVIRONMENTS OF THE ANTEBELLUM SOUTH

K. David Patterson

The health of antebellum southerners reflected the region's harsh disease environment. This chapter, a reconnaissance of a complex subject that requires much detailed research, suggests three major hypotheses. First, and most readily documented, the South carried a heavy burden of the infectious and noninfectious diseases common to the North and to Europe, somewhat exacerbated by the region's climate and social conditions. Second, the presence of three formidable diseases of African origin, falciparum malaria, hookworm, and yellow fever, gave the South an epidemiological distinctiveness that strongly influenced medical theories and techniques. Finally, the distribution of these imported diseases provides a tentative basis for dividing the region into four more or less distinct epidemiological subregions: the Appalachian Mountains, the Atlantic Coastal Plain, the Gulf Coast, and the Interior.

Health conditions in the South, as elsewhere, have always been profoundly influenced by both natural and human factors. Most of the region has a moist, warm climate and a short, mild winter, and parts of the Gulf Coast and much of Florida are almost subtropical. Favorable conditions for mosquitoes, which transmitted diseases, for worm eggs and larvae, and for a host of waterborne protozoa, bacteria, and viruses, existed for much of the year, in sharp contrast to the colder North. Economic and social conditions were equally important. The South remained predominantly rural; indeed, extensive areas were still being settled in the prewar decades. Despite the growth of commercial agriculture and the acquisition of considerable wealth by some whites, the vast majority of southerners, black and white, were poor.

The South was, by almost any economic, social, or educational index, an "underdeveloped" region. Massive poverty and warm climates produced a disease environment in the Old South similar in many ways to those prevailing in "developing" countries today. Mortality was high for all age groups, appallingly so for infants and children, and the major causes of death were infectious diseases.[1]

It is very difficult to quantify morbidity and mortality or to evaluate the incidence and impact of specific diseases and their changes over time in the antebellum South, partly because of lack of information and partly because so little historical research has been done. Doctors, often poorly trained and not always consulted by the sick, were often unable to assess the local situation. Medical knowledge was still rudimentary, and, with very few exceptions, vital statistics were not collected. Spectacular epidemics tended to be better documented than chronic or endemic diseases. These problems are, of course, hardly unique to the South, but the data are far inferior to those available for, say, Massachusetts, England, or Sweden during the same period.

Four major types of sources provide information about antebellum health conditions: contemporary medical and lay accounts for particular areas, towns, plantations, and so forth; statistical reports on small, closely observed, but atypical groups, such as soldiers; broad but poorly controlled surveys, such as those included in the mortality returns collected in the 1850 and 1860 decennial censuses; and extrapolation from later medical knowledge. Since none of these sources has as yet been fully exploited, the following sketch is unavoidably general and preliminary.

Although the South was a distinct epidemiological region, it shared many "cosmopolitan" diseases with the North and with Europe. Respiratory and gastrointestinal infections, childhood diseases, the ubiquitous helminths (worms), and noninfectious conditions such as cancer, heart disease, stroke, diabetes, and trauma all took their toll on health and life. Census data provide a useful basis for discussing these common problems. Table 1, compiled from the 1850 returns, shows leading causes of death for two southern states, Mississippi and North Carolina.[2] In the 1850 census, enumerators' schedules included a question about any deaths during the previous year. Where there had been

1. Abdel R. Omran, "Epidemiologic Transition in the United States: The Health Factor in Population Change," *Population Bulletin*, XXXII (May, 1977), 1–42.
2. These diseases are classified according to the scheme in Todd L. Savitt, *Medicine and Slavery: The Diseases and Health Care of Blacks in Antebellum Virginia* (Urbana, 1978), 143–45.

TABLE 1.
LEADING CAUSES OF DEATH IN TWO STATES, 1850

Cause	Number	% of All Deaths
(N = 122)	Mississippi	(N = 8,721)
1. Fevers, unclassifiable	1,105	12.7
2. Respiratory diseases	709	8.1
3. Cholera	617	7.1
4. Diarrheal diseases	573	6.6
5. Nervous system diseases	502	5.8
6. Diphtheria	398	4.6
7. Tuberculosis	383	4.4
8. Accidents	365	4.2
9. Digestive system diseases	344	3.9
10. Dropsy	302	3.5
11. Worms	298	3.4
12. Scarlet fever	270	3.1
13. Typhoid fever	257	2.9
14. Whooping cough	242	2.8
15. Old age	125	1.4
Total	6490	74.4
(N = 114)	North Carolina	(N = 10,165)
1. Respiratory diseases	1017	10.0
2. Fevers, unclassifiable	839	8.3
3. Dropsy	724	7.1
4. Tuberculosis	617	6.1
5. Nervous system diseases	505	5.0
6. Digestive system diseases	421	4.1
7. Old age	409	4.0
8. Accidents	379	3.7
9. Typhoid fever	335	3.3
10. Diarrheal diseases	329	3.2
11. Diphtheria	324	3.2
12. Childbirth	175	1.7
13. Scarlet fever	170	1.7
14. Worms	166	1.6
15. Measles	112	1.1
Total	6522	64.2

SOURCE: Seventh Census, 1850, Mortality Returns, 151–155; 199–201.

deaths, the enumerators then asked for such details as age, sex, place of birth, and cause of death.

As Todd L. Savitt has pointed out, since such responses were subjected to all the uncertainties of recall and lay diagnosis, the seductively tabulated census returns must be used with great caution.[3] Because the returns cover only one year in ten, they may reflect unusual epidemiological conditions. Some of the alleged causes of death, such as "old age" and "dropsy" (which included, among others, many cardiac conditions), are hopelessly vague and meaningless in the context of modern terminology. In some cases, many different "causes" were combined under very broad general categories. Among these are "nervous system disease," which included strokes and a host of ill-defined disorders, and "fevers," a confusion of symptoms for diseases that embraced malaria and other infections. Even apparently clear-cut diseases like "scarlet fever" or "cholera" may not conform precisely to modern diagnosis. We should also remember that mortality returns do not necessarily reflect endemic diseases that caused suffering and economic loss but did not kill.

Some generalizations can, however, be drawn from these census data, as shown for two examples, Mississippi and North Carolina. The patterns of death for the two states were very similar, which is not surprising considering their size and topographical diversity. Much of the mortality was caused by infectious diseases associated with poverty and lack of sanitation; spectacular epidemics of diseases like smallpox and yellow fever were less important than the ubiquitous endemic infections. Typhoid fever, diarrheal diseases, and "digestive system diseases," which reflected poor water supplies and sanitation, were important causes of mortality and presumably responsible for an enormous amount of ill health. Dysentery sometimes occurred in epidemic form, as in eastern North Carolina in 1857.[4] The returns show the uneven impact of the cholera epidemic of 1849–1853: Mississippi suffered heavily, but few deaths were ascribed to cholera in North Carolina. Worms were probably not as significant a primary cause of death as the census data indicate, but *Ascaris, Trichuris*, and tapeworm infections were very common and familiar to both lay and medical persons. Two other worms, trichina and hookworm, were not recognized at the time, but were doubtless very common.[5] Given the low sanitary stan-

3. Savitt, *Medicine and Slavery*, 135–39.

4. N. J. Pittman, "On the Diseases of Edgecomb County," *Transactions of the Medical Society of North Carolina*, VIII (1857), 36–37.

5. The beef tapeworm (*Taenia saginata*) and the pork tapeworm (*T. solium*) were both present. The ubiquity of swine favored the latter, more clinically dangerous species and

K. DAVID PATTERSON

dards, helminths were responsible for much ill health and contributed indirectly to many deaths ascribed to other conditions. Respiratory diseases (mostly listed as "pneumonia") were major killers, and the prevalence of tuberculosis (mostly listed as "consumption") was surprising, given the low level of urbanization. Measles, diphtheria, and whooping cough took a heavy toll of children. Accidents included a large number of deaths from burns and scalds, not surprising in an era when cooking was done over an open fire and women wore long dresses.

Many other diseases killed southerners in smaller numbers—or just made them sick. Chickenpox, smallpox, tetanus, colds, influenza, syphilis, mumps, ringworm, and a host of other infections, deadly and trivial, afflicted people. Cuts, puncture wounds, and scrapes were inevitably common and frequently became infected. Many southerners, then and now, suffered from allergies to local pollens and mildews, as well as from rheumatism, arthritis, cancer, diabetes, cardiovascular conditions, and other noninfectious diseases, many of which were associated with aging.

Nutrition played a major but not entirely clear role in the health of antebellum southerners. Poor nutrition retards growth, lowers productivity, and at times produces clinical disease and death. A person's nutritional status also affects, often profoundly, his or her resistance to infectious and other diseases. The relationship is often circular; many parasitic and other infections contribute to malnutrition. The historical study of nutrition is very difficult, in part because many of the complexities of the field remain unknown. In addition, food and its preparation varied regionally and between social groups; individuals and races had different nutritional requirements. Pregnant and lactating women and young children were especially vulnerable to the effects of poor nutrition.

Although our historical knowledge about such matters is still incomplete, enough good research has been done, especially on blacks, to allow some generalizations to be made. Antebellum southerners depended heavily on pork and corn as staples, but the warm climate also permitted extensive cultivation of a variety of fruits and vegetables, which were available for more months of the year than in the North. The rural, often undeveloped, landscape was exploited extensively for hunting, fishing, and gathering of wild plants. In general,

---

ensured that trichinosis (*Trichinella spiralis*) was widespread. However, contrary to Savitt's assertion (*Medicine and Slavery*, 66), the fish tapeworm (*Diphyllobothrium latum*) did not occur in the South.

TABLE 2.

INFANT AND CHILD DEATHS AS PERCENTAGES OF TOTAL DEATHS IN
TWO STATES, 1850

State	% Deaths 0–1 year	% Deaths 1–5 years	% Deaths 0–5 years	Total Deaths all ages
Mississippi	21.4	25.4	46.8	8,721
North Carolina	19.2	17.8	37.0	10,165

SOURCE: Seventh Census, 1850, Mortality Returns, 151–155; 199–201.

most southerners had an adequate intake of calories, and, except sea-
sonally for some slaves, enough animal protein. Deficiencies of vi-
tamins A, C, D, and niacin were no doubt common, particularly in
winter and especially among blacks and poor whites. Two vitamin
deficiency diseases, pellagra ("black tongue") and rickets, were listed
in the 1850 census returns as minor causes of death. Iron deficiency
anemia, compounded by malaria and hookworm infection, was probably common. Still, though nutrition was far from the ideal and one
wonders about the impact of the high fat and salt consumption on
cardiovascular health, most prewar southerners, especially the whites,
probably ate about as well as their northern or European contemporaries. Indeed, the region as a whole probably was better fed in 1850
than in 1900.[6]

The severity of infant and child mortality, defined respectively as
deaths before age one and between one and five years, evidences the
real shortcomings in southern nutrition and sanitation. Table 2 lists
infant and child deaths as percentages of all deaths in Mississippi and
North Carolina. Even if we allow for substantial underreporting of
infant mortality, the percentages of antebellum infant deaths are very
high. The percentages representing child and infant deaths combined
are also extremely high and suggest an appallingly effective syner-
gism between malnutrition and infection among toddlers and young
children.[7]

6. Kenneth F. Kiple and Virginia Himmelsteib King, *Another Dimension to the Black
Diaspora: Diet, Disease, and Racism* (Cambridge, England, 1981), 79–95; Savitt, *Medicine
and Slavery*, 86–103; Sam Bowers Hilliard, *Hogmeat and Hoecake: Food Supply in the Old
South, 1840–1860* (Carbondale, Ill., 1972); Joe Gray Taylor, *Eating, Drinking, and Visiting in
the South: An Informal History* (Baton Rouge, 1982). Pellagra apparently did not become a
major problem until late in the nineteenth century.

7. J. E. Gordon, J. B. Wyon, and W. Ascoli, "The Second Year Death Rate in Underdeveloped Countries," *American Journal of Medical Sciences*, CCLIV (1967), 358–64. The
census data are not accurate enough to allow calculation of age-specific death rates.

The overall epidemiological conditions of the antebellum South, including the heavy burden of infectious diseases and high mortality among infants and children, are strikingly similar to those prevailing in many Third World countries today. The disease environment was typical of almost any poor, rural society prior to the advent of modern preventive and curative medicine.

In many respects, at least given our present state of knowledge, the disease environment of the prewar South seems fairly similar to that prevailing in the North or West during the same period. Climate might suggest a higher incidence of respiratory diseases in the North and more diarrhea-dysentery conditions in the South, but these were primarily nonlethal and hence would not necessarily be reflected in the census mortality returns. For example, rural Maine and urban Massachusetts reported percentages of deaths from respiratory diseases comparable to Louisiana, but lower than those reported for portions of Virginia, Tennessee, North Carolina, or Mississippi (Table 3).

The high percentage of deaths ascribed to respiratory diseases in the Virginia mountains (modern West Virginia) compared with the percentages reported for western North Carolina and eastern Tennessee suggests problems in reporting or unusual disease conditions in the census year. Tuberculosis probably was a more important killer in the North. A high rate might be expected for densely populated Massachusetts, but for some reason Maine, which had a scattered population not unlike those of most southern states, suffered from even greater tuberculosis mortality. The higher tuberculosis rate in western Virginia's mountains is also noteworthy, though in Tennessee and North Carolina the mountain counties reported a lower rate of tuberculosis mortality than the lowlands.

Further research is needed to clarify antebellum patterns of morbidity and mortality in the South and the nation as a whole. However, the perception of contemporary and modern observers that the South was "different" is easily defended. The South was an epidemiologically distinct region largely because, unlike the rest of the country, it had massively imported and sustained three African diseases.

The importation of slaves produced a modified West African disease environment throughout the entire Caribbean basin, including the American South. Since Africa shared most of the major infectious diseases of the Eurasian land mass, Africans, like European immigrants, brought such diseases as smallpox, measles, amebic and bacillary dysenteries, gonorrhea, and intestinal helminths to the South, either directly from Africa or via the West Indies. African strains of

TABLE 3.
RESPIRATORY AND TUBERCULOSIS DEATHS IN SEVERAL REGIONS,
1850

Region	Respiratory Diseases (% of all deaths)	Tuberculosis[a] (% of all deaths)	Total Deaths
Maine	3.8	23.1	7,584
Massachusetts	5.0	17.2	19,904
Louisiana	4.4	5.4	11,956
Virginia: mountain counties[b]	22.0	11.7	3,422
North Carolina: coastal counties	9.5	5.7	2,909
North Carolina: mountain counties	7.3	3.6	1,588
Tennessee: mountain counties[c]	5.6	7.7	1,927
Tennessee: western counties[d]	7.7	8.7	3,062

SOURCE: Compiled from Seventh Census, 1850, Mortality Returns.
[a]The vast majority of cases in all regions were "consumption" or pulmonary tuberculosis.
[b]Modern West Virginia.
[c]Eastern quarter of the state.
[d]Western quarter of the state along the Mississippi River.

some of these pathogens might have been particularly virulent, but this would be hard to document. Fortunately, some African diseases, like trypanosomiasis, did not become established in the Americas. A few, such as schistosomiasis and onchocerciasis, became problems in the West Indies and northern South America but were not transmitted within the United States.[8] Others, such as bancroftian filariasis, were only minor local problems in the South.[9] A relatively harsh climate and the absence of the proper insect or snail intermediaries protected the South against these African invaders.

8. The best source on these intercontinental disease transfers is Rudolph Hoeppli, *Parasitic Diseases in Africa and the Western Hemisphere: Early Documentation and Transmission by the Slave Trade, Acta Tropica* Supplement 10 (Basel, Switzerland, 1969).

9. Todd L. Savitt, "Filariasis in the United States," *Journal of the History of Medicine and Allied Sciences,* XXXII (1977), 140–50.

Three African diseases, however, flourished in the southern climate and made the South a distinct disease zone. Falciparum malaria (malignant tertian, aestivoautumnal) was far more deadly than the vivax malaria (benign tertian) long familiar to northern Europeans, which was widespread in the North and Midwest as well as the South. The hookworm *Necator americanus*, which should more properly be called *Necator africanus*, has always been much more common in the South than the European species (*Ancylostoma duodenale*). Yellow fever clearly originated in Africa and reached North America via the Caribbean in the late seventeenth century. None of these three diseases of African origin is specifically named among the major killers of Mississippians and North Carolinians listed in Table 1. However, "fever, yellow" can be found among the "fevers," and malaria appears under the names "fever, intermittent" and "fever, remittent" in the 1850 nosology. Hookworm had not been discovered.

Vivax malaria, which can thrive in cool climates, was imported into the Americas by early European settlers and flourished in the South as well as much of the Northeast and upper Midwest in the antebellum period. Agricultural development and rising standards of living resulted in a gradual retreat of vivax malaria from the North in the late nineteenth century, but it remained entrenched in the South until the 1940s.[10] The most dangerous species, *Plasmodium falciparum*, did not reach the North American mainland until the last decades of the seventeenth century, when it arrived in the bodies of African slaves.[11] Because *P. falciparum* requires warm temperatures to complete the mosquito phases of its life cycle, it remained restricted to the South.[12] A local mosquito, *Anopheles quadrimaculatus*, already ranged over most of the South and soon proved to be an efficient transmitter. This insect prefers to breed in sunlit pools, so its habitat was extended when forests were cleared and dams and rice fields constructed. Contemporary observers soon became well aware that malaria spread with agricultural development.[13] Although the severity of infection fluctuated

10. Ernest Carroll Faust, "Clinical and Public Health Aspects of Malaria in the United States from an Historical Perspective," *American Journal of Tropical Medicine and Hygiene,* XXV (1945), 185–201.

11. Peter H. Wood, *Black Majority: Negroes in Colonial South Carolina from 1670 through the Stono Rebellion* (New York, 1974), 87; Darrett B. Rutman and Anita H. Rutman, "Of Agues and Fevers: Malaria in the Early Chesapeake," *William and Mary Quarterly,* 3rd ser., XXXIII (1976), 42–43.

12. Leonard J. Bruce-Chwatt, *Essential Malariology* (London, 1980), 132–33; George C. Shattuck, *Diseases of the Tropics* (New York, 1951), 15.

13. Thomas E. Evans, "On the Medical History of the Eastern Part of Mississippi, etc.," *New Orleans Medical and Surgical Journal,* VI (1849), 741–45.

annually, especially near the northern frontiers of *P. falciparum*'s range, malaria was a permanent problem throughout the areas in which it became established.

Most blacks had an almost absolute genetic immunity to *P. vivax* malaria. Because of sickle-cell trait, a large portion, perhaps as many as a quarter, were immune to falciparum malaria as well; but this immunity was gained at the cost of the deaths from sickle-cell disease of one fourth of the children of parents with the protective trait.[14] Thus, though blacks could and did suffer from malaria, whites were far more vulnerable. Recovery from malaria conveyed a temporary, strain-specific immunity, so "fever" was most lethal among the "un-seasoned," such as newcomers to the region and the very young. Still, probably a majority of southerners suffered from malarial chills and fevers each summer and autumn, unless they were wealthy enough to flee to more salubrious regions in the North, the hills, or the piney woods.[15]

The impact of malaria on life and health is impossible to quantify, but it was enormous. Malaria was most prevalent along the Atlantic and Gulf coastal plains and in the Mississippi Valley, but it was found almost everywhere in the South.[16] Malaria was a killer, particularly of the young and the weak, and a serious hazard for pregnant women and babies. Many of the deaths ascribed to "fever, not specified" were caused by malaria and, because the symptoms of the disease are quite variable, malaria was undoubtedly the primary cause of many deaths recorded under other categories. Malaria was even more significant as a secondary cause of death. Year in and year out, it sapped the mental and physical strength of southerners and increased their vulnerability to other diseases.

The second in our trio of African diseases, the species of hookworm afflicting the South, was not discovered until 1902, but its symptoms were already well known in the early nineteenth century. Like malaria, this nematode causes anemia and weakens many more people than it kills. Heavily infected persons tend to be lethargic, and children often have retarded growth. The disease is acquired by walking barefoot over soil contaminated with the feces of infected people;

14. Kiple and King, *Another Dimension*, 17–22; H. M. Mathews and J. C. Armstrong, "Duffy Blood Types and Vivax Malaria in Ethiopia," *American Journal of Tropical Medicine and Hygiene*, XXX (1981), 299–303.

15. Charles F. Kovacik, "Health Conditions and Town Growth in Colonial and Antebellum South Carolina," *Social Science and Medicine*, XII (1978), 131–36.

16. August Hirsch, *Handbook of Geographical and Historical Pathology* (3 vols.; London, 1883), I, 223–50.

thus it is clearly associated with poverty and poor sanitation. Larval hookworms develop most readily in warm, moist, sandy soils rich in humus. *Necator americanus* is not found north of the Ohio River. Surveys done in the early twentieth century revealed widespread infections over the entire southern region and especially high prevalences in the coastal plain of the Atlantic and Gulf states.[17] These surveys, along with some older medical accounts, indicate that the disease was also widespread during the antebellum period.[18]

Yellow fever was the most spectacular and terrifying component of the southern disease environment. It was not, however, permanently established in the United States but was introduced by ships from the Caribbean at irregular intervals. This fact, plus the proclivity of the mosquito vector, *Aedes aegypti*, for urban breeding, made yellow fever primarily a disease of port cities. In the eighteenth century yellow fever struck cities as far north as Philadelphia and Boston, but after 1822 the disease rarely appeared north of the Virginia coast. Charleston, Savannah, and other Atlantic ports were frequently hit in the pre–Civil War years, but yellow fever was most destructive on the Gulf Coast and occasionally penetrated into the lower Mississippi Valley.[19] On both coasts, epidemics were especially numerous from the late 1840s to 1858. New Orleans, as John Duffy has related, suffered terribly in the 1850s, when almost 20,000 people died.[20] Yellow fever was a catalyst for acrimonious debates between miasmatists and contagionists and became the single most important stimulus for public health reform in the antebellum South.[21] It caused heavy mortality among newcomers to the region; local people gained permanent immunity by surviving the disease. Those who did so as children were particularly fortunate because yellow fever attacks are usually mild or even subclinical in the young. Blacks apparently had some genetic

17. Shattuck, *Diseases of the Tropics*, 544; Harold W. Brown, *Basic Clinical Parasitology* (4th ed.; New York, 1975), 125–26.

18. Hirsch, *Handbook*, II, 313–15; Charles Wardell Stiles, "Early History, in Part Esoteric, of the Hookworm (Uncinariasis) Campaign in Our Southern United States," *Journal of Parasitology*, XXV (1939), 283–89.

19. John Duffy, "Yellow Fever in Continental United States During the Nineteenth Century," *Bulletin of the New York Academy of Medicine*, 2nd ser., XLIV (1968), 687–701. Hirsch has a useful table of Caribbean and North American epidemics in *Handbook*, I, 328–31.

20. John Duffy, *Sword of Pestilence: The New Orleans Yellow Fever Epidemic of 1853* (Baton Rouge, 1966); Duffy, "Yellow Fever," 689.

21. See, for example, David R. Goldfield, "The Business of Health Planning: Disease Prevention in the Old South," *Journal of Southern History*, XLII (1976), 557–70.

resistance to yellow fever; even American-born blacks had lower case mortality rates than whites.[22] Yellow fever seriously affected economic life and killed tens of thousands of southerners, but it was geographically restricted and by no means the most important disease in the region. However, because it struck in deadly, unpredictable epidemics, yellow fever terrorized the public and attracted much more medical and historical attention than more mundane endemic causes of sickness and death such as dysentery, worms, or pneumonia.

Although the South, with its yellow fever, hookworm, and falciparum malaria, clearly differed epidemiologically from the North and West, it was still a very large and diverse area. Health conditions, and attempts to explain and control them, thus varied enormously in human and natural environments as different as the Louisiana bayous, the rice fields of coastal South Carolina, the Virginia Piedmont, and the mountains of eastern Tennessee. Accurate delineation of subregions will be possible only after much more research. Mortality data from the census will be of limited help, even where state totals can be disaggregated into smaller regions, because of the limitations discussed earlier and because they do not concern nonfatal illnesses. However, even though the census data grossly understate malaria incidence, ignore hookworm, and do not include yellow fever epidemics in noncensus years, our knowledge of the ecology of the three African diseases provides a basis for provisionally delineating four major epidemiological subregions.

The Appalachian subregion was, in terms of health as well as climate, an extension of the North. Long, relatively severe winters made morbidity from respiratory diseases especially serious in the mountains, but the short summers gave diarrheal diseases less time to flourish. Heavy soils ensured that *Ascaris* and *Trichuris,* not hookworm, were the dominant nematodes in most places. Yellow fever did not occur, and the summers were too cool for *P. falciparum* to develop in mosquitoes; thus in those pockets where malaria existed, it was the milder vivax variety.

The Atlantic Coastal Plain, from Tidewater Virginia to northern Florida, constituted a second subregion. Warm summers and short winters favored the transmission of both falciparum and vivax malaria and provided an excellent climate for the various viruses, bacteria, and protozoa that cause diarrheal diseases. Low, often swampy terrain and

22. Kiple and King, *Another Dimension,* 29–49.

K. DAVID PATTERSON

rice cultivation favored mosquito breeding, and the light soils were excellent for hookworm larvae. The black population was large in this subregion, in contrast to the mountains, which ensured that *P. falciparum* and hookworm would be introduced. Yellow fever also occurred in the Atlantic Coast subregion, but only as a sporadic scourge of such ports as Norfolk, Charleston, and Savannah.

The third subregion embraced the Gulf Coast and extended into the lower Mississippi Valley. Sparsely populated Florida should probably be included in it as well. A very warm, moist climate with a short period of possible frost favored the transmission of malaria and diarrheal diseases over most of the year. On the other hand, morbidity from respiratory diseases was probably lower than in the other subregions. Hookworm and other nematodes abounded, and beginning in the eighteenth century, leprosy occurred in Louisiana. It was the West Indian connection, however, that made the Gulf subregion distinctive and that allows us to project it as far inland as Memphis. Ships from the islands and southern Mexico introduced yellow fever to ports from Texas to Florida, and some outbreaks spread north along the Mississippi. Dengue fever, another mosquito-borne viral disease, was probably more common in this region than elsewhere and probably shared a Caribbean connection with the much more conspicuous and lethal "yellow jack." Epidemiologically as well as commercially, New Orleans and Mobile could appropriately be thought of as Caribbean cities.[23]

The fourth subregion, the Interior, accounts for the remainder of the South. This loosely delineated geographical area lay between the mountains and the coasts. In general, the climate was cooler and the soils heavier than on the coasts, so malaria and hookworm were less severe. Yellow fever was absent. Disease conditions varied with latitude, altitude, soil type, and human geography, and these conditions tended to blend into the patterns of the other, better-defined subregions. Conditions in the Alabama black belt may well have been closer to those of the Gulf or Atlantic zones, while the Carolina Piedmont's health problems were probably more like those in the Appalachian Mountains.

Whatever their ecological differences, the southern subregions were all linked, to a greater or lesser extent, by a common fatal involvement with the epidemiological heritage of the slave trade. From the begin-

23. James D. Goodyear, "The Sugar Connection: A New Perspective on the History of Yellow Fever," *Bulletin of the History of Medicine,* LII (1978), 5–21.

164

nings of this trade until the early nineteenth century, some 600,000 Africans were brought into what is now the United States. These blacks had evolved some resistance to the trinity of virulent pathogens that they brought with them as by-products of the slave trade. The whites and Indians, however, found these diseases extraordinarily lethal and debilitating. The effect was a deadly, if unintentional, form of biological revenge. Even discounting the smallpox transmitted from slave ships and the "fluxes" caused by West African strains of bacteria or amoebas, the slave trade proved to be the very opposite of a demographic bargain. The human costs were staggering. From the beginning of slave imports until 1860, we may safely infer that the South lost far more whites directly or indirectly from the biological consequences of the trade than it acquired by importing its 600,000 involuntary immigrants. Indeed, the demographic implications of the slave trade indelibly marked the South well into the twentieth century. Southern whites of the antebellum period paid a heavy price in life and health for their "peculiar institution." The world the slaveholders made, as Eugene D. Genovese has called it, was literally, as well as figuratively, a very unhealthy place.[24]

24. Eugene D. Genovese, *The World the Slaveholders Made: Two Essays in Interpretation* (New York, 1964).

CHAPTER 8

MEDICAL MEN AND THE ECOLOGY OF THE OLD SOUTH

James H. Cassedy

From the colonial period onward, southern physicians, like their peers elsewhere, believed that various components of the physical environment—the geographical and topographical habitat, the weather and climate, the flora and fauna—somehow, individually or together, greatly influenced both the incidence of specific diseases and the general level of salubrity around them. These convictions deepened as knowledge of environmental factors expanded and as the social and economic environment interacted with the physical in increasingly complex ways. In fact, by the antebellum period, the environmental concerns of the learned tended to be broader in scope than they usually are among ecologists of the 1980s. In their efforts to understand the ecological circumstances of health and disease, southern as well as northern and European analysts extended their inquiries beyond medicine to such fields of knowledge as sociology, anthropology, biology, and political economy, as well as to geology, geography, meteorology, and demography. Southern medical studies thus evidenced serious concern for the hygienic role played by the region's vast dark forests and great bodies of water; endless birds, insects, and wild animals; extremes of heat, humidity, and rainfall; and wealth of earth and minerals. And, as time went on, they also became concerned about the medical implications of such human-centered phenomena as slavery, the plantation culture, and the South's slowly growing urban life.

The physical environment of the antebellum South had many similarities to that of the North. The differences are summarized in the one word, latitude. However, in that age of Humboldt, scientists and physicians came to realize that latitudinal differences were not always as significant as, for instance, the mean temperature differences indicated by isothermal lines drawn between sites with comparable readings. Whichever term was used, there were significant differences in heat, humidity, precipitation, flora and fauna, and other factors, and hence presumably also in the impact of certain of the principal diseases in the respective regions.

Literate eighteenth- and nineteenth-century southern physicians sometimes appeared to be as interested in exploring environmental matters as in taking care of their patients. The pattern was set in Charleston, South Carolina, which, from the 1740s onward had a succession of intellectually curious practitioners who made significant contributions to the growing literature on medical topography. These men—John Lining, Lionel Chalmers, George Milligen, and David Ramsay in the eighteenth century; Joseph Johnston, John Shecut, P. C. Gaillard, F. Peyre Porcher, Robert Gibbes, and others in the antebellum decades—like a numerous coterie of European and northern physicians, were in the mainstream of a vigorous neo-Hippocratic environmentalism, which gained in strength and adherents with every discovery in geology and mineralogy; every refinement in meteorology, botany, and zoology; every improvement in scientific instruments. These physicians avidly recorded temperature, wind, precipitation, and humidity; made notes on marshes and swampland; counted the aboriginal populations of the region; explored the electrical equilibrium of the atmosphere; scoured the countryside for knowledge about plant growth and rock formations; and attempted to correlate their scientific findings with the incidence of disease, especially of the great fevers.

Some observers used such information to estimate differences between environmental influences on the settled populations and on newcomers.[1] Certain physicians tried to associate environmental conditions, particularly climate, with differences in skin color.[2] Some used data to determine the general salubrity of towns and their attractiveness for commerce, as well as to support claims about the virtues of health resorts and mineral springs.[3] To refute European detractors of the American environment, other physicians related their data on cli-

1. By 1805 Savannah and other coastal cities already had high enough mortality among newcomers to noticeably deter further immigration (J. E. White, "A Few Remarks on the Weather and Diseases of 1805," *Medical Repository*, XI [1808], 23).

2. Hugh Williamson, *Observations on the Climate in Different Parts of America* (New York, 1811).

3. Charles F. Kovacik, "Health Conditions and Town Growth in Colonial and Antebellum South Carolina," *Social Science and Medicine*, XII (1978), 131–36.

mate and weather to information about such matters as the growth and diversity of animal species, the girth of trees, the size of crops, and the fecundity of women, though none proved as thorough and effective in this as Thomas Jefferson had been in his *Notes on the State of Virginia*.[4] And still others were able to document in some degree the appallingly rapid decline of native Indian tribes in a southern environment rendered hostile by the white and black men's diseases, bad habits, and relentless efforts to take over the land.

Southern physicians as well as northern became at least vaguely aware at an early stage that many of the settlers in this new land had to undergo a process of personal "seasoning" before they could expect to be at least relatively free of the debilitating fevers that seemed endemic. They also learned that the processes of settlement, such as cutting down trees and turning over virgin soil, somehow stirred up insalubrious qualities in the new environment. This unhealthfulness seemed to persist in many areas until crops were planted, fields were drained, and streams were dammed. Despite such measures, however, the summers continued to be marked by devastating fevers on more than a few Tidewater plantations. To avoid these, white families that were able retreated from June to November to northern states, or to close-to-home summer sites on higher ground. These latter sites were typically located in pineland, which the planters learned to leave clear of gardens and vegetation "to ensure the healthfulness of the place." Ultimately, however, even these asylums sometimes proved vulnerable to the insidious intermittent fevers, maladies which the planters rightly identified as "the bane . . . of every portion of America south and west of the Hudson River."[5] The immediate morbidity and mortality from these maladies was bad enough. But in addition the fevers, particularly malaria, left a constant enormous residue of debilitation throughout the southern populace, thus imposing a grave collective handicap upon the development of all areas of human activity, including the further settlement of the region.

By the second and third decades of the nineteenth century, several other events had occurred that, in combination, markedly affected the human ecology of the Atlantic Coast states. The end of the slave trade, for one, put a premium upon slaves already in the United States, while the opening up of new territories and states in the lower South created

4. Gilbert Chinard, "Eighteenth Century Theories of America as a Human Habitat," *Proceedings of the American Philosophical Society*, XCI (February, 1947), 27–57.

5. Quoted in H. Rawling Pratt-Thomas, "Plantation Medicine," *Journal of the South Carolina Medical Association*, LXVI (1970), 153–55.

a ready market for surplus slaves. At the same time, the exhaustion of land in the coastal states made migration to the lower South increasingly attractive to planters. Finally, the multiplication of reports in the outside world about alleged southern insalubrity, together with the deterrent effect of slave labor, kept substantial new populations of white immigrants from taking the places of whites who had left the coastal states.

By the 1850s it was apparent that such trends were profoundly affecting not only the population, wealth, and political power of the older coastal states, but their salubrity. In parts of middle Georgia, wasteful agricultural practices had left "a desolate picture for the traveller to behold. Decaying tenements, red, old hills stripped of their native growth and virgin soil, and washed into deep gullies, with . . . patches of Bermuda grass, and stunted pine shrubs struggling for a subsistence on what was once one of the richest soils in America."[6] Similarly, Virginia's continuing obsession with the single crop of tobacco had, according to Henry C. Carey and Frederick Law Olmsted, led not only to the exhaustion and abandonment of huge acreages of land but to "constantly increasing unhealthiness": "The entire country is full of the ruins of gentlemen's mansions . . . and noble old churches. . . . The splendor, indeed, which filled all the countries of Lower Virginia has departed. Why? Because the whole country is miasmatic, and is suffered to remain so."[7] A Virginia physician, reflecting in 1858 on the widespread inertia throughout the region, noted that his medical peers around the state had become so "listless and indifferent" that almost none were even making the effort any more to undertake the meteorological observations that were deemed necessary to measure the state's insalubrity.[8]

This progressive physical deterioration of the land did not extend very far from the coast, at least not prior to the nineteenth century. In 1800 vast expanses of the interior were still wilderness. By 1860, however, many of those tracts had been peopled. The interim years saw the interior landscape overrun by settlers, many of them from older states.

During the early decades of these migrations, the antebellum inte-

6. E. M. Pendleton, "General Report on the Topography, Climate and Diseases of Middle Georgia," *Southern Medical Reports*, I (1849), 316–17.

7. Henry C. Carey, *Principles of Social Science* (3 vols.; Philadelphia, 1858–65), I, 144–45; Frederick Law Olmsted, *A Journey in the Seaboard Slave States, with Remarks on their Economy* (New York, 1856), 164–73.

8. J. Stanley Beckwith, "On Climatology," *St. Louis Medical and Surgical Journal*, XV (1857), 449.

rior environment remained a crude one, fully as rough and ready as the western frontier in many respects, and the medical scene substantially mirrored the general backwoods character. The untrammeled individualism; the dangerous occupations and violent recreation; the knives, guns, and hard liquor all tended to spawn frequent injury and simple medicine. The unlettered democracy of the region that was so receptive to bawdy humor, tall tales, and superstition also proved highly hospitable to almost the entire pantheon of nineteenth-century medical sects.

J. Y. Bassett noted some scenes from the medical life near Huntsville, Alabama, in the 1830s: a man stabbed in a brawl and operated on with a bowie knife by a rank pretender to surgical skill; a "political doctor" trying uncertainly to deal with a bullet wound of the stomach; and so on. Along with the violence, according to Bassett, "there was a wild, speculating, and gambling spirit abroad"; he recalled one physician who charged a patient $500 for ten days of treatment involving bleeding and administration of stimulants and then proceeded to lose the entire fee back to the patient at a card game.[9]

According to S. C. Farrar, Jackson, Mississippi, had a similar medical environment in the early 1830s. Jackson was then a town of 150 to 200 inhabitants, many of whom lived in ramshackle houses devoid of comfort. Little gardening was done, and food was hauled in from Vicksburg by wagons. Bars or "dogeries" clustered at every crossroad. The ravines that cut through the town were filled with mud, garbage, and excrement, and all drained into the main source of drinking water, the Pearl River, with predictable results. Medical observers thought, however, that the unusual incidence of serious fevers between 1833 and 1837 was not so much due to these conditions as to the clearing of vast tracts of new land, the scantiness and spoilage of food supplies, and the arrival of large numbers of unacclimated newcomers. With the business depression of 1837, speculation fell off abruptly, the clearing of new fields halted, and the tide of immigration became a wave of emigration. As a result, an "almost complete cessation of endemic diseases" occurred in the area, a phenomenon that continued for several years into the early 1840s.[10]

Edward Delony felt that the numerous new settlers in Talbot County, Alabama, were generally unhealthy on arrival in the mid-

9. J. Y. Bassett, "Report of the Topography, Climate and Diseases of Madison County, Alabama," *Southern Medical Reports,* I (1849), 260–62.

10. S. C. Farrar, "General Report on the Topography, Meteorology and Diseases of Jackson, the Capital of Mississippi," *Southern Medical Reports,* I (1849), 349–54.

1830s. The increase in bilious diseases among them, however, was essentially felt to be the result of opening up new land. Meanwhile, in Delony's opinion, the very large numbers of gynecological problems among the female immigrants were the direct result of the arduous labor and fatigue accompanying the settlement process.[11]

The plantations were more typical of the later antebellum interior than its often scraggly towns. Indeed, here as in the rest of the South, the plantation was a central element in the physical and social universe of most people, white and black. Owners did not always give much thought to ecological factors in locating and operating their plantations; they seemed to be too "absorbed in that insatiable desire to make cotton and buy negroes." It was left to a few neo-Hippocratic physicians with an appreciation for environmental influences to suggest guidelines for the salubrity of these centers of life.

One of them, John Douglass, advised building the plantation house and other dwellings as high as possible above nearby streams and swamps. A preferred site would be one surrounded by sandy hills that would provide shelter from strong winds and "preserve a more equitable temperature of the air." He urged planters not to locate slave quarters in the woods.

Douglass and H. A. Ramsay agreed that, once a site was occupied, it was necessary to institute a "proper system of culture of soil, building, drainage, ditching, and manure making" to maintain the salubrity of the plantation. Slave quarters should be well built, roomy, elevated, thoroughly ventilated, and kept clean. Stables should be at a distance from habitations. Ditches should be kept clear and deposits of decaying leaves or other debris burned frequently. Ramsay, assuming that pneumonia and malaria were both caused by decomposing matter, claimed that those plantations "who make most manure, and have their lots closest to their houses, have most cases of pneumonia."[12]

Antebellum physicians came to agree that water should not be allowed to accumulate near plantation dwellings and that marshes had to be drained. Trees should be left standing along streams and mill ponds to provide barriers to deadly disease emanations from the water. Meanwhile, the health of slaves could be enhanced by giving

11. Edward Delony, "Topography and Diseases of Talbot County, Ga.," *Southern Medical and Surgical Journal*, I (1836–37), 602–606.

12. John Douglass, "A Brief Essay on the Best Mode of Preserving Health on Plantations," *Southern Journal of Medicine and Pharmacy*, II (1847), 216–19; H. A. Ramsay, "A Practical Essay upon the Symptomatology, Etiology, Vital Statistics, and Treatment of Pneumonia," *Charleston Medical Journal and Review*, VI (1851), 16–21.

them strong shoes and clothing, along with plain but good-quality food, especially meat and salt.

This consensus about plantation hygiene emerged in the context of a widespread new wave of medical topographical observation around the South, one that achieved particular force during the late 1840s and 1850s. This development was fueled by, among other things, the launching of geological surveys in some states, the formation of the American Medical Association, the rise of enthusiasm for sanitation in the urban North, and the long-delayed spread of southern medical journalism. E. D. Fenner of New Orleans took a notable initiative in promoting such studies in 1849 and 1850. In response to a questionnaire circulated by Fenner, observers from almost every part of the South sent in medical reports for publication. From these Fenner filled two volumes that provided an unprecedented profile of the medical, topographic, meteorological, and demographic circumstances of the region's diseases.[13]

E. M. Pendleton's report in the first of these volumes epitomized the scientific enthusiasm, the breadth of interest, and the strength of the environmental viewpoint that characterized many or most of the articles. Like many of the other authors, Pendleton gave his report the authority of a fairly large collection of numerical data. He self-consciously pursued the statistical methods of William Farr and Lemuel Shattuck in his analysis of population and disease. And his comprehensive concern for the physical environment reflected the currently popular concepts of Alexander von Humboldt. Pendleton reported on middle Georgia, an area he identified as being "bounded on the south by an isothermal line running diagonally through the State, about 30° south of west from Augusta to Columbus," and on the north by another isothermal line that separated the cotton-growing area of middle Georgia from the grain-growing environment of upper Georgia. Pendleton reviewed the geological, agricultural, and botanical features of the region and provided comparative thermometric, barometric, and pluviometric tables. In the context of this information, his subsequent discussion of the fevers of the region emerges as a prototype of the prevailing environmental or filth theory of disease causation. This he summarized by concluding that "the simultaneous action of a certain amount of heat, moisture and vegetable putrefaction, is essential to the production of periodic fevers. If one be absent, the remaining two are incapable of producing the effect."[14]

13. *Southern Medical Reports*, I (1849); II (1850).
14. Pendleton, "Report on Middle Georgia," 315–25.

Nowhere in the South was the operation of these three factors more pronounced than along the shores of the Gulf of Mexico and the Mississippi River. Much of this area was an alluvial zone sloping gradually down to the Gulf but broken up by sluggish streams and estuaries. In southern Alabama, according to James Harris, a local physician, this particular type of topography, together with the hot sun, created one of the "most extensive hot-beds of malaria known within the geographical limits of the Union." And in it, by Harris' account, there particularly flourished an abundance of "long moss and mosquitoes, the former gradually extending its mournful drapery, and the latter their musical companionship" throughout the area, even more pervasively if possible than in other parts of the South.[15]

Equally flourishing in such a setting was yellow fever, a disease that constituted a constant epidemic threat in the area throughout the antebellum period. The profound ignorance of its source made the threat of yellow fever more difficult to face. There were some, of course, who thought it was imported by ship from not-too-distant hotbeds of disease across the water—Havana and Vera Cruz were particularly notorious. This possibility led to quarantines at some ports and lively debate about that measure in many communities. Many other individuals thought that yellow fever arose out of local topographical and climatic conditions. Edward H. Barton, a prominent New Orleans physician and leader of this anticontagionist group, had no doubt that the city's epidemics of yellow fever grew out of grossly unsanitary conditions. Like Pendleton, he argued that the essential cause was the very particular combination and interaction of three main factors: heat, humidity, and decaying filth. Accordingly, he emphasized the need for elaborate continuing meteorological observations and calculations and simultaneously pushed for the thorough cleansing of the city's physical environment.[16]

A third group, centered in New Orleans, argued that neither the contagionists nor the environmentalists had proved their cases. Members of this group opposed both quarantines and sanitary measures, chiefly on the ground that such actions obstructed the commercial life of the city, and they were scornful of all varieties of yellow fever theorists. Morton Dowler, however, heaped most of his scorn on Barton and the other environmentalists because of their penchant for assum-

15. James C. Harris, "Observations on the Medical Topography, Climate, and Endemic Influences of South Alabama," *Western Journal of Medicine and Surgery*, 2nd ser., VI (1846), 462–64.

16. E. H. Barton, Y. R. Lemonnier, and T. G. Browning, "Annual Report of the Board of Health," *New Orleans Medical and Surgical Journal*, VI (1849–50), 666–73.

ing meteorological determinants in the causation of yellow fever. To try to base public health action on data produced "by our electrometers, our hygrometers, our thermometers, our barometers, our rain gauges, and our river-gauges" was absurd and a waste of taxpayers' money, Dowler observed, especially since the sciences of meteorology and hydrology were still in their infancy.[17]

Such critics had no better opinion of the so-called animalcular hypothesis of yellow fever causation. This theory was maintained by several prominent medical scientists of the region. In Mobile, Josiah Nott argued the hypothesis persuasively during the 1840s and 1850s upon the basis of extended epidemiological observation.[18] And in New Orleans, William P. Hort and John L. Riddell pursued it through the lenses of their microscopes. Riddell in particular, who armed himself with the best instruments of his day, made extensive microscopic observations of organisms found in the atmosphere during the yellow fever epidemic of 1850 and 1851, and he even suggested a plan for inoculating unacclimated persons once the germ of yellow fever was definitely identified. Throughout most of the 1850s, he enthusiastically explored the many different kinds of microscopic life that abounded both in the waters and on land around New Orleans. He ultimately implicated microorganisms in a large variety of pathological conditions. However, at that stage of bacteriological knowledge most people still thought that topographical and climatological factors as well as contagion substantially influenced the origin and spread of most disease germs, particularly those of malaria.[19]

Certain New Orleans physicians found other features of their habitat worth exploring. Bennet Dowler, for one, in company with such nonphysician contemporaries as John James Audubon and Timothy Flint, Mark Twain and J. D. B. De Bow, was fascinated by the awesome Mississippi, the immense river that was such a dominating presence in the lives of the inhabitants of not only New Orleans but the entire Mississippi Valley. Dowler, looking at the river as a physician and scientist, characterized it as "the greatest of all hydrographical sublimities" and "the chief element, whether for good or evil, in [the] medical topography and hygiene" of the region. He agreed with

17. M. Morton Dowler, "On the Reputed Causes of Yellow Fever, and the so-called Sanitary Measures of the Day," *New Orleans Medical and Surgical Journal*, XI (1854–55), 56.

18. J. C. Nott, "The Epidemic Yellow Fever of Mobile in 1853," *New Orleans Medical and Surgical Journal*, X (1853–54), 577–83.

19. John L. Riddell, "Memoir on the Nature of Miasm and Contagion," *New Orleans Medical and Surgical Journal*, XVI (1859), 348–69.

Daniel Drake that the river was "of paramount interest to the medical aetiologist." As such, it had to be fully studied in all of its hydrological, meteorological, and chemical aspects before the endemic fevers of the region could be understood.[20]

Dowler and other valley physicians were all too aware of the prodigious havoc the periodic flooding of the river caused in property destroyed, lives lost, social disruption, and sickness. They were also aware, by the late 1840s, that the river played some role or another in the rapid spread of epidemic disease from the coastal region to the interior towns and plantations. Many were convinced that yellow fever went upstream on the steamboats. John W. Monette, for one, saw that the landing of the steamboats along the river was a key epidemiological circumstance. When it occurred, he observed, and "when any town or city, and especially those south of lat. 35°, contains infectious air [from filthy conditions] that place is in a proper condition for the dissemination of yellow-fever."[21]

Similarly, by the time of the second great onslaught of cholera at midcentury, it had become widely apparent that "the boats from New Orleans . . . scattered cholera patients all over the Valley of the Mississippi." But what happened then was a matter of keen ongoing debate. By 1849 some were persuaded that the disease had been spread by the contact of these sick people with the well. But many others still felt it more likely that the disease rose out of unsanitary local conditions.[22]

Investigations of such matters around the South not infrequently had very direct economic implications. And, from the 1840s onward, the investigations began to take on political and social implications as well. Not surprisingly, the studies of the region's disease environment thus increasingly incorporated various of the elements of southern regional chauvinism, including the perceived need of southerners in many walks of life to defend the institution of slavery. In the effort to attract students to newly opened medical schools and readers to newly established medical journals in the Deep South, medical spokesmen

20. Bennet Dowler, "Researches on Meteorology," *New Orleans Medical and Surgical Journal*, IV (1847–48), 425; Bennet Dowler, "Contributions to the Hydrographical Thermology and Hygiene of the Mississippi River," *New Orleans Medical and Surgical Journal*, XV (1858), 453; Bennet Dowler, "Psychological and Hygienic Observations and Reflections on Rivers," *New Orleans Medical and Surgical Journal*, XVIII (1861), 59.

21. John W. Monette, "Observations on the Epidemic Yellow Fever of Natchez, and of the South-west," *Western Journal of Medicine and Surgery*, V (1842), 423.

22. "Cholera," *Western Journal of Medicine and Surgery*, 3rd ser., III (1849), 177–78.

began to stress a characteristically *southern* medicine. Southern diseases, including those of the blacks, were so distinctive, the argument went, and appeared in such a complex setting of unique environmental factors, that they required very special handling, the niceties of which could only be learned in the South and taught by southern physicians trained in the region.[23]

Medical regionalism was far from existing solely in the South; a comparable version flourished in the Midwest at the same time. But southern advocates brought special ingenuity to their arguments. Samuel Cartwright, one of the most ingenious, founded his rationale for a separate southern medicine upon his consideration of the classical doctrines of Hippocrates, which, he felt, had been badly distorted over the centuries by medical men trying to adapt them to northern climes. Those doctrines, he pointed out, had been written in and for a southern climate, specifically the Aegean island of Cos, which lies between the 36th and 37th parallel of latitude. He went on to say that isothermal lines revealed the mean temperature and climate of Cos to be virtually the same as in much of the Deep South. Both places differed significantly in climate from Edinburgh and Philadelphia, the centers of "northern" medical teaching. Accordingly, Hippocrates could be properly understood and his doctrines applied only by physicians who lived in a climate comparable to that of Cos, notably the southern states of the United States.[24]

Not all southern physicians fully agreed on the details of a geographically justified southern regional medicine. Josiah Nott, for instance, complicated the rationale by extending his belief in the separate creation of the races into a theory of acclimation in which racial characteristics were at least as important as climatic factors in determining a person's susceptibility to the endemic diseases of a region. But E. D. Fenner found that the great majority of southern physicians and planters, whatever their views about the creation of the races, strongly believed in the traditional environmental concept of acclimation.[25]

23. See, for example, the manifesto issued by E. D. Fenner in his "Introductory Address," *New Orleans Medical Journal*, I (1844–45), i–iv. Similar sentiments had been expressed earlier, however, as in "Introduction," *Southern Medical and Surgical Journal*, I (1836–37), 1–4.

24. Samuel A. Cartwright, "Cartwright on Southern Medicine," *New Orleans Medical and Surgical Journal*, III (1846–47), 259–72.

25. J. C. Nott, "Acclimation," in Josiah C. Nott and Geo. R. Gliddon (eds.), *Indigenous Races of the Earth* (Philadelphia, 1857); E. D. Fenner, "Acclimation; and the Liability of Negroes to the Endemic Fevers of the South," *Southern Medical and Surgical Journal*, n.s., XIV (1858), 452–60.

Whatever the differences on this point, southern medical spokesmen throughout the 1840s and 1850s generally united in defending their region, both against outside (northern) criticism of their medical and social institutions and against allegations that the southern climate was less salubrious than the northern. Samuel Forry, who in 1840 examined the experience of U.S. Army troops with disease and mortality in various climates and regions over a twenty-year period, had concluded that the ratio of mortality to the number of cases of sickness was four times greater in the South than in the North. Figures for individual diseases varied: remittent and intermittent fevers in the South were found to be five times as numerous as in the North, while deaths from intemperance were ten times greater at certain southern army posts than at northern posts. In most cases, Forry concluded that the differences in morbidity and mortality were due to differences in climate and other environmental conditions.[26]

Southern medical spokesmen deeply resented Forry's claim that sickness and death increased "in proportion as southern latitudes are reached," or, in other words, as one went south down the Mississippi River. Moreover, as Bennet Dowler argued, the army statistics were not a fair representation of southern healthfulness. Based as they were "on a small number of troops, mostly of foreign birth, of irregular habits and unacclimated, and who seldom remain an entire year at the same post, [they] cannot be regarded as affording conclusive evidence of the inherent salubrity or insalubrity of a climate or civic population."[27]

Another source of the bitter contention over comparative regional healthfulness was the federal census. Southern spokesmen took great satisfaction from early antebellum census data, which showed much greater proportions of deaf, dumb, and insane blacks in the North than in the South. They publicized these figures widely as proof that the social environment provided by the institution of slavery was more salubrious than that of the North's free society. Northern observers claimed statistical error and tried in vain to get the data corrected. Later censuses showed that mortality from tuberculosis, too, was far greater in the northern climate than in the southern. Regarding this finding, northern analysts again urged that southern methods of identifying and accounting for their diseases were faulty. Some claimed, moreover, that even if it were true that death from tuberculosis "decreases

26. Samuel Forry, *The Climate of the United States and Its Endemic Influences* (New York, 1842).

27. Dowler, "Thermology and Hygiene of the Mississippi," 481–84.

from North to South," this adverse finding was offset by the mortality from the great fevers, which measurably decreased from South to North.[28]

The various arguments about regional environmental salubrity became so bitter that they effectively hampered and delayed the medical and scientific community's efforts to investigate environmental factors in disease. Clearly the acrimony added a further poisonous component to the already hostile atmosphere surrounding the relations between the antebellum South and North. Here we may draw an analogy between Barton's and Pendleton's formulae of disease causation and the outbreak of the Civil War. The two physicians argued that it took more than a single element to bring about an outbreak of yellow fever; they specified a very particular combination of extreme heat, high humidity, and unsanitary conditions. Similarly, it can be argued that the Civil War was not caused either by slavery, state's rights, or southern expansionism acting alone, but by a peculiar combination of all three acting together with such other factors as regional medical rivalries and perceived environmental differences. In any case, it is evident that, as the antebellum period came to its unfortunate climax, the isothermal lines of the scientific physicians became, politically if not ecologically, progressively less important even to themselves than the Mason and Dixon Line.

28. Augustus A. Gould, "Climatology of Consumption, No. II," *Boston Medical and Surgical Journal*, LXXI (1864–65), 449–51.

CHAPTER 9

THE IDEA OF SOUTHERN MEDICAL DISTINCTIVENESS: MEDICAL KNOWLEDGE AND PRACTICE IN THE OLD SOUTH

John Harley Warner

T he historian seeking to assess in what ways medical knowledge and practice in the Old South differed from that in the North must inevitably come to terms with the fact that antebellum southern physicians themselves assertively proclaimed that their region was indeed medically distinctive. The argument for southern medical particularity pervades the medical literature and archival records that constitute the historian's primary texts. Yet the ubiquity of this argument does nothing to clarify how it should be read or interpreted. Was it primarily a political manifesto representing the physician's contribution to southern nationalism, a reflection of invidious economic motives, a normative statement made to promote professional reform, or a prudent medical assessment of existential regional differences? I have elected herein to locate the argument for the distinctiveness of southern knowledge and practice within the context of national medical thought as the inescapable prerequisite to evaluating the extent and meaning of the peculiarly southern character of the region's medical practice.

My initial thesis is a simple one. In its underlying premises, logic, and even in the nature of its content, there was nothing inherently

This paper appeared in a different form in Judith Walzer Leavitt and Ronald L. Numbers (eds.), *Sickness and Health in America: Readings in the History of Medicine and Public Health* (2nd ed.; Madison, 1985), 53–70. The paper was supported in part by NIH Grant 03910 from the National Library of Medicine; an award from an Arthur Vining Davis Foundation grant to the Department of Social Medicine and Health Policy, Harvard Medical School; a Charlotte W. Newcombe Dissertation Fellowship; and NSF Grant SES-8107609. I am grateful for this support.

179

distinctive about the argument for southern medical distinctiveness. The sources, substance, and structure of the knowledge that purportedly guided medical practice in the North and South were remarkably similar in ways that are often taken for granted, but which are nonetheless important. At the same time, the social production and dissemination of the argument for regional medical singularity in the South did take on characteristics that set it apart from its conceptual analogues in other regions. The South was distinctive not in possessing medical knowledge and practice avowedly molded to its peculiarly regional needs, but rather in the fervor with which physicians exploited and proselytized the region's medical particularity.

Southern physicians, especially from the early 1830s onward, pointed to a variety of factors that distinguished the South's medical character and that dictated modifications in the medical knowledge and practice appropriate elsewhere. Historians have identified these influences upon southern practice and analyzed their implications.[1] Geographic patterns of disease distribution, virulence, and classification; the large population of blacks and relatively small proportion of recent European immigrants in the South; and regional peculiarities in climate, topography, and diet purportedly necessitated distinctively southern rules for diagnosis, prognosis, and treatment.

Physicians most often drew these diverse factors together into a coherent argument for southern medical distinctiveness when they were establishing the premises for institutional separatism. If southern knowledge and practice were necessarily different from those elsewhere, their reasoning went, then southern medical schools, literature, and societies were the necessary forums for generating and transmitting knowledge matched to the needs of southern medical practice.[2] But though such uses of the argument for southern medical

1. Among the most useful studies are James O. Breeden, "States-Rights Medicine in the Old South," *Bulletin of the New York Academy of Medicine,* LII (1976), 348–72; John Duffy, "Medical Practice in the Ante Bellum South," *Journal of Southern History,* XXV (1959), 53–72; Duffy, "A Note on Ante-Bellum Southern Nationalism and Medical Practice," *Journal of Southern History,* XXXIV (1968), 266–76; James Denny Guillory, "Southern Nationalism and the Louisiana Medical Profession, 1840–1860" (M.A. thesis, Louisiana State University, 1965); Mary Louise Marshall, "Samuel A. Cartwright and States' Rights Medicine," *New Orleans Medical and Surgical Journal,* XCII (1940), 74–78; and Richard Harrison Shryock, "Medical Practice in the Old South," *South Atlantic Quarterly,* XXIX (1930), 160–78.

2. On the use of this argument to support medical schools, see John Duffy, "Sectional Conflict and Medical Education in Louisiana," *Journal of Southern History,* XXIII (1957), 289–306; and John Harley Warner, "A Southern Medical Reform: The Meaning of the Antebellum Argument for Southern Medical Education," *Bulletin of the History of Medicine,* LVII (1983), 364–81.

distinctiveness resembled calls for separatism in other realms of southern life, such as creative literature, liberal education, agriculture, and religion, the meaning of the argument must be discerned within the contexts not only of southern culture and its values but also those of medicine.

John McCardell has noted that antebellum calls for southern cultural distinctiveness in such endeavors as liberal education rarely engendered concrete proposals regarding the form such beliefs should take in practice,[3] and this was not infrequently the case in medicine as well. Southern physicians, however, often were explicit about the ways their region's peculiarities should alter behavior at the patient's bedside. This was especially true in medical therapeutics. For example, the climate and topography of the South encouraged the production of noxious miasmata or malaria by the action of solar heat on decaying animal and vegetable matter, particularly in low, damp, swampy areas. The malarial influence in some parts of the South purportedly altered the character of all diseases occurring in these regions and necessitated concomitant modifications in treatment. "Periodicity is frequently smuggled into the system," a Louisiana physician noted, and therefore in miasmatic regions if periodicity was *"even* suspected, the *experiment* of giving quinine should be fairly tried."* Not only was the southern physician to use quinine more readily than his northern counterpart, but he was also to be guided by different dosage rules adjusted to his patients' constitutions. Thus, a Virginia medical professor could claim that individuals "fetched up" on malaria required larger doses of quinine to effect a cure than similarly afflicted patients who had recently arrived in a malarious district.[4]

The southern environment, physicians maintained, affected in a like fashion dosages and frequency of use of calomel, a mercurial purgative thought to stimulate the liver's activity. In the South both

3. John McCardell, *The Idea of a Southern Nation: Southern Nationalists and Southern Nationalism, 1830–1860* (New York, 1979), 204–205.

4. W[illia]m A. Booth, "Observations and Remarks upon the Action of the Sulphate of Quinine," *New Orleans Medical and Surgical Journal,* V (1848–49), 16; William Octavius Eversfield, Notes from Lectures on Therapeutics and Materia Medica by Dr. [John Staige] Davis, University of Virginia, 1859–60, lecture of May 12, 1860, in William Octavius Eversfield Notebooks, Manuscripts Department, Alderman Library, University of Virginia, Charlottesville. On therapeutic thought and practice in nineteenth-century America, see Charles E. Rosenberg, "The Therapeutic Revolution: Medicine, Meaning, and Social Change in Nineteenth-Century America," in Morris J. Vogel and Charles E. Rosenberg (eds.), *The Therapeutic Revolution: Essays in the Social History of American Medicine* (Philadelphia, 1979), 3–25; and John Harley Warner, *The Therapeutic Perspective: Medical Practice, Knowledge, and Identity in America, 1820–1885* (Cambridge, Mass., 1986).

malaria and heat from the sun continually stimulated the liver, a student attending medical lectures in Charleston in the late 1830s typically reasoned, exhausting that organ and leaving it debilitated. To therapeutically arouse torpid southern livers, calomel was given "in the treatment of the diseases of the South generally . . . because the liver is virtually the 'scape goat' for almost all the affections of the other organs . . . in Southern latitudes." A Georgia student attending the same school several years earlier explained in his thesis that because southerners' livers were so dulled, calomel was "required to be administered in doses nearly twice as large in the south as in the north" in order to elicit the same physiological response. "We are," he continued, "compelled to resort to what would be considered by northern practitioners, enormous doses of calomel, without which, we would be continually foiled in our attempts to cure the biliary disorders of the south." Northern judgments on calomel use, grounded upon northern experience, were irrelevant, for "a larger dose of any medicine will be required in a southern climate to produce a given effect in a disease where the liver is deeply implicated than in a northern, in consequence of the continued excitement—to which this organ is subjected in southern latitudes."[5]

The place southern physicians assigned to venesection in their practice, compared to that of the North, presented an inverted image of the patterns exhibited by quinine and calomel. "The general experience of physicians," one southern practitioner commented on pneumonia, "is, that the loss of much blood is not so well borne, nor its curative influence so favorably exerted in this as in Northern climates." Both plethora and systemic overstimulation, conventional indications for therapeutic depletion by venesection, were identified with cold climates, and therefore bloodletting was regarded as more appropriate for northern constitutions and diseases. A physician in Monroe, Louisiana, typically noted in his diary in 1819 that the fevers prevailing in his region were sufficiently debilitating so "as not to admit the cure of the Lancet except in very few cases and those of persons who had lately arrived from the North and were very robust." Eli Geddings, lecturing on the institutes and practice of medicine at the Medical College of South Carolina in 1861, told his students that not only

5. Quotations from John P. Caffry, "A Thesis on Calomel in Southern Fevers" (M.D. thesis, Medical College of the State of South Carolina, 1839), and Jeremiah Butt, Jr., "A Dissertation on the Influence of Climate" (M.D. thesis, Medical College of the State of South Carolina, 1835), both in South Carolina Room, Main Library, Medical University of South Carolina.

venesection but antiphlogistic therapies in general were ill-suited to the conditions of southern practice. But he cautioned his pupils that if they moved to another region, its environment could well demand the use of the lancet. "I wish you to understand," he told them in a lecture on pneumonia, that "the treatment, I am now to recommend is not designed for the disease, as it occurs now. But as many of you may practice in other parts of the world, it is my duty to state to you the management of the inflammatory variety. The treatment of the latter is in the main antiphlogistic."[6]

Not all categories of medical knowledge were affected by such regional considerations in the same way. Physicians were very selective in the aspects of medicine they identified as regionally variable and premised their judgments upon a fundamental division of medicine into knowledge about medical practice on the one hand and about the basic sciences on the other. Even the most strident proponents of a distinctive southern medicine held that the principles of anatomy, chemistry, and physiology, as well as the mechanical manipulations of dentistry and surgery, were not modified by local conditions and were therefore universal in their generation and validation. But this was not true of region-specific knowledge about medical practice, which encompassed diagnosis, prognosis, and medical therapeutics; physicians claimed that these were distinctively southern. Edward Hall Barton, a Louisiana spokesman for southern medical distinctiveness and the case for educational separatism it supported, could state with conviction in 1835 that "southern practitioners *must* be taught in the south"; yet he was innocent of duplicity when he qualified this claim in his next sentence, saying, "These remarks are not at all intended to deny that the principles of medicine are universal, and that they are, in general, the same every where; but the very nature of man is so modified by the diversities of climate, that it is often indispensible to have a personal experience of them to make successful applications."[7]

William W. Cozart, a North Carolina student attending medical lectures in Charleston, developed this theme in his thesis entitled "The

6. "Dr. Ames on the Treatment of Pneumonia," *New Orleans Medical and Surgical Journal*, X (1853), 423; R. F. McGuire, Diary, 1818–52, entry for December 18, 1819, in Department of Archives, Louisiana State University Library, Baton Rouge; Simon Baruch, Notes on Lectures of E[li] Geddings, Institutes and Practice of Medicine, delivered at the Medical College of South Carolina, 1860–61, lecture of February 18, 1861, in Special Collections, Robert W. Woodruff Library, Emory University, Atlanta.

7. Edward H. Barton, *Introductory Lecture on the Climate and Salubrity of New-Orleans, and Its Suitability for a Medical School* (New Orleans, 1835), 21; see also Barton, *The Application of Physiological Medicine to the Diseases of Louisiana* (Philadelphia, 1832).

Place Where Southern Students Should Acquire Their Medical Knowledge" (1856). "The general principles of Medicine may be communicated by teachers that are competent without regard to locality," he asserted.

> But the case is different in respect to particular ones, and their application to practice; those differing wherever the peculiarities of localities differ. And it is well known by the medical profession that diseases are modified by these places, and other circumstances; and in order that these indications should be met successfully, the adaptation of the treatment must be varied accordingly. The faculties of every institution teaches what they have observed of diseases, and the plan they pursued in the treatment of them, during their own practice. In fact, their practice is their teaching. And as the northern diseases differ materially in their characters from the southern, the advantages therefore, southern students have by attending southern Colleges are no doubt considerable.

The southern graduate of a Philadelphia or New York medical school, Cozart claimed, "returns home in high spirits and with bright anticipations, 'sticks out his shingle,' ready and very willing to go to work." But however thorough his knowledge of medical science, he was destined to fail in practice when he treated his first patients, in accordance with northern teachings, with general bloodletting and sedative medicines that produced dire results. "Now his bright anticipations are clouded; disappointments discourage him; and a sad experience teaches him that the instructive lessons of a northern institution will not answer, in the treatment of southern diseases. He cannot now under the circumstances establish an extensive practice," Cozart concluded, "the confidence of the people in him is shaken, he is neglected; despised, and soon forgotten."[8]

The plain fact that the precepts informing medical practice were region-specific, as well as southern physicians' inclination to stress the dissimilarities between medicine in their region and elsewhere, tend to overemphasize the fractionalization of medical knowledge during the antebellum period. Underlying the regionally variable character of medicine as a body of knowledge was the basic assumption that the attributes of knowledge in the North and South were identical. The same fundamental rules directed the generation and validation of medical knowledge in both the North and South. This is crucial for

8. William W. Cozart, "An Inaugural Dissertation on the Place Where Southern Students Should Acquire Their Medical Knowledge" (M.D. thesis, Medical College of the State of South Carolina, 1856), South Carolina Room, Main Library, Medical University of South Carolina.

assessing the argument for southern medical distinctiveness, for it means that those physicians who vigorously affirmed the particularity of southern medical knowledge at the same time unwaveringly maintained that a single epistemology governed knowledge regarding medical practice in all regions.

The basis for the southern physicians' argument for regional medical distinctiveness, the idea that the knowledge best suited to southern practice had to be produced and tested in the South to match southern circumstances, therefore was fundamentally grounded upon an aspect of medical knowledge, its epistemology, that they shared with American physicians elsewhere and deemed to be universal. The growing allegiance to empiricism that began to dominate clinical epistemology from the 1820s implied that the knowledge most appropriate to guide practice was that gained within a context closely resembling the one in which it was to be applied in both type of patient and physical and social environments. By closely observing the effects of treatments on a patient with particular symptoms, habits, constitution, and surroundings, the physician derived therapeutic precepts that would be reliable under similar conditions, but whether or not these precepts were transferable to other conditions had to be ascertained independently. Knowledge befitting southern medicine was, accordingly, most suitably acquired through direct experience with southern practice. This was not an oddly southern perception: physicians in all parts of the United States drew similarly localistic conclusions from the same epistemological precepts. Moreover, by avowedly sharing the assumptions about the nature of medical knowledge held by other American physicians, southern practitioners were constrained to construct a distinctively southern body of knowledge and practice within the limits imposed by this epistemology. It was precisely because an epistemology that could justify the existence of distinctive local knowledge dominated regular medical thought in all regions of America, and because it plainly supplied the premises for erecting and legitimizing a singularly southern medicine, that the southern argument for regional medical distinctiveness was in itself not at all distinctive.

In fact, the notion that there must be a separate body of medical knowledge for the South was only one expression of the principle of specificity, a principle central to the belief system of American physicians of all regions. Medical treatment was not specific to disease (indeed, disease-specific treatment implied a routinism that was a stigma of quackery), but did have to be sensitively matched to the specific characteristics of individual patients and the peculiarities of the environments in which they became ill and were treated. Typically, a student attending medical lectures at the University of Michigan recorded in his class notes on therapeutics the "circumstances which modify indications" for treatment: "Age of patient. The sex. . . . A good constitution. . . . The Temperament. The disease going on in the organ. Idiosyncrasies, or personal peculiarities. Variation of the pulse. Habits of the patient. Tolerance of medicines. Climate. The prevailing epidemic influence. Race. Profession. Severity of disease."[9] Therapeutic principles that aptly directed the treatment of immigrants might be invalid as guides to the treatment of native-born patients, and analogous discriminations were based upon age, gender, social class, and moral status. It was entirely in keeping with the doctrine of specificity that physicians were able to develop notions about the peculiarity of Negro physiology and Negro therapeutic requirements that were sustained by prevailing medical theory.

Medical management was similarly specific to such idiosyncrasies of place as climate, population density, and topography. For example, American physicians commonly held that the physical and social environments of a city molded the constitutions of its inhabitants and their diseases in ways that required treatments unlike those for rural populations. In 1843 a Boston practitioner pondering the greater malignance of fevers in the surrounding countryside wondered "whether the stronger febrile tendency in places which have so much the advantage of the city in purity of air, &c., may not depend somewhat upon the more stimulating and gross diet made use of in the country, especially in the excess of animal food?" Medical literature often depicted conventional images of the robust farmer and the debilitated city dweller, applying these caricatures to pathological conditions and to the therapeutic measures they required. "The peculiar mode of living in large cities," a professor of medicine in Lexington, Kentucky, told his students in 1838, changed the type of inflammation found in urban residents. "Their diseases," he proposed, "are much more of a nervous character than sanguinous. The treatment of the same disease, Erysipelas for instance, in one of those large towns and here would be entirely different[;] in one case you would stimulate[,] in the other debilitate."[10] Knowledge gained through urban practice was of dubious

9. John B. Rice, Notes on Lectures of Prof. Alonzo B. Palmer, Materia Medica and Therapeutics, University of Michigan College of Medicine and Surgery, December 4, 1855, in John B. Rice Papers, Rutherford B. Hayes Library, Fremont, Ohio.

10. L. C., "Prevailing Fevers in Country Towns," *Boston Medical and Surgical Journal,* XXIX (1843), 359; R. T. Dismukes, Notes on Lectures of B[enjamin] W[inslow] Dudley,

relevance for the country physician, for it might, as in this instance, dictate the opposite of the treatment actually required by the individual case.

Similar considerations informed American physicians' attitudes toward European therapeutic knowledge. A western practitioner visiting London in 1845 was impressed by the extent to which treatment for inflammatory affections differed from the therapeutic strategy that would have been pursued in the United States. "A course of practice which with us would prove successful," he wrote to the readers of the *Western Lancet*, which he edited, "would necessarily be fatal here from its very activity." Particularly surprised by the success achieved in London with very limited therapeutic use of calomel and bloodletting, he attributed the former to "the debilitated and broken down constitutions so commonly met with here," and said of the latter, "That bleeding should be tolerated here to a less extent than in the United States, is not surprising; and that tonics and stimulants should find an extensive and appropriate application, is what might be anticipated from the habits and other modifying circumstances that so powerfully influence the constitutions of the inhabitants of London; and hence it is that iron, quinine, porter, wine &c., are frequently employed, when an American physician would resort to depletion." Instruction given in American medical schools reflected these perceptions. A South Carolinian attending medical lectures at Transylvania University in 1828 recorded in his class notebook that inflammation was "modified by a variety of circumstances. . . . [L]ocation or situation modified [it]. In *Paris* we would stimulate by Porter, Bark &c—In Kentucky we would bleed & purge."[11]

The sorts of factors that made urban knowledge suspect for rural patients and European knowledge suspect for American patients also

Professor of Anatomy and Surgery in the Medical Department of Transylvania University, Lexington, Kentucky, 1838–39, in Manuscript Department, Perkins Library, Duke University, Durham. Although fully sustained by medical theory, some statements of such perceptions were clearly propelled by proprietary interests as well.

11. L[eonidas] M[oreau] Lawson, "Foreign Correspondence," *Western Lancet*, IV (1845–46), 150–51; [Lawrence] Jefferson Trotti, Notebook (MS bound with catalog from Transylvania University, 1828, in Special Collections and Archives, Frances Carrick Thomas Library, Transylvania University, Lexington, Ky.). On the notion that American medical knowledge and practice must be distinct from that of Europe, and the changing course of this idea, see Ronald L. Numbers and John Harley Warner, "The Maturation of American Medical Science," in Nathan Reingold and Marc Rothenberg (eds.), *Scientific Colonialism, 1800–1930: A Cross-Cultural Comparison* (Washington, D.C., 1987), 191–214.

led physicians in all regions of the United States to maintain that therapeutic and prognostic knowledge suitable for one part of the country might be inapplicable or even dangerous in another. A type of perception common during the first two thirds of the nineteenth century is reflected in the class notes of a medical student in Cincinnati who, summarizing his teacher's comments in 1834, wrote: "Says 10 grs. of calomel is as effectual in Pennsylvania, as 50 in the Valey of the Mississippi." Knowledge about practice could not be freely transferred from one region to another, but rather had to be revalidated for use in a context other than that in which it was produced. "It may be proper to state my practice has been chiefly within the city of Boston," a physician of that city noted as a prefacing caveat to reporting his own experiences using the lancet and leeches in treating scarlatina. "As the situation of the place, and of course, its climate and soil, the customs and manners of the inhabitants, may have great influence in varying the type of acute diseases, a difference in the mode of treat[ment elsewhere] may not only be proper, but required."[12] There was no fundamental difference between the assumptions about medical knowledge underlying his remarks and those supporting the argument for southern medical distinctiveness.

One of the most persistent misconceptions about medical practice in antebellum America is that treatment was generally rote; this is belied by surviving casebooks and other indicators of actual practice. While physicians' commitment to specificity dictated in principle that treatment be varied according to circumstances, among the most striking features of records of practice from the period are the complexity and diversity of prescribing habits. Like their counterparts in other regions of the country, most southern practitioners were not doctrinaire in their therapeutic practices and did not routinely bleed or give calomel, quinine, or opium. As the principles articulated by the theorists of southern medicine predicted, calomel and quinine were undeniably among the most widely prescribed drugs; however, even these medicaments were not given as a matter of course. Venesection, on the other hand, was practiced on only a small fraction of the South's sick. These usage patterns are evident in the records of practice of a dozen

12. John Leonard Riddell, Manuscript Volumes, vol. 26, Minutes of Lectures Delivered at the Medical College of Ohio, in the Winter of 1834–5, Lecture of Dr. [Jesse] Smith, November 5, 1834, in Special Collections Division, Howard-Tilton Memorial Library, Tulane University, New Orleans; "Extract from Dr. Ingalls's Letter on Scarlatina," *Boston Medical and Surgical Journal*, XVII (1837), 239.

antebellum southern physicians selected for their geographic and temporal diversity. Venesection, for example, although declining in the South as elsewhere between 1810 and the Civil War, was never used by these physicians on more than about 6 percent of their visits. These ledgers and practice books, far from reflecting a minimalist reading of the *Pharmacopeia*, present impressive variety within each physician's armamentarium. Further evident is a striking diversity among practitioners, some with characteristic penchants reflecting in part the fact that similar therapeutic ends could sometimes be attained through a variety of means.[13]

The widespread application of the principle of specificity to medical practice and to the assessment of medical knowledge both within and without the South plainly demonstrates that the conceptual bases of the southern argument for regional medical distinctiveness were in no way singular. It is further possible to establish the lack of southern particularity in the premises and character of the content of the argument by displaying its didactic origins. Not only were the assumptions underlying this argument shared by northern physicians, but to a large extent the argument was actually acquired in the North, and through northern institutions, by southerners who brought it back to the South and exploited it.

The notion that the characteristic attributes of place modified disease and indications for treatment had been a part of medical thought for over two millennia, embodied most prominently in the Hippocratic treatise *On Airs, Waters, and Places* and in Sydenham's formulation of the epidemic constitution and its influences. But in late eighteenth- and early nineteenth-century America, a dual impetus mobilized energies to establish the particularity of American nature, including its diseases. In part, Americans were driven by an ideal of cultural independence, a desire to free themselves intellectually, as politically, from their colonial status. At the same time, they were responding to European disparagements of the New World as a habitat and charges of the inherently valetudinarian character of American nature. The late eighteenth-century French Buffon–de Pauw thesis in particular, which postulated the physical degeneracy of animal life in the New World, elic-

13. The records upon which this is based are described in John Harley Warner, "The Idea of Southern Medical Distinctiveness: Medical Knowledge and Practice in the Old South," in Judith Walzer Leavitt and Ronald L. Numbers (eds.), *Sickness and Health in America: Readings in the History of Medicine and Public Health* (2nd ed.; Madison, 1985), 67, n. 21.

ited a concerted effort by the Jeffersonians to vindicate their continent by demonstrating that American nature was indeed distinctive, but decidedly superior.

In medicine, the case for the exceptionalism of American nature was expressed most forcefully in the endeavor to establish that the American environment, both physical and social, shaped disease and medical need in ways that demanded the existence of a distinctively American medical practice. This position was expounded particularly in Philadelphia, the geographic epicenter of the Jeffersonian circle. For example, Benjamin Rush, professor of the theory and practice of medicine at the University of Pennsylvania from 1789 to 1813 and the most prominent medical member of the cadre of men who best represented Jeffersonian philosophy, believed that political and social organization, the physical environment, and health were all linked, making disease and treatment functions of both place and culture. Rush fully embraced the implications of this posture for medical regionalism and nationalism. Benjamin Smith Barton, another member of the Jeffersonian circle, succeeded Rush in the Pennsylvania chair and held it until his death in 1815. He shared Rush's allegiances to medical nationalism and regionalism, and sought to further a distinctively American medicine by his own investigations on the uses of American plants in the treatment of American diseases. Barton's successor, Nathaniel Chapman, who occupied the chair from 1816 to 1850, disagreed in many respects with Rush, his preceptor, but resolutely shared the elder physician's belief in the adaptation of medicine to place. Chapman's medical nationalism, which was of an aggressively chauvinistic bent, was objectified in his founding of the *Philadelphia Journal of the Medical and Physical Sciences* in 1820 as a forum for developing an American medical culture to rival that of Europe.[14]

All three men urged in their lectures that American conditions produced more energetic diseases that demanded more forcefully sedative treatments than the diseases of Europe. This idea that American diseases were singularly vigorous, like Jeffersonian claims that live mammoths still roamed somewhere on the North American continent,

---

14. Daniel J. Boorstin, *The Lost World of Thomas Jefferson* (New York, 1948); [Nathaniel Chapman], "Prospectus," *Philadelphia Journal of the Medical and Physical Sciences*, I (1820), vii–xii; Gilbert Chinard, "Eighteenth Century Theories on America As a Human Habitat," *Proceedings of the American Philosophical Society*, XCI (1947), 27–57; Antonello Gerbi, *The Dispute of the New World: The History of a Polemic, 1750–1900*, trans. Jeremy Moyle (Pittsburgh, 1973); George Rosen, "Political Order and Human Health in Jeffersonian Thought," *Bulletin of the History of Medicine*, XXVI (1952), 32–44.

helped refute the Buffon–de Pauw thesis by demonstrating the vitality of organic life in America on a scale unmatched in Europe. A North Carolina student attending Rush's lectures in 1811 copied in his notebook, "More attention is necessary to the natural history of the United States than would strike you at first, as our diseases differ so much from those of Europe." In most diseased conditions, he recorded, "the Citizens of the United States will require . . . [copious depletion] more than the Natives of Europe." Barton echoed this view in his lectures four years later. A student transcribing Barton's lectures wrote that the stimulant cinchona bark "has not been infrequently employed in Erysipelas particularly in Europe. But in the U. States the disease differs essentially from what it is in Europe. In Europe it is in general attended [by] prostration of strength and debility, and requires the invigorating method of cure. But in the U. States this disease is in general one of the Phlegmasia of an inflammatory character and requires the antiphlogistic method of cure." The same pattern held in other diseases; chorea, for example, assumed a debilitated form "in the enervated and enfeebled inhabitants of Europe. But in the U. States where the Blessings of Liberty are combined with the numerous other causes in developing the Physical man, this disease is usually of the tonic and sthenic character," which called for bleeding and purging.[15]

The Philadelphia faculty's allegiance to medical nationalism and regionalism was of seminal importance to the argument for southern medical distinctiveness. From the start of the century through the end of the antebellum period, Philadelphia was the most influential center for the formal training of southern physicians. Many southern medical students attended lectures in Philadelphia before, and even after, the emergence of southern medical schools. Moreover, when medical schools were established in the South, their faculties were substantially Philadelphia trained; when the region's first medical school opened in Charleston in 1823, nearly all its faculty members had received their formal medical education in Philadelphia. A very large proportion of the most vocal advocates of southern medical distinctiveness had attended medical lectures in Philadelphia, among them Edward Hall Barton, Daniel Warren Brickell, Samuel Adolphus Cartwright, Samuel Henry Dickson, Paul Fitzsimmons Eve, and Josiah

15. James P. Miller, Notes on Doctor Rush's Lectures Delivered 1811–12 in the University of Pennsylvania, lecture of November 24, 1811, in Manuscripts Department, William R. Perkins Library, Duke University; James Rackliffe, Notes on the Lectures of Benjamin S. Barton, Philadelphia, lecture of November 1, 1815, in Trent Collection, Duke University Medical Center Library, Durham.

Clark Nott. The links to Philadelphia teachings among other leading proponents of southern medical distinctiveness are less direct but nonetheless clear. For example, Erasmus Darwin Fenner, the most articulate exponent of a distinctive southern medical education, received his M.D. degree in 1830 at Transylvania University, where he studied with Charles Caldwell, a former pupil of Rush at the University of Pennsylvania, where Caldwell had taught for several years prior to an altercation with his former mentor. Caldwell not only stressed in his lectures at Transylvania (and, later, at Louisville) the necessity of regional and national variations in medical knowledge and practice, but Fenner also credited him with being the first to use the recognition of medical regionalism as the basis of a coherent case for the propriety of regional medical education.[16]

The fact that in the years before the Civil War literally hundreds of southern medical students annually elected to go to Philadelphia was in no sense a denial of the singularity of southern medical practice. Just as American physicians traveled to the hospitals of Europe in growing numbers during the antebellum period to gain knowledge about medical science despite their doubts about the applicability of European practice to American patients, so too southern students could seek medical knowledge in Philadelphia while remaining wary of the practical precepts taught there. Thus when a South Carolina physician considering going to Philadelphia for further professional study wrote to Josiah Nott for advice in the mid-1830s, Nott counseled that advantages for professional improvement in Philadelphia were unmatched elsewhere in the United States, but cautioned him against placing too much faith in northern practice. Nott especially recommended the opportunities for gaining pathological knowledge and studying physical diagnosis with the clinician William Wood Gerhard, adding, "You will see I think much to object to in Gerhard's practice—but he is a profound pathologist."[17]

One southerner studying in Philadelphia confidently asserted that "as for learning the theoretical part of Medicine and studying those branches on which we must found our practice (as Anatomy & Physiology) Philadelphia presents as many advantages perhaps as any

16. E. D. Fenner, "Introductory Lecture Delivered at the Opening of the New Orleans School of Medicine, on the 17th Nov., '56," *New Orleans Medical News and Hospital Gazette*, III (1856–57), 597; *Autobiography of Charles Caldwell, M.D.* (1855; rpr. New York, 1968), 358–59.

17. [Josiah Clark Nott] to James M. Gage, March [1837], in James M. Gage Papers, Southern Historical Collection, University of North Carolina at Chapel Hill.

other place in the united states." But at the same time he recognized the advantages of home education in practice itself, and applauded a fellow North Carolinian's decision to attend medical lectures in Charleston rather than outside the South, commenting that "the practice there will correspond better with that of our country." Similarly, a North Carolina physician who had received his medical training at the University of Pennsylvania and proudly referred in later years to "my old master Dr. Rush" not only named his son Benjamin Rush Norcom but also sent him to the University of Pennsylvania for medical lectures after he had completed an apprenticeship with his father. Yet despite his overt, genuine allegiance to the Philadelphia school, the father did not question the superiority of southern therapeutic knowledge for treating patients in that region. He noted in a letter to his son in Philadelphia, "We know better, here, how to manage carolina constitutions than the Physicians of Philadelphia."[18]

One message that was crystalline in the lectures delivered at the University of Pennsylvania and attended by many of the southerners who led the drive for regional medical distinctiveness was that medical practice necessarily differed in the North and South. Rush told his students that such differentiae of the regions as climate, miasmatic exhalations, diet, dress, work habits, and social structure altered the symptoms of diseases and appropriate therapeutics, stating unambiguously that "diseases of warm & cold climates require different treatment." Chapman, acknowledging the same fact, at times explicitly qualified therapeutic dicta in his lectures by saying that they might be inapplicable in hot climates. "Do not prescribe for the name of the disease," a southern student attending Chapman's lectures in Philadelphia copied into his notebook.

> The same disease varies at different seasons and in different parts of the Country. In no one is this more illustrated than in bilious Fever[.] In this City and section of the Country it is a disease very different in its nature and requiring different treatment from what it is farther to the South. Here it is almost uniformly inflamatory, exacting for its management the very constant and profuse use of the lancet, but in the Carolinas and Georgia this must be wholly laid aside, or sparingly & discriminately employed.

18. James K. Nisbet to N[athaniel] E. McCleeland, February 26, 1830, Nisbet to McCleeland, September 18, 1830, both in McCleeland Family Papers, Southern Historical Collection; Ja[me]s Norcom to Benjamin Rush Norcom, February 21, 1832, in Dr. James Norcom and Family Papers, North Carolina State Archives, Raleigh. James Norcom wrote on Rush in a letter to his son John Norcom, February 18, 1846, in Dr. James Norcom and Family Papers.

In another lecture Chapman noted that "the mercurial treatment of dysentery is much more called for in warm climates, where the liver is generally affected." Indeed, prevailing southern judgments on the necessary peculiarities of the use of venesection, calomel, and quinine in that region are all apparent in Philadelphian teachings.[19]

Lecturers at other northern schools where southern students matriculated conveyed a similar message. David Hosack, who had received his M.D. degree at the University of Pennsylvania in 1791, routinely drew attention to regional diversity in medical practice in his lectures at the College of Physicians and Surgeons in New York, where he taught from 1807 to 1826. "As each climate produces particular diseases," he observed, "attention should be paid to it. In warm climates, most disorders arise from debility." But, he continued, "in cold climates there is considerable vigour in the system, together with nervous energy. The inhabitants of the North* are for the most part exempt from those bilious disorders, consequent to warm climates, but they are subject to Inflammatory affections and bear copious depletion, and are also more able to undergo the operation of medicine than those of a warmer region." Regional variations in individual therapeutic practices, such as the use of cinchona bark, were accounted for within his framework. "In hot climates," Hosack explained, "the bark is resorted to because they have to counteract the putrescent tendency but in this climate it is injurious and useless."[20]

In saying that medical knowledge and practice in their region were distinctive, southern physicians were, then, not unique. Nor was there

19. Quotations from John Austin, Notes on the Lectures of Benjamin Rush, 1809, Historical Collection, Rudolph Matas Medical Library, Tulane University Medical Center, New Orleans; Benjamin Huger, Notes on Materia Medica from Lectures Delivered by Nathaniel Chapman, 1816, vol. 1, in Waring Historical Library, Medical University of South Carolina, Charleston; Samuel Barrington, Notes on the Practice of Medicine Taken from the Lectures of N. Chapman, M.D. Professor of the Institutes & Practice of Physic &c., in the University of Pennsylvania, 1818–19, 1820–21, 1821–22, in History of Medicine Division, National Library of Medicine, Bethesda. And see P. Washington Little, Notebook of Lectures by Rush 1805–06, Notes on Physiology, Pathology, &c &c &c Delivered at the University of Pennsylvania, Trent Collection, Duke University Medical Center Library; and Samuel Murphy, Notes from Doctor [Nathaniel] Chapman's Lectures, 1830, vol. 1, in University of Pennsylvania Archives, Philadelphia, Pennsylvania.

20. Buckner Hill, [Notes on Hosack's Lectures, vol. 1], commenced November 1, 1824, in Buckner Hill Notebooks, North Carolina State Archives; John Barratt, Lecture Notes [on Lectures of Dr. Hosack], 1822, in South Caroliniana Library, University of South Carolina. The asterisk in the quoted comments led to the following addition at the bottom of the page: "*Inhabitants of the North, do not require the same treatments (of tonics) as those in southern climates."

anything in its essence idiosyncratic about the premises underlying their case for regional distinctiveness or about the rules they used in its formulation. Yet, in one respect, the argument for southern medical distinctiveness was singular—not in its content, nor in its assumptions about medical knowledge and practice, but in the emotion, the force, the stridency that informed the way it was argued.

The stridency of the argument for southern medical distinctiveness is revealed by the tenor of its rhetoric, which was characterized by an urgency seldom so persistently expressed in regular medical literature, save for denunciations of unorthodox medical sectarians. Physicians frequently cast their case for the individuality of southern practice in language that evoked the crusading sense of a sociopolitical movement, as when the editors of a New Orleans journal urged that in medical education, "it is the 'manifest destiny' of the South to become each year more and more independent." "Too long has the South been slumbering in inactivity," charged a Georgia medical editor urging the same point. "Hitherto she has been the passive pupil of science, content to draw her knowledge from foreign sources; but the voice that drives away her slumbers shall arouse her to emulation, and the South shall disdain to borrow what she can herself so copiously supply." It was not accidental that the advocates of southern medical distinctiveness often chose agricultural metaphors to present their case in ways calculated to produce emotional resonance in their readers or listeners; as Drew Gilpin Faust has shown, the images of agriculture offered exceptionally potent symbols through which southerners could better understand and express the sources of stress within the social order. "The most scientific farmer in England will not be equal to the Southern planter in growing cotton, sugar, rice, maize, [or] tobacco," asserted Bennet Dowler, a New Orleans physician and physiologist. Similarly, he claimed, "The British physician may know more of the typhus fever among the paupers of his native land, than the Southern physician; but the former might not be equal to the latter in the medical treatment of negroes and whites in the Southern States." As a Tennessee practitioner argued, "Medicine, like disease, must spring from the very elements, soil, sunshine, moisture, etc., that produce disease."[21]

21. Quotations from "Medical Sectionalism," *New Orleans Medical News and Hospital Gazette*, IV (1857–58), 158; B. Dowler, "A Review of Medical Literature, Including Critical Remarks on Professor Palmer's Report on That Subject, As Published in the Transactions of the American Medical Association, Vol. XI," *New Orleans Medical and Surgical Journal*, XVI (1859), 446; S. P. Crawford, "Southern Medical Literature," *Nashville Medical and*

The fact that southern physicians saw the case for southern medical distinctiveness as an inspiration for medical activity further evidences the peculiar strength of this idea in the South. This is best demonstrated by the express modeling of southern schools and literature in conformity with the ideal of a distinctive southern practice, but it is also illustrated by other forms of action less arguably motivated by economics. Medical societies used regional specificity as a rationale for investigating the peculiarities of climate, disease, and treatment in their locales, and the products of this enterprise offer the best counterexample to the largely correct assertion that antebellum medical societies were sociopolitical organizations void of serious scientific activity.[22] Physicians claimed that they must study diseases in their local milieu to determine their etiology and behavior. Such local knowledge would direct prudent activity in the face of epidemics, for example, and thereby protect the health and commerce of their region.

Reports on the topography, meteorology, diseases, and therapeutics of a single county or district abounded in late antebellum southern medical journals, and many medical theses were of the same genre. "It is a fact which reason would suggest, and which experience has verified, that the varied circumstances of soil, climate & local peculiarities presented by a country, do in numerous ways engender and modify diseases," a student at the Medical Department of the University of Nashville began his thesis in 1851. "Hence the necessity of investigating these circumstances and peculiarities, that we may be able . . . to treat disease more successfully." A student at the Medical College of the State of South Carolina, who wrote a thesis entitled "The Topography of South Alabama and the Diseases Incident to Its Climate" (1843), similarly noted that a proper physician was obligated to study the modifying influences of a particular region.[23] Such local studies were

Surgical Journal, XVIII (1860), 198. See also Drew Gilpin Faust, "The Rhetoric and Ritual of Agriculture in Antebellum South Carolina," *Journal of Southern History*, XLV (1979), 541–68; and Dorse Harland Hagler, "The Agrarian Theme in Southern History to 1860" (Ph.D. dissertation, University of Missouri, 1968).

22. See, for example, J. P. Barratt, "Transactions of the South Carolina Medical Association," *Charleston Medical and Surgical Review*, XI (1856), 180, 183; A. H. Buchanan, "Address Delivered at the First Annual Meeting of the Nashville Medical Society," *Nashville Medical and Surgical Journal*, XVII (1859), 199; and P. H. Lewis, "A Medical History of Alabama," *New Orleans Medical and Surgical Journal*, III (1846–47), 691–706, and IV (1847–48), 3–34, 151–177.

23. James A. Briggs, "An Inaugural Dissertation on the Medical Topography and Diseases of Warren County, Ky." (M.D. thesis, Medical Department of the University of

of course common in the North and especially the West as well, but their pursuit in these regions did not display the extent of openly sectional ardor that animated investigations in the South. That the argument for southern medical distinctiveness often explicitly informed such endeavors demonstrates that the force empowering it was sufficient to direct action as well as to engender rhetoric.

Northern physicians who denounced the political drive for southern medical independence ordinarily did not question the underlying premise that southern medical distinctiveness was a reality ordained by nature. When the Philadelphia medical author and editor John Bell assailed pleas for peculiarly southern medical literature and education as "states-rights medicine," for example, it was the strident use of the argument for southern distinctiveness to support rigid institutional separatism and not the assumed need for regional specificity to which he objected. He defended the pertinence to southern practice of northern teachings (and especially his own recent treatise on practice) by affirming that northern authors and professors recognized the individuating factors that characterized various regions and took them into account. "It should be remembered, that our northern lecturers and writers on systematic medicine still continue the old fashion of pointing out the modifications in fevers and other diseases arising from the difference of locality and climate in general, as well as from manner of living, age, and sex," he asserted. "They are not quite like moles, whose purblind vision prevents their seeing beyond their own habitations; but, on the contrary, they extend their investigations over the whole habitable world, making collections from all quarters, which they afterwards arrange and place on the altar of science; as an offering to their countrymen throughout the whole United States."[24] Bell's well-known term "states-rights medicine" was a damning epithet created by a self-interested critic of the movement for southern medical separatism, not an objective appraisal of the animus or intellectual integrity of claims about regional medical distinctiveness.

Medical theory prevalent during the antebellum period and the

---

Nashville, 1851), Special Collections, Medical Center Library, Vanderbilt University, Nashville; Thomas Hunter, "A Dissertation on the Topography of South Alabama and the Diseases Incident to Its Climate" (M.D. thesis, Medical College of the State of South Carolina, 1843), South Carolina Room, Main Library, Medical University of South Carolina.

24. "Dr. Cartwright's Address—States-Rights Medicine," *Bulletin of Medical Sciences,* IV (1846), 212.

unmistakable diversity presented by the American habitat and peoples plainly were sufficient to make inevitable the serious discussion of regional differences by physicians. But they do not explain why southern physicians so energetically took up the case for regional specificity and aggressively pleaded its cardinal importance in directing southern medicine. Southern physicians recognized that the doctrine of specificity, duly applied to the environmental variation existing within the South, pointed to the need for substantial fluctuations in medical practice in different sections of their region. Yet, while they acknowledged the importance of this diversity (hence the abundance of local studies), southern physicians placed far greater emphasis upon those modifying circumstances that characterized the South as a discrete unit. Further, they proselytized the idea of southern medical distinctiveness with a vigor unmatched in other regions of America in analogous contexts; neither northern attention to America's dissimilarities to Europe nor western emphasis upon the disparities between that region and the Northeast exhibited such zeal. That emotion, that force, is what must be explained to understand what was uniquely southern about the argument for southern medical distinctiveness.

Much of the force that impelled the case for southern medical particularity must be ascribed to the same engines that drove southerners from a variety of occupations in their rising defense of the southern way of life. It was patently not by happenstance that the growing preoccupation with regional distinctiveness in southern medicine chronologically paralleled the larger movement in the South that began in the early 1830s toward economic, cultural, and political sectionalism and nationalism. Tensions inevitably engendered by the South's colonial agrarian economy, reliance upon slavery, and diminished political power, augmented by a regional sensibility piqued by external charges of immorality, intellectual sloth, and social retrogression, imbued all questions of the region's particularity with a strong emotional vibrancy. Further, southern medical editors and educators, functioning within a medical marketplace in which competition for subscribers and students was acute, had a potent economic incentive for using the argument for southern medical distinctiveness to underscore the advantages of regional medical literature and schools. All of these considerations are cogent and important. Nevertheless, implying that southern physicians promoted their arguments for southern medical distinctiveness simply because they were southerners, or because they were driven by invidious economic incentives, explains away as much as it explains.

The force that propelled the argument for southern medical distinctiveness was in large measure a product of anxieties experienced by southern physicians whose identities, and not just livelihoods, were bound up with both their region and profession. The pivot upon which these anxieties turned was the low, marginal status of the medical profession in the South, a phenomenon expressed in several interrelated ways. To begin with, physicians in the South, as elsewhere in the United States, routinely lamented the low esteem in which their profession as a whole was held by the public, despite the fact that many individual physicians enjoyed high prestige in their own communities.[25] The notorious difficulty of maintaining a financially successful practice, they maintained, reflected a dearth of public faith and support for regular physicians, a circumstance encouraged by sectarian competition and displayed by sectarian successes. Moreover, southern physicians were acutely aware of the disparaging judgments pronounced upon the medical endeavor in their region by prominent members of the medical profession in the North. Authoritative northern assertions of the inferiority of southern practices and theories were made more grating by southern practitioners' undeniable institutional and intellectual dependence upon the North. Finally, thinking southern physicians plainly perceived intellectual lethargy to be characteristic of the medical profession in their region and regarded the lack of an active professional community to appreciate and reward medical enterprise as both a cause and illustration of the region's professional degradation.

Many southern physicians saw in the celebration of southern medical distinctiveness a means of alleviating anxieties that stemmed from the low status of the medical profession in the South. The singular force that drove this argument and linkages that southern physicians perceived between it and both the sources and solutions of the profession's distress may be discerned in a reconstruction of medical history that became common in the late antebellum South. During the 1840s and 1850s, such self-proclaimed leaders of southern medicine as Cartwright, Dowler, Fenner, and Nott fashioned a Whiggish reconstruc-

25. See Barbara G. Rosenkrantz, "The Search for Professional Order in 19th-Century American Medicine," in Leavitt and Numbers, *Sickness and Health in America*, 219–32. The comparatively high standing of individual southern physicians in their communities tends to be supported by E. Brooks Holifield's survey of preachers, lawyers, and physicians in the urban South in 1860, which revealed that the mean wealth of physicians was greater than that of the other groups (*The Gentlemen Theologians: American Theology in Southern Culture, 1795–1860* [Durham, 1978], 32).

tion of professional history that took on the role and form of a distinctively southern professional myth. Constructed to explain the low status of medicine in the South and the means of its elevation, this mythologized history was driven by the same animus that imparted such force to the argument for the distinctiveness of southern medical practice.

The "true regular science of medicine," this history held, originated in a southern climate, the Greece of Hippocrates, and in this southern cradle it approached perfection. Erected from observations of southern climates, constitutions, and diseases, the principles of this medicine were matched to southern needs and were still suited to many of the medical needs of the American South. But southern medicine, boasting an unrivaled intellectual vitality at a time when, according to Fenner, "London and Paris, Edinburgh, Dublin and Vienna, were in a state of barbarism," did not retain its dominance. Medicine flourished in the southern latitude of Rome "until," as one Atlanta professor told an entering class of medical students, "the floods of vandal barbarism poured down upon the doomed city, from the plains of the North, and bore off upon their dark and turbid bosom, almost every trace of learning and refinement."[26] A variation of the same theme illustrated the deterioration of southern medicine by contrasting not ancient Greece and Rome with Edinburgh and Philadelphia, but instead the colonial South with the mid-nineteenth century South.[27] The looted remnants of superior southern medicine were taken to cold latitudes, and there they were distorted to meet northern needs.

The objective of this historical account was to show that the medicine some regular southern physicians practiced in mid-nineteenth-century America, and learned through northern institutions, was not true regular medicine, but rather a "reformed" system suited to the climate of the northern parts of America and Europe. According to the historical narrative, which was cast in a loose temporal framework typical of myth, medical sovereignty passed almost directly from Rome to Edinburgh, a city characterized as a cold, desolate outpost on the northernmost boundary of civilization. There, medicine was reformed to suit the peculiar requirements of the Edinburgh environment; according to Cartwright, "a new nomenclature was there made to em-

26. Fenner, "Introductory Lecture," 587; Alexander Means, "An Address to the Second Course of Lectures in the Atlanta Medical College," *Atlanta Medical and Surgical Journal*, I (1855–56), 708.

27. Fenner, "Introductory Lecture," 587, 597; E. D. Fenner, "Introductory Address," *Southern Medical Reports*, I (1850), 8–9.

brace the new order of diseases observed, new theories invented, and a new practice adopted to suit the diseases in that little hyperborean corner of the globe." This reformed system of medicine was transplanted to America when pupils of the Edinburgh school established what Cartwright called a "branch school" in Philadelphia, at the University of Pennsylvania, and taught Edinburgh medicine until it attained national dominance.[28]

However, this reformed system was fundamentally inappropriate for southern medical practice. Treatment, transformed as it was to suit a northern climate "under the auspices of Cullen and his followers," an Alabama physician told the delegates to the state medical association's annual meeting in 1855, "became quite too frigid for the ardent temperament and more relaxed system of our 'Sunny south.' "[29] Northern lecturers and writings therefore taught a reformed system of medical knowledge and practice fitting for their regions, but deceptive and dangerous for the southern practitioner. Much of the uncertainty and want of confidence that did exist in southern practice was due to the reliance of some southern physicians upon improper northern authority, a continual source of corruption, rather than upon their own experience at southern bedsides or the observations of other physicians practicing in the South. The underlying message this version of medical history bore was that physicians of the South could elevate their professional standing and regain for the South its position of leadership in medicine by throwing off the hegemony of a reformed system of medicine never designed for use in the South, by observing southern diseases and treatments for themselves, and by restoring true regular medicine.

The same historical framework was also used to account for the flourishing state of medical sectarianism in the South. The Edinburgh reform, in Cartwright's assessment, "was all well enough for that little place on the globe, but it went farther and imposed the same reformed physic on the rest of the world." To meet Edinburgh's sthenic, inflammatory fevers, the diseases of "a climate that almost forces the red blood through the skin," northern reformers had properly relied principally on the lancet and antiphlogistic drugs. However, this treatment was harmful when applied to southern fevers, which were often of a

28. Samuel A. Cartwright, "Malum Egyptiäcum, Cold Plague, Diphtheria, or Black Tongue," *New Orleans Medical and Surgical Journal,* XVI (1859), 380, 815.

29. W. Taylor, "Annual Oration," in *Transactions of the Medical Association of the State of Alabama at Its Eighth Annual Session . . . Mobile, February 5,–6,–7, 1855* (Mobile, 1855), 120.

more debilitated or asthenic character, and led to unsuccessful thera-peutic management that encouraged public disillusionment with the regular profession and fostered the rise of quackery. Moreover, Cart-wright argued, stimulants and hot, fiery drugs such as peppers, ap-propriate for diseases in the South, had been cast out from the re-formed armamentarium because they were not useful in treating the diseases of Edinburgh. Cayenne pepper, a mainstay in the practice of the unorthodox Thomsonian sect, was therefore more appropriate to the needs of southern patients than were many of the remedies of the reformed system of medicine practiced by regular physicians, a situa-tion that accounted for Thomsonian successes. The regrettable alle-giance of some physicians to medical knowledge of European and northern provenance blinded them to the value of drugs such as red pepper and lobelia in treating southern diseases, Cartwright confided in a letter to a nonphysician friend, driving many patients to embrace Thomsonianism and reject the regular profession.[30]

The use of history as a tool for explanation, legitimation, and affir-mation of links with tradition certainly was commonplace in nine-teenth-century American medicine. For some southern physicians, though, the retelling of this particular account of the historical course of southern medicine went so far as to assume the cadence of a ritual. A stylized narrative recounted as a preface to calls for professional vigor and improvement in southern medicine, the story served functions conventionally attributed to myth. It explained why medicine in the South occupied its present degraded status and how this had come to be. Further, it exemplified proper values for the professional culture, clarifying what was important, and set role models. For example, Hip-

30. Quotations from Sam[uel] A. Cartwright to Rezin Thomson, June 15, 1856, *Nashville Medical and Surgical Journal*, XI (1856), 214; and see Cartwright, "Malum Egyp-tiäcum," 380–88, 800–17; Cartwright, *The Pathology and Treatment of Cholera: With an Appendix, Containing His Latest Instructions to Planters and Heads of Families (Remote from Medical Advice) in Regards to Its Prevention and Cure* (New Orleans, 1849); and Samuel A. Cartwright to John Francis Hamtramck Claiborne, April 26, 1856, in John Francis Hamtramck Claiborne Papers, Southern Historical Collection. Attributing southern problems to northern sources became a convention in southern medical literature. When the editors of the *New Orleans Medical and Surgical Journal* referred to sectarians as "the Goths and Vandals of empiricism," the point that these were tribes of barbarian north-erners who swept down to loot and destroy a superior southern civilization was unam-biguous. See editors' introduction to Samuel A. Cartwright, "Address Delivered before the Medical Convention, in the City of Jackson, January 13, 1846," *New Orleans Medical and Surgical Journal*, II (1845–46), 729. Similarly, southerners pointed again and again to the facts that Samuel Thomson was a New Englander and Samuel Hahnemann a European.

pocrates was the archetypal southern physician, for rather than relying on established wisdom he observed for himself southern diseases, peoples, and environments, thereby developing morbid natural histories and therapeutic strategies appropriate to southern patients. Emulation of his allegiance to the careful observation of southern nature was the foundation upon which a Greek revival medicine singularly suited to the needs of the American South should be fashioned. Moreover, this story aided the legitimation of a self-conscious effort to develop, or redevelop, a distinctive southern medicine by demonstrating its ancient roots and modern corruption. The repetition of this narrative was also a source of creative power and control. It projected a model of professional redemption bearing the message that to elevate in their region what Paul F. Eve called "this much abused, but little comprehended, this neglected and now degraded, this noble, this God-like Profession,"[31] southern physicians needed to follow the Hippocratic example, recognize the distinctive character of southern medicine, and liberate themselves from northern and European authority.

Regarded within the context of this reconstruction of professional history and the functions it was designed to serve, the argument for southern medical distinctiveness clearly had taken on attributes that Clifford Geertz has ascribed to ideologies. "The attempt of ideologies to render otherwise incomprehensible social situations meaningful, to so construe them as to make it possible to act purposefully within them," he suggests, accounts for "the intensity with which, once accepted, they are held."[32] Geertz's model of an ideology as a response to social, cultural, and psychological strains helps clarify the physicians' strident advocacy of the idea of southern medical distinctiveness, which made understandable the degraded status of the medical profession in the South. The specific contours of these strains as southern physicians experienced them are plainly identified by the problems this reconstructed professional history sought to explain and begin to resolve. Southern physicians had developed a minority consciousness like that of their region. Aware of their collective loss of status, south-

31. Paul F. Eve, "Address to the Class, on Opening the Course of Lectures in the Medical College of Georgia, the 17th of October, 1837," *Southern Medical and Surgical Journal*, II (1838), 11.

32. Clifford Geertz, "Ideology as a Cultural System," in David Apter (ed.), *Ideology and Discontent* (New York, 1964), 64. Aptly for the historian's purposes, Geertz quotes Talcott Parsons' observation: "The concept of strain is not in itself an explanation of ideological patterns but a generalized label for the kinds of factors to look for in working out an explanation" (p. 54).

ern physicians saw themselves located on the periphery of creative activity and institutional power in medicine, and their rhetoric lucidly reveals their experience of marginality, isolation, and alienation. Assessing their position vis-à-vis the North, thinking physicians in the South perceived a disturbing dependency, inferiority, and consequent humiliation.

A fervently argued case for southern medical distinctiveness represented one means of alleviating these burdens. As I have suggested elsewhere, the preoccupation of some southern physicians with their region's peculiar medical problems, and with the need for a singularly southern body of medical knowledge and practice that this implied, was driven by a reform animus.[33] Medical men in the South saw in the argument for southern medical distinctiveness a platform for energizing and thereby elevating the medical profession in their region. A distinctive southern medicine promised to remedy the low standing of the profession in the South by raising the public's regard for the healing abilities of regular physicians, thereby scotching sectarian competition; by releasing southern practitioners from their dependence upon the North and Europe, thereby making possible scientific and institutional parity; and by activating the medical community, thereby augmenting both its cognitive and social power. This argument was of special importance to the southern physician with intellectual aspirations, for it offered an avenue to the justification and vitalization of the intellectual life of the southern medical community.

Thus while the basic assumptions about the nature of medical knowledge that underlay the argument for southern medical distinctiveness were shared by physicians outside the South as well as within it, the energetic promulgation of the argument was at once a response to the epidemiological, ethnic, and climatic realities of the southern environment; a tool in southern competition for economic advantage and social influence with the traditional loci of professional power, northern medical institutions; and a contribution to the growing impulse toward southern nationalism. But at the most fundamental level, the case for the particularity of southern medical practice was driven by anxieties and needs that pertained especially to the situation of the thinking physician who practiced in the South. In the idea of a

33. Warner, "A Southern Medical Reform." My understanding of the position occupied by the physician with intellectual aspirations in the antebellum South owes much to my reading of Drew Gilpin Faust, *The Sacred Circle: The Dilemma of the Intellectual in the Old South, 1840–1860* (Baltimore, 1977); and Faust, "A Southern Stewardship: The Intellectual and the Proslavery Argument," *American Quarterly*, XXXI (1979), 63–80.

distinctively southern medicine such physicians saw a motivation for action, a catalyst for the realization of their aspirations for the medical profession in the South, that accounts in large measure for the intensity with which they asserted their region's medical singularity. In this respect, the argument for southern medical distinctiveness was distinctively southern.

At the core of this judgment of distinctiveness, though, is an inescapable irony. There can be no doubt that the collective experience of physicians in the antebellum South is properly characterized by their self-perceived marginality, isolation, low professional status and lack of community appreciation, economic uncertainty, and dependence upon external sources for innovation and external institutions for the dissemination of knowledge, as well as by defensiveness rooted in a consciousness of inferiority. But in varying degrees, and with due regard to the cultural diversity existing within the profession, these same attributes precisely characterize the experience of the American physician during the same period. Isolated from the medical centers of Europe yet dependent upon them for both new knowledge and synthetic instruction; working in a profession accorded a dubiously high standing in American society; competing for uncertain financial security with irregular practitioners whom society granted equal legal, and often social, status; alienated from European physicians on the cutting edge of medical science and within an American culture known for its valuation of practice over learning; and conscious of their inferiority to Europe in medical institutions and the pursuit of medical science, American physicians, taken as a whole, mirrored an image of the problems of southern physicians that was dimmer but nonetheless whole. The argument for southern medical distinctiveness was in its essence a southern response to problems felt in varying degrees by medical practitioners in all regions of America. Regarded in this way, the experience of the physician in the Old South, embodying in exaggerated form the anxieties of their professional counterparts in other regions, may best epitomize the experience of the antebellum American physician.

CHAPTER 10

A SOUTHERN MEDICAL REFORM: THE MEANING OF THE ANTEBELLUM ARGUMENT FOR SOUTHERN MEDICAL EDUCATION

John Harley Warner

From the 1830s through the end of the antebellum period, many southern physicians argued with growing conviction that southern medical practice was distinctive and that, therefore, southern practitioners ought to be educated through southern medical institutions. The utility of this argument as a socioeconomic and political doctrine that could be cited in support of a case for regional separatism is apparent. But beyond this, energetic elaboration and proselytization of the argument by physicians makes it clear that professional consciousness of the centrality of medical education to the standing and success of the medical enterprise in the South had become acute. The meaning of regional education must be understood in terms of physicians' aspirations, identity, and anxieties, and therefore it is necessary to consider those practitioners who supported southern medical education in their professional role as physicians and not merely as southerners.

The leading proposition underpinning the case for southern medical education was belief in southern medical distinctiveness, the conceptual bases of which are described in Chapter 9 of this volume.[1]

A different form of this paper appeared in the *Bulletin of the History of Medicine*, LVII (1983), 364–81, and is reprinted here with permission. I am grateful to Barbara Gutmann Rosenkrantz for her criticisms and suggestions. The paper was supported in part by NIH Grant LM 03910 from the National Library of Medicine, and by NSF Grant SES-8107609.

1. I also give a fuller analysis of the issues mentioned in this paragraph in "A Southern Medical Reform: The Meaning of the Antebellum Argument for Southern Medical Education," *Bulletin of the History of Medicine*, LVII (1983), 364–66; and *The Therapeutic Perspective: Medical Practice, Knowledge, and Identity in America, 1820–1885* (Cambridge, Mass., 1986), 58–80.

Medical theory fully sustained this belief. In particular, the principle of specificity dictated that treatment had to be matched not to disease (the same disease might require opposite treatments under different circumstances) but to the individual characteristics of a patient and of his or her physical and social environments. But while medical theory underlay arguments for southern medical distinctiveness and regional education, it did not compel them, as its failure to generate movements for regional medical education of comparable force in other areas of the country illustrates. There were also powerful social, political, and economic incentives for fashioning a distinctive southern medicine with its own educational institutions. But to view southern physicians' support for regional medical education merely as one facet of rising sectionalism describes the movement without explaining it.

The argument for southern medical education is better understood by recognizing the function it served for southern physicians. It was the chief expression of a movement for southern medical distinctiveness that many physicians, especially those having intellectual aspirations, saw as the most promising means of elevating the profession in the South. Although they diverged widely in many of their specific medical beliefs, such disparate southern physicians as Edward Hall Barton, Samuel Adolphus Cartwright, Bennet Dowler, Paul F. Eve, Erasmus Darwin Fenner, and Josiah Clark Nott were united in their allegiance to southern medical distinctiveness. By carving out an important realm of medical knowledge in which they were uniquely able to excel, a territory demarcated by both cognitive and geographic boundaries, such physicians sought to overcome their personal feelings of marginality and alienation, and those they shared with other intellectuals of their region. Thus the movement for southern medical particularity gained impetus both from the emphasis on specificity in medical practice, which the southern physician shared with his northern and western counterparts, and from the particular position occupied by the physician in the South who valued intellectual activity. The institutions of medical education—schools, hospitals, textbooks, and journals—offered physicians a concrete context within which their commitment to southern medical distinctiveness could be objectified and thereby became a vehicle for the vindication, vitalization, and reformation of medicine in the South.

Physicians in the antebellum South were especially aware of the losses of status experienced by their region and profession since early in the century. By the early 1830s the South had developed a minority consciousness through its colonial agrarian economy, dependence upon slavery, and loss of political power. Physicians shared with other southerners a sensitivity to the charges brought against their region of economic and political inferiority, immorality, and social backwardness.[2] At the same time, the decline in status of the American medical profession as a whole, marked by such signs as the abolition of medical licensing laws, loss of public confidence and esteem, and growing strength of unorthodox medical sects, was felt in the South as much as in other sections of the country. The low standing of intellectual inquiry in the South further exacerbated the sense of marginality that thinking southern physicians experienced as a result of their regional and professional anxieties about status and identity. Drew Gilpin Faust has pointed out the plight of antebellum southern intellectuals striving to define their place within "a culture known for its inhospitality to letters" and their shared perception of "the sorry state of intellectual endeavor in the region."[3] Physicians who valued intellectual enterprise actively participated in the southern man of mind's search for legitimacy that Faust has deftly detailed.

Southern physicians were aware that they were working on the periphery of medical inquiry and creative activity. "I have been living twenty years in the woods," John Young Bassett, Sir William Osler's "Alabama student," wrote from Huntsville to the Boston theologian Theodore Parker in 1849, "and when I want a book, I have to write to Paris, Bremen, or London for it and generally find it out of print; I am consequently not even a literary man." Yet many southern medical intellectuals suffered from an isolation more profound than that imposed by geography alone: they perceived themselves as intellectually isolated within a southern professional community that was inactive, slothful, and apathetic. Erasmus Darwin Fenner, a New Orleans medical educator and editor, was typical in his chiding of the South's physi-

2. Jesse T. Carpenter, *The South as a Conscious Minority, 1789–1861: A Study in Political Thought* (New York, 1930). General reviews of separatist thinking in the South during this period are Avery O. Craven, *The Growth of Southern Nationalism, 1848–1861* (Baton Rouge, 1953); John McCardell, *The Idea of a Southern Nation: Southern Nationalists and Southern Nationalism, 1830–1860* (New York, 1979); and Charles S. Sydnor, *The Development of Southern Sectionalism, 1819–1848* (Baton Rouge, 1948).

3. Drew Gilpin Faust, "A Southern Stewardship: The Intellectual and the Proslavery Argument," *American Quarterly,* XXXI (1979), 63, 68. See also Faust, *The Sacred Circle: The Dilemma of the Intellectual in the Old South, 1840–1860* (Baltimore, 1977). My understanding of the position of southern physician-intellectuals has been greatly crystallized by the insights Faust has drawn from a more diverse array of intellectuals whose shared anxieties and efforts to dissipate them were not informed by a shared professional role.

cians for their "silent indolence."[4] Josiah Clark Nott, who placed the development of a medical school in Mobile above his far more renowned anthropological pursuits, complained in a letter to a Charleston colleague that southern physicians placed little value on learning, recording with disgust that a successful Mobile practitioner had recently boasted to him of not having read a book in two decades.[5]

To the minds of this group of thinking southern physicians, professional indolence was inseparably bound to the region's dependence upon northern and European institutions of medical education. Southerners argued that northern authorities, who were profoundly ignorant of southern conditions, condemned practices that were in fact sensitively gauged to the needs of the South and thereby perpetuated an image of the region as medically backward. For example, defenders of southern therapeutic acumen resented northern writers' rejection of the proposal made by southern practitioners that large doses of quinine were called for in a variety of fevers. "The heroic doses of this drug in vogue among Southern practitioners," a Mississippi physician charged, "are among the marvels of medicine. Our Northern brethren hear of them with a smile of incredulity, if not with the sneer of derision. In this case ridicule is certainly no test of truth." Southerners widely believed that northern assumptions of southern inferiority were further expressed in a disparaging estimate of the southern profession as a possible source of new knowledge. Thus when Samuel Cartwright, a leading exponent of the medical distinctiveness of blacks, presented before the Natchez Medical Society a new method of reducing dislocations, he bitterly predicted that it "will be received with less inclination to examine into its merits than to ridicule it in

---

4. Quotations from John Young Bassett to Theodore Parker, December 15, 1849, in John Young Bassett Papers, Southern Historical Collection, University of North Carolina at Chapel Hill; and E. D. Fenner, "Introductory Address," *Southern Medical Reports,* I (1849), 9. Similar examples are "Editorials and Miscellaneous Articles," *Medical Journal of North Carolina,* I (1858), 89; and "Northern Schools and Southern Students," *New Orleans Medical Journal,* I (1844–45), 121. William Osler recounted Bassett's career in "An Alabama Student," in *An Alabama Student and Other Biographical Essays* (London, 1908), 1–18.

5. J. C. Nott to James M. Gage, July 28, 1838, in James M. Gage Papers, Southern Historical Collection. Nott, who had traveled to Europe in the previous year to put together a cabinet for the new school, wrote to the French surgeon and anthropologist Paul Broca (October 6, 1860) saying that he had chosen to spend his time teaching surgery rather than doing anthropological research. I am indebted to Joy Harvey for providing a copy of this letter; the original is in the archives of the Societé d'Anthropologie de Paris, deposited at the Musée de l'Homme, Paris.

advance. The medical world are not looking to the far distant Mississippi for any discovery in surgery."[6]

In the appraisal of some southern physicians, much of the uncertainty and lack of confidence that did exist in southern practice could be attributed to excessive reliance on external authority. Northern and European diagnostic and therapeutic directives were often inappropriate to the management of diseases in the South. Adherence to such directives, especially by young practitioners still guided by what they were taught by books and in schools rather than by their own observation, limited the success of southern physicians in their efforts to heal. "Who is to blame?" asked one North Carolina physician.

> Assuredly we of the South! Studying the works almost solely of British and continental writers, which, however perfect in all points for these regions, are sadly deficient for us, we force the form of our diseases to bend [to] their descriptions, and blindly follow a treatment intended for varieties of diseases we never witnessed. Consummate and fatal folly! Yet, year passes year only to note its repetition, whilst we, reclining in inglorious ease or censurable indifference, view the perpetuation of the error, knowing too that hundreds are yearly added to our ranks who will have to pass through the same trials and difficulties, and experience the same disasters we encountered, before they will be enabled to diagnose correctly, or treat successfully any diseases, save those common to all countries, without a warning, a sign or explanation from us to guide the neophyte through the labyrinth before him.[7]

The inadequacy of northern educational authority for practice in the South, southerners held, coupled with many physicians' persistent dependence upon it, misdirected the southern practitioner, imperiled public confidence in the profession, and encouraged quackery.

The underlying cause to which physicians attributed the South's medical degeneracy was the lethargy of the southern medical profes-

6. S. L. Grier, "Is Typhoid or Epidemic Pneumonia Identical with Periodic Fevers?" *New Orleans Medical and Surgical Journal*, IX (1852–53), 435; Samuel A. Cartwright, "Some Account of a New Method of Reducing Dislocations, Applicable Both to Recent and Ancient Cases," *New Orleans Medical Journal*, I (1844–45), 43. Typical objections to northern judgments are J. H. Bernard, "Inaugural Dissertation on Pneumonia" (M.D. thesis, Medical Department of the University of Nashville, 1857), Special Collections, Medical Center Library, Vanderbilt University, Nashville; Bennet Dowler, "Illustrations of Fever," *New Orleans Medical and Surgical Journal*, XVI (1859), 217–28; and "[Review of] George B. Wood (U. Penn.), 'A treatise on the practice of medicine,'" *New Orleans Medical and Surgical Journal*, IV (1847–48), 704–706.

7. "Report of Otis Frederick Manson, M.D., on Malarial Pneumonia," *New Orleans Medical News and Hospital Gazette*, IV (1857–58), 402.

sion, which by leading them to follow uncritically the authority of northern medical dogma, had permitted the rise of quackery and the concomitant degradation of their profession's standing. "From indolence and neglect," observed Fenner, "our profession has in some degree lost caste in society, and consequently its legitimate domain has been exposed to incursions of the vilest imposters and the most ignorant pretenders to science." This problem indicated its own solution, which was also the most immediate objective of the movement for a distinctive southern medical education, namely, to energize the physicians of the South, rousing them to a vigorous cultivation of the opportunities and obligations inherent in the region's medical particularity. This was a persistent editorial theme in southern medical literature. "Surely North Carolina has incurred the reproach of slothfulness long enough," the opening volume of one journal of that state pleaded, calling for physicians to awake from their "protracted slumber with fresh energy, redoubled strength, and broader, nobler, and more comprehensive aspirations."[8]

Fenner, for example, who was one of the leading advocates of southern medical education, plainly saw his *Southern Medical Reports* (1849–50) principally as a medium for invigorating medical activity in a listless South. He stated in the preface to the first volume that his motivation was "a desire to stimulate the physicians of the South to a more zealous and energetic prosecution of the noble science to which they have devoted their lives." In several letters written to John Young Bassett, Fenner openly explained his posture toward the publication. "In my Editorial capacity I shall take a pretty bold & independent stand respecting the *status* of the Profession in the South & shall have to rely greatly upon the respectable physicians of the Country for support," Fenner wrote. "I shall commence *cleaning up, at home.* . . . I shall take liberal views of all things & endeavor to avoid sectional feelings as much as the nature of the subject will admit. I hate every thing like *bigotry* & *sectionalism.*" If southern physicians persisted in their apathy, he complained to Bassett, it would be to the dishonor of southern medicine. "I am a *volunteer* in the cause of Medical Science in the

8. Fenner, "Introductory Address," 12; "Editorials and Miscellaneous Articles," *Medical Journal of North Carolina,* I (1858), 89. See also "Editorial and Miscellaneous," *Stethoscope and Virginia Medical Gazette,* IV (1854), 284; George R. Grant, "An Introductory Address, Delivered at the Opening of the Session of 1847–1848, to the Students of the Memphis Medical College, November 1, 1847," *South-Western Medical Advocate,* I (1847), 145–62; and Joseph LeConte, "On the Science of Medicine and the Causes Which Retard Its Progress," *Southern Medical and Surgical Journal,* n.s., VI (1850), 457.

South," he wrote. "If I do fail, I mean to make a *splendid failure* of it—one that shall stand as a *pronouncement of shame* against the physicians of my time."[9]

Energetic celebration of the South's medical distinctiveness offered physicians an opportunity not only to alleviate anxieties about their own intellectual standing, but also to generate the knowledge necessary for southern students and practitioners. "We cannot believe that the north is either morally or intellectually superior to the south," a student at the Medical College of South Carolina in Charleston urged in his thesis, which he wrote as an argument for the southern education of southern physicians. "We have all the elements . . . in our midst, and it will be a direct suicidal act, if we make this the land 'where genius sickens and where fancy dies.'" The educational needs of southern medicine could be met only if southern physicians would observe the region's diseases, formulate their own theories, and publish their pathological and therapeutic discoveries. "This task," Fenner asserted, "is imposed upon *Southern* physicians, and must be performed by them, or remain unaccomplished." Bennet Dowler, who in his own physiological investigations made use of native southern materials through his vivisectional experiments on alligators, argued further that unlike most other sciences, medicine, because ot its regional specificity, could not be imported. "In the science of medicine," a Mississippi practitioner similarly claimed, "there is no choice between a foreign supply and home production. Our medical literature cannot be *manufactured* for us abroad." Stimulus for the southern medical endeavor and validation of its products also had to come from within. Therefore, he concluded, "it behoove[s] Southern practitioners to be a law unto themselves. Verily the gods on our medical Olympus will do little for the man who cannot put his shoulder to the wheel and help himself."[10]

9. Fenner, "Introductory Address," 9; Fenner to John Young Bassett, October 24, 1849, in Bassett Papers; Fenner to Bassett, December 6, 1850, in Bassett Papers. See also Fenner to Bassett, August 8, 1849, September 18, 1849, and July 13, 1850, all in Bassett Papers.

10. William W. Cozart, "An Inaugural Dissertation on the Place Where Southern Students Should Acquire Their Medical Knowledge" (M.D. thesis, Medical College of the State of South Carolina, 1856), Waring Historical Library, Medical University of South Carolina, Charleston; E. D. F[enner], Review of James Johnson and James Ranald Martin's *The Influence of Tropical Climates on European Constitutions*, in *New Orleans Medical and Surgical Journal*, III (1846–47), 384; B. Dowler, "A Review of Medical Literature, Including Critical Remarks on Professor Palmer's Report on That Subject, As Published in the Transactions of the American Medical Association, Vol. XI," *New Orleans Medical and Surgical Journal*, XVI (1859), 441–51; S. L. Grier, "The Negro and His Diseases," *New Orleans Medical and Surgical Journal*, IX (1852–53), 763, 753.

As a consequence of the region's lethargy, physicians maintained, the singular natural resources of the South were largely unexploited. This circumstance both reflected the need for medical knowledge of southern provenance and pointed to the intellectual opportunity offered to the southern physician, for only those laboring within the region could develop its natural wealth. Staking out and exploiting this uniquely southern medical realm was crucial; as one Tennessee practitioner noted, "The Medical salvation of the man who aspires to success and usefulness depends upon it. No one can assist us in anything more than drawing the landmarks." An inward focus upon their own region was the most promising avenue for southern physicians to gain recognition and esteem. "Let us," urged Fenner, "endeavor to reciprocate . . . the obligations annually conferred by our brethren of the North and of Europe. We have a richer and more varied field for observation than they have, and, with equal industry, would be able to contribute more [than they] to the archives of medicine."[11] Southern medical investigators also sought through their work to alter the purportedly unfounded appraisal by outsiders of the South as an unhealthy region.[12]

The task of those who saw themselves as the artificers of southern medical reform was twofold. Beyond validating their endeavor and galvanizing the southern medical profession, they had to produce specific medical accomplishments that at once actualized and symbolized their personal and regional aspirations for intellectual legitimacy. As they perceived it, this latter aspect of their duty encompassed both concrete contributions to medical knowledge and especially the elevation of southern medical institutions.

Although the program for southern medical reform extended to all the various institutions for the production and dissemination of medical knowledge and promotion of professional unity, the largest portion of reformist energies focused upon the instruments of medical education. Of these, medical schools offered the most potent symbol of professional uplift. While a degraded condition of southern schools plainly represented the dependency of the South on northern sources of knowledge, at the same time the changing status of these institu-

11. S. P. Crawford, "Southern Medical Literature," *Nashville Medical and Surgical Journal*, XVIII (1860), 197; Fenner, "Introductory Address," 11–12. See also "Introduction," *Southern Medical and Surgical Journal*, I (1837), 3.

12. See J. C. Nott, "An Examination into the Health and Longevity of the Southern Sea Ports of the United States, with Reference to the Subject of Life Insurance," *Southern Journal of Medicine and Pharmacy*, II (1847), 2; and "[Review of] Southern Medical Reports . . . edited by E. D. Fenner," *Charleston Medical Journal and Review*, V (1850), 531.

tions offered an index by which the progress of the envisioned medical renaissance in the region could be measured. Not only were northern teachings viewed as misleading for southern practice, but the fact that many southern students were sent by their preceptors to places such as Philadelphia for medical lectures encouraged the public to place the medical profession in what one Virginia medical editor called "the inferior position we have ourselves chosen to assume," for it entailed a tacit confession of the South's inability to train its own physicians. "The annual pilgrimage of Southern young men to the medical schools of the North," a New Orleans physician charged, "is an unnatural and humiliating sight, yet we have but ourselves to blame for it." Southern medical schools could redress the imbalance, an Alabama physician asserted, "leading us out of the bondage entailed upon us by the schools of Europe and the North."[13]

The notion that southern medical education was an imperative imposed by nature was a point emphasized again and again in the literature arguing for a distinctive southern medicine. Southern physicians maintained that differences between regions and their medical sects were ordained by the natural order of things; they were not artificial products of political or social choices, and therefore patterning institutions to take these differences into account was not only proper but necessary. "As surely as there is a distinction between foreign and American medicine, so surely is there a distinction between Northern and Southern medicine," a New Orleans physician argued. "Nature alone is the sectionalist, and we are but her humble interpreter." Fenner reiterated these words when he assertively denied a northern charge that the movement for southern medical education was politi-

13. "The Medical Department of the University of Virginia," *Virginia Medical and Surgical Journal*, IV (1855), 160; "The New Orleans School of Medicine," *New Orleans Medical News and Hospital Gazette*, III (1856–57), 163; W. Taylor, "Annual Oration," in *Transactions of the Medical Association of the State of Alabama at Its Eighth Annual Session . . . Mobile, February 5,–6,–7, 1855* (Mobile, 1855), 127. See Sam[ue]l Cartwright, "Philosophy of the Negro Constitution," *New Orleans Medical and Surgical Journal*, IX (1852–53), 207–208; P. H. Lewis, "Reply to Dr. W. M. Boling's Review of Doctor Lewis' Medical History of Alabama, with Some New Facts and Remarks, in Relation to the Diagnosis and Identity of the Fevers of the South," *New Orleans Medical and Surgical Journal*, IV (1847–48), 639; John W. Monette, "Observations on the Pathology and Treatment of the Endemic Fevers of the Southwest, Commonly Called 'Congestive Fever,'" *New Orleans Medical Journal*, I (1844–45), 126; and the resolutions regarding southern medical education by the state medical associations of Alabama and Mississippi, in "Proceedings of the Medical Association of the State of Alabama—Mobile, December, 1850," *Southern Medical and Surgical Journal*, n.s., VII (1851), 311; and in "Mississippi Medical Convention," *New Orleans Medical and Surgical Journal*, II (1845–46), 684.

cally motivated and represented "States Rights Medicine": "If this be *sectional medicine,*" he retorted, "I cannot help it. It was not made so by me, but by Nature."[14]

Physicians' allegiance to specificity, which provided the theoretical foundation for a distinctive southern medicine, meant that the core of any intellectually compelling program for southern medical education had to be personal experience with southern practice. Underlying this link between specificity and the pedagogical emphasis placed upon practical experience was an assumed distinction between region-specific and universal categories of medical knowledge. "As to the study of the *rudiments* of the science of medicine (Anatomy, Physiology, and Chemistry,)," explained an Alabama practitioner, "they can be learned North, as well as South, for *they* are the same everywhere." But he contrasted the universality of medical principles with the regional specificity of practice, which was best learned by "observation at the bedside" in the locality where the student intended to practice. "Our practice here," he continued, "is entirely different from that taught in northern institutions, and by northern writers."[15] Thus it was commonly stressed that a medical graduate of a northern school who migrated to the South would have to unlearn many of his teachers' precepts in realms such as therapeutics and prognosis and replace them with rules of practice developed from his own experience at the bedside.[16]

Accordingly, the pivot upon which southern schools' claims to a singular ability to educate southern physicians turned was clinical instruction. Incorporating those branches of medicine that *were* region-specific, clinical training both gave southern medical education its

14. "Medical Schools, No. 1," *New Orleans Medical News and Hospital Gazette,* III (1856–57), 678; E. D. Fenner, *Introductory Lecture, Delivered at the Opening of the New Orleans School of Medicine, on the 17th November, 1856* (New Orleans, 1856), 23. See also W. M. Carpenter, "Introductory Lecture Delivered before the Medical Class of the Louisiana Medical College on the 20th Nov. 1844," *New Orleans Medical Journal,* I (1844–45), 367; and "Medical Sectionalism," *New Orleans Medical News and Hospital Gazette,* IV (1857–58), 158.

15. Jas. C. Billingslea, "An Appeal on Behalf of Southern Medical Colleges and Southern Medical Literature," *Southern Medical and Surgical Journal,* n.s., XII (1856), 400, 399. See also "Medical Lectures for 1857–58," *Southern Journal of Medicine and Pharmacy,* VI (1857), 225–28.

16. See Fenner, "Introductory Address," 10; "Editorials and Miscellaneous," *Virginia Medical and Surgical Journal,* III (1854), 86; and H. V. M. Miller, "Valedictory Address to the First Graduating Class of the Medical College of Memphis, Delivered on the 5th Day of March, 1847, and Published at the Request of the Class," *South-Western Medical Advocate,* I (1847), 49–67.

identity and drew attention to the inadequacies of northern schools. The student trained in Philadelphia who returned South would "find himself deficient in that education of the senses which observation alone can give," a New Orleans physician maintained, and as a practitioner would have to reject northern precepts and "set about to acquire that knowledge which he should have derived from clinical instruction when a student." Thus for knowledge about medical practice, "that a student can learn any more in Philadelphia or Paris than he can in Nashville, Charleston or New Orleans is all a farce, an idle whim," the editors of the *Georgia Blister* asserted. "Medicine is only successfully learned by practical and personal experience. . . . It is the greatest piece of folly imaginable," they continued, "for Southern students to be going to Paris and Philadelphia to learn Southern medicine."[17]

While such claims were based upon a genuine belief in the necessity of regional medical training, they plainly were informed by economic motives as well. Commitments to reform and professional uplift in no way exempted southern schools from the pressures of a competitive market. Physicians in the South, as elsewhere, created and operated medical schools to secure financial profit and prestige, the measure of which was largely determined by the number of students they could enroll. Many of the physicians who most vocally supported southern medical education, including the New Orleans practitioner and Georgia editors quoted above, had proprietary interests in a medical school, and fashioned increasingly impassioned appeals to convince southern students who persisted in studying in the North to change their ways. But it would be a mistake to regard their rhetorical commitment to southern medical education as merely an invidious guise for economic self-interest. Physicians who urged regional education had not necessarily been suborned by proprietary interests, for not only individual profit but also regional medical betterment were to be gained by persuading students to remain in the South.

The faculties of the South's various medical schools were, of course, competing not only with northern teachers but also among themselves for paying students. Southern medical schools were enormously diverse in their structures, facilities, and orientations. When a Virginia medical journal urged in 1852 that professional elevation demanded "a great Southern medical institution," it cogently observed that "a con-

17. J[ohn] H[arrison], "[Review of] *Annual Announcement of the Jefferson Medical College.* (Philadelphia, 1848)," *New Orleans Medical and Surgical Journal*, V (1848–49), 346–47; "Southern Medical Schools—Southern Toadyism," *Georgia Blister and Critic*, I (1854), 34–35.

test is soon to commence—if it has not already begun—which will decide *where* this college shall be situated."[18] What each school elected to emphasize in eliciting the profession's support and attracting students had as much to do with the limitations and strengths of the resources at hand as it did with any notion of a model institution's attributes. Atlanta, Knoxville, Mobile, Nashville, New Orleans, and Richmond, among others, each claimed to have the location most favorable for the development of a center for southern medical education. Richmond's advocates argued that any city farther south would be too warm for anatomical instruction; Mobile's supporters charged that other cities, such as New Orleans, were too frequently attacked by epidemics for the safety of students; Knoxville's spokesmen pointed out that their city was not only healthy for summer study and anatomical pursuits, but also accessible from all parts of the South.[19]

Yet central to almost all southern discussions about the merits of various cities as locations for a medical school was a preoccupation with clinical education. The spokesmen for cities such as Charleston and Mobile that had substantial clinical facilities stressed their educational value, while physicians of Charlottesville and Knoxville pointed to their communities' potential for clinical instruction.[20] Atlanta's advocates openly acknowledged that their small town's school was at a disadvantage because it could not compete with the clinical opportunities of the New Orleans hospitals, which were "superior in this

18. "The Great Medical Centre of the South," *Stethoscope and Virginia Medical Gazette,* II (1852), 468.

19. "Atlanta Medical College," *Atlanta Medical and Surgical Journal,* I (1855–56), 243–45; Edward H. Barton, *Introductory Lecture on the Climate and Salubrity of New-Orleans, and Its Suitability for a Medical School* (New Orleans, 1835); "Can a Medical College Succeed in Atlanta?" *Georgia Blister and Critic,* I (1854), 120–22; James Conquest Cross, "On the Propriety of Establishing a School of Medicine in the City of Memphis, Tennessee," *South-Western Medical Advocate,* I (1847), 1–47; "The Great Medical Centre of the South," 468–76; "Is Knoxville Eligible As a Site for a Medical School?" *Southern Journal of Medical and Physical Sciences,* IV (1856), 57–62; Taylor, "Annual Oration," 111–29; "Virginia Medical Schools," *Stethoscope and Virginia Medical Gazette,* I (1851), 44–45.

20. "The Great Medical Centre of the South," 469; "Is Knoxville Eligible," 61–62; "The Medical College of the State of South Carolina," *Charleston Medical Journal and Review,* XIV (1859), 858; "The Medical Department of the University of Virginia," *Virginia Medical and Surgical Journal,* IV (1855), 161; "Mobile Medical Association," *Montgomery Daily Message,* March 10, 1857, clipping in Alabama Medical Society Papers, Maps and Manuscripts Division, State of Alabama Department of Archives and History; Paul F. Eve, "Address to the Class, on Opening the Course of Lectures in the Medical College of Georgia, the 17th of October, 1837," *Southern Medical and Surgical Journal,* III (1839), 5; Taylor, "Annual Oration," 125.

respect to any other city in the Union." However, they pointed out "some counterbalancing advantages which lie at the very foundation of the usefulness of the medical man." Unlike New Orleans, their town was conducive "to an avoidance of excesses, the indulgence in which too often, during a residence in large cities, lays the foundation for a life of dissipation and degradation." Nevertheless, nearly all southern physicians recognized the superiority of New Orleans for hospital instruction. "What can not be furnished by Charleston, Richmond, Augusta, Savannah, Atlanta, Mobile or Nashville," claimed the editors of a Georgia medical journal, "can be found in New Orleans, where immense hospital facilities, and the greatest possible variety of disease, are spread out without obstruction to the enquiring student." "New Orleans," they asserted, "*must* and *should* become the great centre of medical teaching in the South."[21]

In the late antebellum period, the New Orleans School of Medicine, founded in 1856 by Fenner and a group of assertively progressive physicians who characterized themselves as "Young Physic,"[22] was perhaps regarded as the school best suited to fulfill physicians' aspirations for southern medical education. In this school, the variety of commitments that animated the movement for southern medical distinctiveness and the use of education as a professional leaven clearly intersected. The school's faculty shared a concern about the low standing of the medical profession in the United States, and especially the South, and regarded educational reform as the principal means of professional improvement. By lengthening the term of study, appointing additional professors, and requiring substantial clinical work, they were self-consciously fulfilling the American Medical Association's program for educational reconstruction. They regarded their school not merely as an instrument for training physicians, but also as an objectification of needed reforms that would serve as an exemplar for other schools. Fully in keeping with their professed objectives, they sought to compete successfully for students, not by lowering their requirements, as many proprietary schools did, but by elevating their standards. Moreover, the faculty was solidly committed to introducing a plan of instruction that celebrated the South's medical distinctive-

21. Quotations from "Atlanta Medical College—Close of the Session," *Atlanta Medical and Surgical Journal*, IV (1858–59), 51; "Southern Medicine," *Atlanta Medical and Surgical Journal*, V (1860), 446–47; "New Orleans School of Medicine," *Atlanta Medical and Surgical Journal*, V (1860), 755.

22. "Editorial and Miscellaneous," *New Orleans Medical News and Hospital Gazette*, II (1855–56), 139.

ness. Their school would exploit southern medical resources, educate practitioners sensitive to distinctively southern medical needs, and further the medical regeneration of the South.[23]

The most striking characteristic of the New Orleans School of Medicine was the central position accorded clinical instruction as the medium through which the faculty hoped to bring its reformation to fruition. In part, this school, like other schools, was making use of the available resources to give it a competitive advantage. But beyond this, the faculty was explicitly emphasizing that portion of medical education, clinical knowledge, that *was* specific to region. In doing so, they were also self-consciously, albeit selectively, drawing upon the epistemology of the Paris clinical school. Indeed, Parisian epistemology, coupled with faith in specificity, provided the most powerful theoretical components of the argument supporting distinctive southern medical education.

The philosophy of the Paris clinical school has commonly been regarded as a source of universalizing tendencies in medical thought. Movements toward universally applicable diagnostic and therapeutic criteria can be found in the Paris school's sharper delineation of diseases into more rigid ontological categories through pathoanatomical correlation with clinical observation, as well as in attempts to discover clinical truth by the application of numerical methods that transcended individual idiosyncrasies in order to set up universal norms. But the thrust of Parisian medical philosophy, as it was used by Americans, cut two ways. Southern physicians took the main methodological message of the Paris school to be a firm emphasis on empirical clinical observation as the principal means of generating and validating diagnostic and therapeutic knowledge. This interpretation fostered the notion that in such realms of medicine as therapeutics, knowledge could best be gathered and transmitted where the patients to whom and place within which that knowledge would ultimately be applied came together. Thus while southern physicians acknowledged Paris as the leading locus of scientific activity and source of knowledge in the basic medical sciences, they could reject Paris as a source of knowledge in areas such as therapeutics by using one interpretation of the Paris

23. D. Warren Brickell, "Introductory Lecture," *New Orleans Medical News and Hospital Gazette*, IV (1857–58), 597; "Health of Our City and Its Prospects—Financial and Educational," *New Orleans Medical News and Hospital Gazette*, VII (1860–61), 620; "Medical Schools, No. 4—The American Medical Association and the Question of Medical Education—How Nearly Has the New Orleans School of Medicine Conformed to the Proposed Standard?" *New Orleans Medical News and Hospital Gazette*, IV (1857–58), 294–301.

school's empirical epistemology to reject the validity of Parisian therapeutic knowledge for southern practice.

The New Orleans School of Medicine actively exploited the abundant clinical resources of Charity Hospital, which admitted 12,192 patients in the year before the school was founded. The curriculum's clinical emphasis was facilitated bureaucratically by policies of the State of Louisiana giving students free access to the wards and physically by the construction of the school's building across the street from the hospital. "The knowledge and treatment of actual existing disease," argued the editor of the school's journal, who later joined its faculty, "can only be understood, only appreciated, by being in its presence. The practice of medicine can only be acquired in hospitals, in dissecting rooms, in being near the body." Fenner told students at the school's opening, "You may study elsewhere the different branches of medical education—anatomy, physiology, materia medica and chemistry; but when you come to study disease, a well-regulated hospital affords the greatest advantages. You go there to convert theoretical into practical knowledge." Through daily clinical instruction at the Charity Hospital, modeled after a plan that the school's catalog identified as "that which has been found so eminently successful in the hospitals of Paris," the student was brought "by daily lessons at the bed-side, into immediate contact with the disease he will be called on to treat." "This institution," Fenner urged, "is of special importance to the Southern Medical Student, on account of its presenting the very types and varieties of disease he will meet with when he goes into practice."[24]

The argument for southern medical education, which began to grow in force in the early 1830s, became strongest in the 1850s when it was

---

24. Quotations from [Editorial on Medical Education], *New Orleans Medical News and Hospital Gazette*, I (1855), 123; E. D. Fenner, "Introductory Address Delivered at the Opening of the New Orleans School of Medicine, on the 17 Nov., '56," *New Orleans Medical News and Hospital Gazette*, III (1856–57), 599; *Annual Report and Circular of the New Orleans School of Medicine* (New Orleans, 1857), 5; *Announcement of the New Orleans School of Medicine* (New Orleans, 1856), 5; Fenner, "Introductory Address Delivered at . . . the New Orleans School of Medicine," 579. On the hospital's clinical resources, see *Rapport du Conseil des Administrateurs de l'Hôpital de Charité à la Législature de l'état de la Louisiane* (New Orleans, 1857), 17. The faculty also set up a free dispensary to recruit patients of different sorts for clinical instruction; see "The Free Dispensary of the New Orleans School of Medicine," *New Orleans Medical News and Hospital Gazette*, III (1856–57), 735–38; and "The Free Dispensary of the New Orleans School of Medicine," *New Orleans Medical News and Hospital Gazette*, V (1858–59), 179–81. The frequently repeated objective of the school's faculty was to make New Orleans "the Paris of America"; see, for example, "The Lecture Season," *New Orleans Medical News and Hospital Gazette*, IV (1857–58), 552.

both objectified and encouraged by the founding of institutions such as the New Orleans School of Medicine. The movement for southern students to favor southern educational institutions seemed to reach a dramatic climax during the 1859–1860 winter term when some three hundred southern medical students attending lectures at the Jefferson College and University of Pennsylvania medical schools seceded and migrated en masse to southern schools, a course soon followed by over fifty students at the New York University.[25] Historians have not distinguished the animus of this movement from that of the case for southern medical distinctiveness, yet such a distinction is crucial to understanding the movement for southern medical education. Assessed within the context of arguments for southern medical distinctiveness, the secession was epiphenomenal. It was a political act driven by political energies and was unambiguously regarded as such at the time.

Motivation for the secession is properly ascribed to what southerners perceived as the invidious political, social, and moral atmosphere of the late antebellum North. Some southerners viewed the North as a source of immoral, dangerous ideas, particularly abolitionism. The proximate stimulus for the secession movement was southern offense at the "moral stench" created in Philadelphia by sympathizers with John Brown after the abolitionist's execution. "This infernal howl from unleashed furies," a Nashville medical journal charged, "seems to have been loudest and longest at Philadelphia. Its atmosphere was literally poisoned by the foul and nauseous exhalations from the ulcerous throats and lungs of these malignant devils." Moreover, south-

---

The methods of clinical instruction in Dublin also provided a model for teaching at the Charity Hospital, as Edward C. Atwater points out in "Internal Medicine," in Ronald L. Numbers (ed.), *The Education of American Physicians: Historical Essays* (Berkeley, 1980), 164–66. On clinical instruction at the New Orleans School of Medicine, see E. D. Fenner, *A Guide: Clinical Instruction, Prepared for Medical Students* (New Orleans, 1858); and Austin Flint, "Clinical Reports on Cases Observed at the New Orleans Charity Hospital, 1858–9," *New Orleans Medical News and Hospital Gazette*, VI (1859–60), 162.

25. On the secession movement, see Harold J. Abrahams, "Secession from Northern Medical Schools," *Transactions and Studies of the College of Physicians of Philadelphia*, 4th ser., XXXVI (1968–69), 29–45; James O. Breeden, "States-Rights Medicine in the Old South," *Bulletin of the New York Academy of Medicine*, LII (1976), 348–72; and John Duffy, "Sectional Conflict and Medical Education in Louisiana," *Journal of Southern History*, XXIII (1957), 289–306. A jaundiced but exceptionally detailed account of the secession is the "Collection of Newspaper Clippings Concerning Secession of Southern Students from Schools in Philadelphia [and New York] in 1859," in Historical Collection, Library of the College of Physicians of Philadelphia.

erners viewed the northern public as hostile toward southern students. "I believe these Yankees here can tell a Southern student as soon as they [see] him," a North Carolina student attending medical lectures at the University of Pennsylvania wrote to his brother in November of 1859. "They will stare at us like we were some terrible monsters." Six weeks later, in the same letter to his father that contained his sympathetic description of the secession agitation among his southern classmates, in which he did not participate, he commented that "the policemen here will arrest a student especially a Southern student for little or nothing."[26]

The abundant literature the secession movement generated was almost entirely devoid of references to southern medical distinctiveness. In the view of southern physicians who wrote about the secession, as well as in the resolutions and speeches of the students themselves, the secessionists' behavior was a response to a threatening sociopolitical situation that held for them weighty moral implications; there is almost no evidence that the students' actions were motivated by medical considerations.[27] In a letter to his cousin, a Virginian studying medicine in New York characterized the secession movement as "the fiery & precipitate impulses of a few ardent and indignant striplings who endeavor on all occasions to make themselves perfect *Nincompoofs* and a laughing stock for the public." He continued:

> I know that they were actuated by the best motives in acting as they did, but it really provoked me to see Southern men exposing themselves to the ridicule of the filthy and corrupt northern press and I frankly and freely told them exactly what I thought of the ridiculous attitude a good many of them had assumed. . . . I spoke in free and open terms, condemnation of their premature action, and endeavoured to impress upon them the utter absur-

26. "Seceding Students," *Nashville Medical and Surgical Journal*, XVIII (1860), 170–71, 174; Thomas J. Badgett to A. Badgett, November 3, 1859, in Badgett Papers, North Carolina State Archives, Raleigh; Thomas J. Badgett to "Dear Papa," December 18, 1859, in Badgett Papers.

27. See, for example, "Return of Southern Medical Students from Northern Colleges," *Southern Medical and Surgical Journal*, XVI (1860), 73–76; "Southern Medical Students and Southern Medical Schools," *New Orleans Medical News and Hospital Gazette*, VII (1860–61), 110–125; "Southern Medical Students," *Medical Journal of North Carolina*, III (1860), 519–22; "Southern Medicine," *Atlanta Medical and Surgical Journal*, V (1860), 445–47; "Southern Students in Northern Medical Colleges," *New Orleans Medical News and Hospital Gazette*, VI (1859–60), 849–51; and "Southern Students Leaving the Medical Schools of Philadelphia," *New Orleans Medical News and Hospital Gazette*, VI (1859–60), 935–37. An exception was the Mississippi physician W. H. H. Williams' address to the entering class at the Medical Department of the University of Nashville; see "Valedictory to the Class," *Nashville Medical and Surgical Journal*, XVIII (1860), 299–306.

dity of the course they were pursuing viz the idea of 3 or 400 Medical Students taking the initiatory steps toward the disruption of the American Union. I told them that no man was more devoted to Southern interests or jealous of Southern honour than myself and when the time came I should be found at the first blast of the trumpet occupying my position 'upon the tented field' aye in the very vanguard defending Southern rights and institutions.[28]

The editors of southern medical journals commonly separated articles on the secession movement from the medical content of their journals by prefaces that identified such articles as awkward items of political interest that merited inclusion in medical journals only because the actors in the secession were incidentally medical students and physicians.

In fact, southern physicians were not reluctant to attack medical men whom they perceived as allowing political commitments to influence the views they formulated about southern medical distinctiveness or education. Southern physicians differed widely in the extent to which they espoused educational separatism, but they held in common the assumptions underlying Samuel Cartwright's arguments that the region's peculiar climate and large population of blacks demanded a distinctive southern medicine. However, while they shared Cartwright's premises, some physicians attacked the extremism of his conclusions, especially his strident pronouncements on the singularity of Negro physiology, as products of Cartwright's political beliefs. "To mingle medicine and politics," a Charleston reviewer charged, "is an unholy contamination of the former, which no wily argument can justify, no apology atone for." The reviewer agreed with Cartwright that the medical needs of blacks were sufficiently distinctive that special chairs of the diseases of Negroes should be set up in southern medical schools, but dissented from the "Cartwrightic-Ethiopian philosophy," holding that "medicine and politics are as incompatible as acids and alkalies, and he who mingles the two is no friend of either." When Cartwright extended his animosity toward abolitionism to an attack on northern medical schools and their professors, one physician dismissed his views as "the impotent effervescence of a mind distracted by political enthusiasm."[29]

28. John W. Lawson to [James DeWitt Hankins], November 28, 1860, in John William Lawson Letter, Manuscripts Department, Alderman Library, University of Virginia, Charlottesville. I am grateful to Thomas P. McPherson for granting me permission to quote from this letter.

29. "[Review of] Cartwright on the Diseases and Peculiarities of the Negro Race," *Charleston Medical Journal and Review,* VII (1852), 92, and see VI (1851), 829–43. See also "Dr.

The reaction of thinking southern physicians to the secession was marked by ambivalence rather than enthusiasm. Typically, the acting dean of the Medical College of Georgia, answering an inquiry from a student considering secession about transferring to that college, pointed out the social and moral superiority of Augusta over Philadelphia, but said nothing about the medical advantages of attending a southern school. "There is but one feeling in our Faculty," he wrote, "a profound paternal sympathy toward students who are subjected to the taunts of vile abolitionists in Northern Cities. We therefore cordially extend an invitation to you & to all southern students who may desire to return south."[30] As a political act, the category to which southern physicians almost universally assigned it, the secession was admissible and perhaps admirable; but as a medical act vitiated by political motivations it threatened violence to the sanctity of southern medical reform. To have endorsed this act with the case for southern education based upon southern medical distinctiveness would have been to risk political debasement of a movement that was crucial to the self-definition of southern physician-intellectuals. The secession implied that choices regarding education should be made according to political criteria, such as a desire to protect students from immoral abolitionist rhetoric, rather than criteria designed to serve medical excellence. It thus partook in the late antebellum South's rising anti-intellectualism, a reaction fundamentally at odds with the reform commitments that animated the case for southern medical education.[31]

Cartwright and Ourselves," *Charleston Medical Journal and Review,* VII (1852), 719–20; and James T. Smith, "Review of Dr. Cartwright's Report on the Diseases and Physical Peculiarities of the Negro Race," *New Orleans Medical and Surgical Journal,* VIII (1851–52), 228–37. Cartwright's article "Report on the Diseases and Physical Peculiarities of the Negro Race" was published in the *New Orleans Medical and Surgical Journal,* VIII (1851–52), 369–73. On Cartwright's views, see especially James Denny Guillory, "The Pro-Slavery Arguments of Dr. Samuel A. Cartwright," *Louisiana History,* IX (1968), 209–27; Guillory, "Southern Nationalism and the Louisiana Medical Profession, 1840–1860" (M.A. thesis, Louisiana State University, 1965); and Mary Louise Marshall, "Samuel A. Cartwright and States' Rights Medicine," *New Orleans Medical and Surgical Journal,* XCIII (1940), 74–78.

30. L. A. Dugas to J. E. Hawkins, December 19, 1859, in J. E. Hawkins Papers, Manuscripts Division, Louisiana State University Library, Baton Rouge.

31. On antebellum southern anti-intellectualism, see Clement Eaton, *Freedom of Thought in the Old South* (Durham, 1940), and Eaton, *The Mind of the Old South* (Rev. ed.; Baton Rouge, 1967), 305. For a brief analysis of the postbellum course of the argument for educational distinctiveness in southern medicine, see John Harley Warner, "Medical Education," in William Ferris and Charles R. Wilson (eds.), *Encyclopedia of Southern Culture* (Chapel Hill, in press).

The argument for southern medical education is best regarded as one among the variety of projects American physicians engaged in to improve the standing of the profession in the mid-nineteenth century. Southern physicians shared with their northern and western counterparts an awareness of the profession's low status. Those physicians who spoke for a distinctive southern medicine, and used the argument to support institutional reform, were the same physicians who, in the South, were especially concerned with the reformation of medical education and elevation of the profession's standing in the United States in general. It was no coincidence that such leading exponents of southern medical distinctiveness as Erasmus Fenner and Samuel Cartwright were among the most vocal in the southern assault upon sectarianism; indeed, to them the vigorous development of southern medical education represented the best means of suppressing quackery. Nor was it a coincidence that the New Orleans School of Medicine, whose faculty as a group was perhaps the most aggressive body of proselytizers for a plan of education built around a recognition of the South's medical distinctiveness, was also among the few schools in the United States to take up the American Medical Association's proposals for medical school reform. To these physicians, the suppression of quackery, the improvement of medical education, and the case for southern medical distinctiveness all represented progressive reforms that would uplift their profession in American society.

Yet the form taken by southern physicians' response to what in part were national anxieties was substantially molded by problems and needs that were peculiarly southern. Through a distinctively southern medical reformation, thinking southern physicians believed that they could constructively respond to the national plight of their profession and at the same time alleviate anxieties that stemmed from their region's status and their own position within it. Southern physician-intellectuals, living in a region that had become a "conscious minority," and which gave little accord to intellectual inquiry, saw in the cultivation of southern medical distinctiveness a platform for uplifting the southern medical profession. Troubled by the stagnancy of the pursuit of medical knowledge in their region and frustrated in their attempts to satisfy their own social and cognitive needs, these physicians looked to the argument for southern medical education and the assumptions upon which it was based for vindication of their own importance and legitimation of the intellectual endeavor in southern medicine.

CHAPTER 11

PUBLIC HEALTH IN THE OLD SOUTH

Margaret H. Warner

By the 1840s both northern critics and southern Jeremiahs were depicting the South as the unhealthiest region of the United States. This combination of outside condemnation and self-reproach drew attention to the notion that the South was peculiarly diseased, a belief that paralleled and augmented the rising tide of southern cultural, political, and social distinctiveness. Southerners, and especially southern physicians, became increasingly concerned about the high mortality levels and the prevalence of deadly disease in their region, factors which formed the basis of its insalubrious reputation. Since the colonial period Americans of both regions had acknowledged morbid differences between North and South, but during the 1840s and 1850s a new anxiety about regional disparities marked the writings of medical southerners. This consciousness was largely occasioned by the retreat of yellow fever from northern cities, where its once-severe visitations had ceased after 1822, and the concomitant rise in both the frequency and malignancy of yellow fever in the South. Like the North and West, the South suffered from cholera, typhoid, and intermittent fevers, but it was yellow fever that distinguished it from the rest of the nation as a region where life and health were particularly endangered. In a period of assertive southern nationalism, this stigma was intolerable. Yellow fever unmistakably dominated public-health thought and activity in the antebellum South,

Research on this paper was supported in part by a predoctoral fellowship from the Educational Foundation of the American Association of University Women. I am especially grateful to Barbara Gutmann Rosenkrantz and John Harley Warner for reading and criticizing the text in its multiple incarnations.

and an analysis of southern efforts to comprehend and control this disease offers the most promising means of understanding the public-health endeavor in this region.

The emerging awareness of the unwelcome distinction conferred upon the South by yellow fever, which first became acute in the two decades before the Civil War, coincided chronologically not only with the efflorescence of southern sectionalism, but also with the well-studied public-health reform movements of the American Northeast, England, and France.[1] Southern physicians concerned about public health shared with their reform-minded colleagues elsewhere the belief that disease was not preordained by some supernatural power, but was the result of physical, often man-made, causes and could be overcome if governmental power were directed against the sources of disease. There can be little doubt that the promotion of urban sanitation in the South was on the whole less energetic and its achievements less impressive than in the Northeast or Europe. But little insight can be gained into the inner workings of southern public health by systematically comparing public health in the South and North to establish the extent of southern inferiority or parity. After all, the South did differ from the North socially, economically, intellectually, demographically, and, not the least, epidemiologically, and the simple fact that these differences affected public-health activity is hardly surprising. Instead, to understand public health in the antebellum South, we must scrutinize the choices that were open to southerners concerned about public health and the decisions they made against the backdrop of the southern environment, an environment forcefully shaped by the reality of yellow fever.[2] My initial task, then, is to explicate the variety of public-health tools that reformers sought to use to control yellow fever and better their singularly insalubrious region. I will next examine the changing structure and evidential foundation of the etiological theory that guided and justi-

1. On these movements, see John Duffy, *A History of Public Health in New York, 1625–1866* (New York, 1968); Barbara Gutmann Rosenkrantz, *Public Health and the State: Changing Views in Massachusetts, 1842–1936* (Cambridge, Mass., 1972); John M. Eyler, *Victorian Social Medicine: The Ideas and Methods of William Farr* (Baltimore, 1979); William Coleman, *Death Is a Social Disease: Public Health and Political Economy in Early Industrial France* (Madison, 1982).

2. In my study "Public Health in the New South: Government, Medicine and Society in the Control of Yellow Fever" (Ph.D. dissertation, Harvard University, 1983), I show that the goals of southern public health officials in the postbellum years were strikingly different from those of their northern counterparts, and the foundations of this disparity were evident in the decades preceding the Civil War.

fied public-health action against yellow fever in the South, constituted the chief focus of research related to public health, and provided the main outlet for the sense of epidemiological crisis.

Because yellow fever flourished in the seaport and inland commercial cities and towns of the South, antebellum public-health activity concentrated on the urban setting. All boards of health established in the Old South were civic in scope, even the so-called Louisiana State Board of Health (1855), which in reality was no more than another New Orleans board. Although city authorities appointed boards of health to battle yellow fever in Norfolk (1800), New Orleans (1804), Charleston (1808), Natchez (1841), and Mobile (1841), such organizations generally had no continuous existence and became active only when an epidemic was imminent or already in force. The boards typically were charged with enforcing quarantine codes that dated from the colonial or territorial periods and frequently had broad sanitary responsibilities as well.[3] Medical members of the boards of health and the port physicians whose task it was to inspect ships in quarantine became the South's first true public-health officials. But their influence was for the most part overshadowed by that of a larger body of physicians, otherwise prominent in the southern medical community, who appointed themselves guardians of the public welfare and spokesmen for the need for public-health reform.

Beginning in the 1840s, the oppressive recurrence of yellow fever epidemics in the South led to intense study of the nature, course, and cause of the disease. Out of this attention to yellow fever, and from the extensive experience with the disease many southern physicians gained during the 1840s and 1850s, came a transformation of etiological theory in the South. By the mid-1850s, in contrast to the anticontagionist consensus of the earlier years of the century, most southern

---

3. The early history of the Louisiana State Board of Health is discussed in John Duffy (ed.), *The Rudolph Matas History of Medicine in Louisiana* (2 vols.; Baton Rouge, 1958–62), II, 160–97; and Gordon E. Gillson, *Louisiana State Board of Health: The Formative Years* (N.p., 1967), 35–76. Duffy and Gillson provide excellent accounts of the complex politics and year-by-year events characteristic of Louisiana public health in the antebellum period. Information on other southern boards of health and quarantines can be found in Wyndham B. Blanton, *Medicine in Virginia in the Eighteenth Century* (Richmond, 1931), 396–99; Blanton, *Medicine in Virginia in the Nineteenth Century* (Richmond, 1933), 224–71; Joseph Ioor Waring, *A History of Medicine in South Carolina* (3 vols.; Columbia, S.C., 1964–71), I, 48–61, 147–59, and II, 30–70; Carey V. Stabler, "The History of the Alabama Public Health System" (Ph.D. dissertation, Duke University, 1944), 1–42; Felix J. Underwood and R. N. Whitfield, *Public Health and Medical Licensure in the State of Mississippi, 1798–1937* (Jackson, Miss., 1938), 13–21.

physicians agreed that yellow fever, whether contagious or not, was importable and hence preventable by quarantine. First widely entertained in the early 1840s, the new theory was supported especially by the spread of yellow fever from New Orleans upriver and also by indications that particular epidemics had originated from clear sources of imported infection. The theory led to the revival of rigid quarantines and a simultaneous campaign for the improvement of urban sanitation. Public-health activists sought both to exclude the "virus" of yellow fever, whatever its nature, and to render sterile its subsequent habitat should it elude quarantine. On the eve of the Civil War, there were few unadulterated quarantinists or sanitationists publishing in the South, and a compromise view that recommended both techniques had come to dominate public-health theory. The transportability doctrine had brought the contending schools together in theory, but it left enough unanswered questions, such as the precise importance of filth and exact nature of the disease germ, to prevent the solid consolidation of public-health reform efforts behind a single, unambiguously defined goal.

Southerners did not ignore the other major epidemic of the period, cholera, but it figured much less prominently in discussions about public health. The cholera epidemic of the 1830s, which proved so deadly to the Northeast, touched much of the South lightly. The epidemic that spanned the years 1848–1855 was more serious in its impact, especially in and around New Orleans, but since the disease struck heavily in the Midwest as well, it did not peculiarly stigmatize the South. Cholera provided the principal inspiration for public-health activity only in cities such as Richmond, Nashville, and Memphis, which were rarely or not at all subject to yellow fever. In response to the threat of cholera the editors of medical journals in these cities promoted civic sanitation and personal hygiene, and temporary boards of health were established to fight cholera in, for example, Richmond (1832), Nashville (1854), and Knoxville (1855). Cholera motivated public-health action in some cities, but it was yellow fever that by and large fostered the South's public-health image and reform activity.[4]

Every year of the two decades before the Civil War brought at least one major yellow fever epidemic in some southern maritime city.

4. Blanton, *Medicine in Virginia in the Nineteenth Century*, 238–43; "Board of Health of the City of Knoxville," *Southern Journal of Medicine and Physical Sciences*, III (1855), 92–95. On cholera in the United States, see Charles E. Rosenberg, *The Cholera Years: The United States in 1832, 1849, and 1866* (Chicago, 1962).

New Orleans, Mobile, Pensacola, Savannah, Charleston, and Norfolk were ravaged with varying frequency during these twenty years, as were numerous inland towns in their shadows. "Yellow Fever," wrote the editor of the *New-Orleans Medical Journal* in its 1844 inaugural volume, "is the *great disease* of our City and region."[5] The disease was becoming an uncomfortably familiar part of the southern landscape, while the North was not similarly afflicted. As southern medical authors repeatedly reminded their readers, Boston, New York, and Philadelphia had been free from yellow fever for at least twenty-five years by 1850, although severe epidemics had attacked the latter two during the first three decades of the nation's history. It was an indictment of southern civilization that a disease which had been conquered in the North was not only becoming more common but also deadlier and more widespread in the 1850s.

During the early settlement of the South, physicians had regarded the country, and not the city, as the region's most unhealthy place to live. The country fever, which appeared under a variety of labels—bilious, congestive, remittent, intermittent, or periodic—was generally attributed to the marsh malaria found throughout the hot, swampy lowlands of the South's rural areas. David Ramsay, a South Carolina physician writing in the late eighteenth century, typically commented that such diseases appeared after land was cleared to make way for settlements and farms, but that as cities such as Charleston grew, the land became progressively better drained, and the city accordingly more healthy. "It has long been observed in the low countries, that they who reside in towns, are more healthy than they who live dispersed in the country," said Ramsay. "The policy of removing on the approach of summer, from the country to Charleston, is therefore wise."[6] A student at the Medical College of South Carolina recalled in 1839 the history of his own area, southern Alabama. "When the country was first settling, bilious and congestive fevers were scarcely known compared to what it is at the present time," he wrote. "[Periodic] fever has become the most frequent and fatal disease of our

5. "Health of the City," *New-Orleans Medical Journal*, I (1844), 94. Likewise, Juriah Harris commented on the widespread reputation southern cities had as yellow fever sites in "Fever in Savannah," *Savannah Journal of Medicine*, I (1858–59), 285. George Augustin (ed.), *History of Yellow Fever* (New Orleans, 1909), 769–780, contains a table showing the years in which yellow fever invaded the seaboard cities of the United States.

6. David Ramsay, *A Dissertation on the Means of Preserving Health, in Charleston, and the Adjacent Low Country* (Charleston, 1790), 30. See also Ramsay, *A Sketch of the Soil, Climate, Weather, and Diseases of South-Carolina* (Charleston, 1796).

country."[7] This experience recurred as the southern frontier was extended.

Although exemption from periodic fevers had made urban areas relatively more salubrious than the country for a time, as southern communities such as Norfolk, Charleston, Mobile, and New Orleans developed during the early nineteenth century, this advantage disappeared. By the 1840s many southern cities had experienced rapid population growth fueled in part by European immigration. Contemporary accounts indicate that the medical profession was aware of the changing demographic characteristics of the region's cities and their impact on public health. For example, the chairman of the New Orleans board of health estimated in 1846 that more than 20,000 Europeans had settled there since '1841. "During the interim between '37 and '39,'" recalled one student of Mobile's medical history, "the city became filled with strangers, particularly Irish and German laborers." Census figures show a fourfold to tenfold increase in the urban populations of, for example, Alabama, Georgia, and Louisiana from 1830 to 1860.[8] The disproportionally small numbers of immigrants coming to the South, in contrast to the other regions of America, nevertheless made a significant contribution to the South's urban population.

As was the case in other American cities, urbanization and immigration brought housing and water shortages and rendered municipal systems for sewage and waste removal grossly inadequate. In the South, these processes also seemed to bring yellow fever, a disease often linked to the urban phenomena of overcrowding, putrefying organic matter, and the excavation of soil for construction. Josiah Clark Nott, the Mobile physician who studied yellow fever and vital statistics, believed that yellow fever inexorably followed the erection

7. John P. Caffry, "A Thesis on Calomel in Southern Fevers" (M.D. thesis, Medical College of the State of South Carolina, 1839), South Carolina Room, Main Library, Medical University of South Carolina, Charleston. On the ubiquity of malarial fevers in the Southeast and Southwest, respectively, see Edmund Ravenel, "On the Medical Topography of St. John's, Berkley, S.C., and Its Relations to Geology," *Charleston Medical Journal and Review*, IV (1849), 697–704; and J. P. Evans, "An Essay on Intermittent and Remittent Fevers," *ibid.*, 675–97.

8. W. P. Hort, "Report of the Board of Health on the Sanitary Condition of the City of New Orleans during the Year 1846, and the Means of Improving It," *New Orleans Medical and Surgical Journal*, III (1846–47), 468; P. H. Lewis, "Sketch of the Yellow Fever of Mobile, with a Brief Analysis of the Epidemic of 1843, in Reply to Inquiries Made by Professor Drake and Others," *New-Orleans Medical Journal*, I (1844), 288; Donald B. Dodd and Wynelle S. Dodd, *Historical Statistics of the South, 1790–1970* (University, Ala., [1973]), 2, 18, 26.

of cities on the southern seaboard. "When the forest is first levelled and a town commenced, intermittents and remittents spring up," he recounted. "As the population increases, the town spreads, and draining and paving are introduced, yellow fever, the mighty monarch of the South, who scorns the rude field and forest, plants his sceptre in the centre, and drives all other fevers to the outskirts."[9] Some physicians predicted that the next natural development in the history of the settlement of southern regions would be the reduction of the malignancy of yellow fever by sanitary improvements, which would lead to its final disappearance. This hope was widely aired in the early 1850s after a few years of mild yellow fever episodes,[10] but the fatal epidemics of the mid-fifties mocked these ambitions and embedded more deeply in the national consciousness the dangers inherent in southern urban life.

In the assessment of alarmed southerners writing in the 1840s and 1850s, yellow fever was greatly damaging their region's interests. Inhibiting immigration and investment, and hence the growth and prosperity of the cities in which it flourished, yellow fever was also very expensive to the South in more direct ways, as those who calculated the cost of major epidemics testified. In loss of labor and capital, claimed one physician who argued that immigrant lives were at least worth the average cost of a slave of similar age and productivity, New Orleans had suffered an average annual debit of almost $10.5 million from 1846 to 1851.[11] In Florida, the yellow fever epidemics of 1841 very nearly delayed the achievement of statehood by drastically reducing the territory's population. On a deeper, but less frequently articulated level, epidemics threatened the security of the southern slaveholding community by weakening the defenses against a black uprising. Because blacks were less liable to yellow fever, whites often maintained that slaves were unafraid of epidemics. Prosperous whites who could afford to flee yellow fever often left household

9. J. C. Nott, "An Examination into the Health and Longevity of the Southern Sea Ports of the United States, with Reference to the Subject of Life Insurance," *Southern Journal of Medicine and Pharmacy*, II (1847), 15.

10. See, for example, Thomas Y. Simons, "A Report on the Epidemic Yellow Fever As It Occurred in Charleston in 1852, with Statistical and Other Observations," *Charleston Medical Journal and Review*, VIII (1853), 364; and an untitled editorial in the *New Orleans Medical and Surgical Journal*, VIII (1851–52), 398.

11. J. C. Simonds, "The Sanitary Condition of New-Orleans, As Illustrated by Its Mortuary Statistics," *Charleston Medical Journal and Review*, VI (1851), 700–709. Henry E. Sigerist discussed Simonds' work in "The Cost of Illness to the City of New Orleans in 1850," *Bulletin of the History of Medicine*, XV (1944), 498–507.

slaves under minimal supervision, while free Negroes were thrown out of work by the absence of their employers. A Louisiana physician's diary reveals that the scenario of a slave revolt was not entirely unrealistic. In 1833, he recorded that during one yellow fever epidemic "the slaves took advantage of the sickness at Alexandria & the absence of many planters & formed a plan of insurrection which was discovered 2 or 3 days before the massacre."[12] The South's wealth, prosperity, and security were all imperiled by the repeated yellow fever epidemics of the antebellum period.

It was in a way ironic, and southerners would probably have said unfair, that yellow fever was the disease primarily responsible for their region's unhealthy reputation. American historian Carl Degler has summarized those characteristics of the antebellum South that have become accepted as distinguishing it from the North. The South was distinctively rural, agricultural, slaveholding, and populated by an ethnically homogenous people derived chiefly from English and Scottish stock.[13] In contrast, yellow fever was an urban disease, one that primarily killed non-southern newcomers. It was well known that people long resident in a southern city became acclimated and were in little danger during an epidemic. Blacks also possessed a degree of immunity, a fact used to support the peculiar appropriateness of blacks for southern working conditions. The South thus gained its notoriety from a disease that was primarily urban; associated not with agriculture but with the radical upturning of soil for railroads, streets, and construction; only tenuously relevant to the institution of slavery; and that struck in large part the urban poor. The distinctively southern disease was not, in this sense, southern at all.

Southern physicians recognized that their efforts to control yellow fever rested upon their knowledge of its etiology, a subject about which little was known with certainty. According to southerners seeking to improve the health of the South, it was the responsibility of all southern physicians who witnessed a yellow fever epidemic to

12. Barbara Elizabeth Miller, "Tallahassee and the 1841 Yellow Fever Epidemic" (M.A. thesis, Florida State University, 1976), 5; Diary kept by Dr. [R. F.] McGuire at Monroe, La., 1818–52 (typescript in the Special Collections Division, Howard-Tilton Memorial Library, Tulane University, New Orleans). The original manuscript of this diary is in the collections of Louisiana State University, Baton Rouge. It is difficult to judge the pervasiveness of this fear, which was probably strongest in, or near, yellow fever centers such as New Orleans, Mobile, and Charleston, and nonexistent in the rural areas of the South never threatened by yellow fever.

13. Carl N. Degler, *Place over Time: The Continuity of Southern Distinctiveness* (Baton Rouge, 1977), 27–97.

observe and record carefully information about the disease that so damaged their region. Studies of yellow fever were pursued with new vigor and purpose during the 1840s and 1850s. Such data would purportedly shed new light on the origins of yellow fever, support etiological theory with the certainty of facts, and end the harmful squabbling that had so diminished the profession in the public's estimation.[14] Yellow fever research was part of the broader southern medical renaissance Erasmus Darwin Fenner called for in the opening pages of his *Southern Medical Reports*. He urged physicians to investigate southern diseases by observing the topography, climate, demography, and peculiar symptoms characteristic of their practices. Southern physicians alone could study southern diseases and discover the knowledge necessary for the salvation of their professional and regional integrity.[15]

Urban southern physicians concerned about public health also advocated the collection of vital statistics, the registration of births, marriages, and deaths. In part, the statisticians sought to show that except for yellow fever, southern cities were fundamentally healthy; the apparent high mortality said nothing about the quality of life of the acclimated resident. Since yellow fever was the only serious danger and it was confined predominantly to what Nott called the "unwashed democracy,"[16] the better sort had little to fear in a southern city. The editors of the *New Orleans Medical and Surgical Journal*, for example, described their city as healthy unless an epidemic was actively prevailing.[17] The explicit motive behind Nott's investigations of the implications of mortality and longevity for life insurance in the South was the rebuttal of criticisms of the South's health. He argued for the longevity of the "better class" of people, those most likely to buy life insurance, and concluded that rates for southerners should not be higher than those in the rest of the country.[18] Nott's explana-

14. "Sanitary Surveys and Hygiene," *Charleston Medical Journal and Review*, VI (1849), 478; "Quarantine," *New-Orleans Medical Journal*, I (1844), 83.

15. [E. D. Fenner], "Introductory Address," *Southern Medical Reports*, I (1849), 7–13. John Harley Warner analyzed the reform animus of this effort in "A Southern Medical Reform: The Meaning of the Antebellum Argument for Southern Medical Education," *Bulletin of the History of Medicine*, LVII (1983), 364–81.

16. J. C. Nott, "Sketch of the Epidemic of Yellow Fever of 1847, in Mobile," *Charleston Medical Journal and Review*, III (1848), 4.

17. John Duffy described the extent of this attitude toward New Orleans' health in *Sword of Pestilence: The New Orleans Yellow Fever Epidemic of 1853* (Baton Rouge, 1966), 6–9.

18. Nott, "Health and Longevity," 145.

tion of the high southern mortality figures as an aberration caused by the vicious poverty of the transient population was a common one. In Norfolk the Irish slums were burned by an angry mob that blamed that town's yellow fever epidemic on the conditions surrounding and engendered by "the dirty Irish."[19] To blame the victims of yellow fever was to say that the distinctive southern disease was an unwelcome and unsolicited foreign import of the lower classes of Europe, who were not a part of the southern tradition.

Other southern physicians, who recognized the genuine unhealthiness of southern cities and were concerned about the toll from both yellow fever and the region's more deadly endemic diseases, sought in vital statistics one pathway to the improvement of public health in the South. Following the lead of British and French hygienists, as well as the resolutions of the 1847 National Medical Convention held in Philadelphia, southern sanitarians such as Edward Hall Barton and Fenner of Louisiana and P. C. Gaillard and Thomas Simons of Charleston held that the effort to control the disorder of death and disease that characterized the urban South had to include gathering statistical evidence that would demonstrate the extent of disease and guide its amelioration.[20] Accordingly, the New Orleans Board of Health stressed in its 1849 report the need for both vital statistics and accompanying sanitary surveys, arguing that if "a city or country is ignorant of the diseases fatal to its population, if it does not know the age at death, sex, color, length of residence, occupation, and in what part of the city, death took place; it must be ignorant of one of its most important duties; that which is dearest to every human being, *its sanitary condition*." Such knowledge was necessary to inform public-health action and gauge its effectiveness. The report concluded that "all laws intended to benefit the sanitary condition without a previous knowledge of *what that sanitary condition is,* are deficient in the basis of all wise legislation and trifle with common sense."[21]

While the movement supporting the collection of vital statistics

19. A. B. Williman, "An Account of the Yellow Fever Epidemic in Norfolk during the Summer of 1855," *Charleston Medical Journal and Review,* XI (1856), 163.

20. The concern of Barton, Fenner, Gaillard, and Simons about endemic urban health problems is evident in their respective contributions to the *First Report of the Committee on Public Hygiene of the American Medical Association* (Philadelphia, 1849), which contains reports on public hygiene from a number of American cities.

21. E. H. Barton, Y. R. Lemonnier, and T. G. Browning, "Annual Report of the Board of Health," *New Orleans Medical and Surgical Journal,* VI (1849–50), 665–66.

was inspired by a broader vision of urban public health than that encompassed by the scope of epidemic disease control, reformers nevertheless felt constrained to associate their cause with yellow fever prevention, an issue certain to command the attention of those accountable to the public. Even so, southern legislators were for the most part unconvinced that vital statistics were of any value in alleviating the South's diseased condition. Only in South Carolina (1853), Virginia (1853), and Kentucky (1853) was statewide registration of vital statistics required in the antebellum South. Some mortality data based on interment and hospital records were available in certain cities, but it appears that only Charleston (from 1842) had a registration plan that included births and marriages as well. In Louisiana, agitation for the registration of vital statistics surfaced again and again in the 1850s, but to no avail.[22]

Students of southern health statistics hoped that their researches would vindicate the healthiness of their unfairly maligned localities. Instead, they were appalled by their findings. "The *motive* which led me to the investigation of our Vital Statistics," a Memphis physician who explored his city's health confessed in 1851, "was the conviction . . . that Memphis is one of the healthiest places on the Mississippi river; and that a comparison of our sanitary condition with other places in this great valley, and also with other cities in the Union, would conclusively establish the truth of this opinion." Rather than refuting those who claimed Memphis was an insalubrious place, he found a higher mortality rate, "1 death in every 25 living" per year, than in any other city in the country, except New Orleans, which it nearly equalled. In like manner, J. C. Simonds began his statistical researches on New Orleans planning "to convince the world, by an array of unquestionable statistical details and impregnable arguments, that . . . our city was not the Golgotha which it was every where represented to be." Unhappily, he concluded, "So far as I have been able to obtain complete data, New-Orleans has manifestly been the most unhealthy city in the civilized world." While New Orleans was clearly perceived as the unhealthiest spot in the South, other southern cities were also branded, if to a lesser

22. Waring, *South Carolina*, II, 67, 104; Blanton, *Medicine in Virginia in the Nineteenth Century*, 9; Gillson, *Louisiana State Board of Health*, 97. J. C. Simonds, "A Memorial to the Legislature of the State of Louisiana, from the Louisiana State Medical Society, and the Physico-Medical Society of New Orleans—with Reference to the Registration of Births, Marriages and Deaths," *New Orleans Medical and Surgical Journal*, VIII (1851–52), 606–20, is the product of one such futile Louisiana initiative.

degree. Mobile was healthier than Memphis, and Charleston more so than New Orleans, but the figures that could be collected indicated to contemporaries the clearly superior health of northern cities.[23]

Critics of the statistical studies displaying the South's unhealthiness went beyond refutation to impugn the patriotism and personal morals of southerners who defamed their cities' reputations and damaged their commerce. But it would serve no purpose, statistical advocates responded, to conceal their cities' condition, for the facts were well appreciated abroad. The immigrants lost to New Orleans were of great value, greater than its supposedly vulnerable foreign trade, argued Simonds. The only solution was to reform the city, to base the prosperity of New Orleans on the solid, secure foundation of good health, and for that purpose statistics and information were vital in providing the knowledge and spirit needed for the work.[24] Elsewhere in the South public-health reformers called for an end to dishonesty, a recognition of the South's unhealthiness, and a campaign to resolve the South's health problems and so elevate its image to the rest of the country. Statistical studies revealing the high mortality of southern cities unrelated to yellow fever did not by themselves create a sense of crisis, but coupled with the incessant return, year after year, of yellow fever to the region, they contributed to the overall sense among southern medical reformers that action had to be taken to remedy the South's unhealthy situation.

23. George R. Grant, "The Vital Statistics and Sanitary Condition of Memphis, Tenn.," *New Orleans Medical and Surgical Journal*, VIII (1851–52), 690, 692, 696; Simonds, "Sanitary Condition," 677–78, 726. Simonds provided the following comparison of average urban mortality rates (*ibid.*, 687; "Contributions to the Vital Statistics of New-Orleans," *Charleston Medical Journal and Review*, V [1850], 280):

City	Deaths per 100 Population	Time Period
New Orleans	8.1	1846–50
Savannah (whites only)	4.1	1840–47
Charleston	2.6	1822–48
Baltimore	2.5	1836–49
Philadelphia	2.5	1807–40
Boston	2.2	1830–45

24. G. A. Smith attacked Grant in "On the Sanitary Condition of Memphis, Tenn.— Being a Reply to Dr. Grant's Paper, Preceding This," *New Orleans Medical and Surgical Journal*, VIII (1851–52), 706. Simonds answered his critics in "Sanitary Condition," 679.

Bolstered by the teachings of European hygienists, southern physicians committed to the improvement of public health had few doubts about the surety of one avenue to that end. To be made healthy, their cities needed to be paved, drained, and cleaned. Physicians such as Fenner and Simons were active spokesmen for the near-universal belief that the miasmata arising from the animal and vegetable wastes that filled southern streets and saturated urban soil shortened the lives of southern city dwellers. "The great object," declared Barton in a report to the Louisiana State Medical Society, "is to remove filth of all kinds as soon as possible, before it contaminates the air we breathe and the water we drink."[25] His list of recommendations was similar to that approved by the Charleston Medical Society in 1849 and others frequently found in editorials of southern medical journals. Sewers were needed to carry away human wastes; the streets should be paved and efficiently cleaned; pure water for drinking and bathing should be supplied cheaply to the populace; no stagnant water should be allowed to stand in the city to generate noxious air; privies should be regulated; and selling putrid food should be forbidden.[26]

The authors of these reform directives aimed their writings not only at other physicians, but also at the municipal and state authorities who controlled the legislatures that could institute such measures. As physicians, they asserted, they had both the special knowledge and the responsibility to guide public-health action. When John Harrison, professor of physiology and pathology at the Medical College of Louisiana, published on the etiology of yellow fever and its relation to sanitary police, he began, "My whole object is to put the subject in detail before the minds of the citizens generally, and of those who have control over municipal affairs, and who only have the power of applying the proper correctives."[27] He self-consciously phrased his explanations in lay language to accomplish this educational purpose.

A strain of optimism ran through physicians' discussions about the prevention of yellow fever during the two decades preceding the Civil

---

25. E. H. Barton, *Report to the Louisiana State Medical Society on the Meteorology, Vital Statistics, and Hygiene of the State of Louisiana* (New Orleans, 1851), 38.

26. Joseph Johnston, "Some Accounts of the Origin and Prevention of Yellow Fever in Charleston, S.C.," *Charleston Medical Journal and Review*, IV (1849), 154–69. The recommendations of the Charleston Medical Society are on pp. 160–61.

27. John Harrison, "Speculations on the Cause of Yellow Fever," *New Orleans Medical and Surgical Journal*, III (1846–47), 563. See also E. H. Barton, "Recommendations," in Barton, *The Cause and Prevention of Yellow Fever, Contained in the Report of the Sanitary Commission of New Orleans* (Philadelphia, 1855), 240–49.

War. The South might be plagued with this horrible disease, and as a result have a distinctively high mortality rate, but it was within the power of medical science to remedy the evil. Barton, who believed that filth was the crucial agent in the production of yellow fever, proclaimed boldly, "Man has control over all!" since cleansing cities was undeniably within his reach. More particularly, that man was the southern physician. "We have now the public ear, let us pour into it wholesome truths," admonished the editor of the *Virginia Medical and Surgical Journal* after the disastrous Norfolk epidemic of 1855 in an essay entitled "What We Have to Do about Epidemics." "Let us avail ourselves of the interest now manifested in such questions, which the recent affliction of our sister cities of Portsmouth and Norfolk has spread throughout the whole Union, to tell the people what steps can be taken, and to enforce upon them the faithful employment of the means divine providence has placed at our disposal, to mitigate, if not to subvert the calamity." Physicians had to explode the myth that disease could not be averted by human agency. The editorial called upon physicians to push for sanitary reform, so that yellow fever would be "furnished with no appropriate matrix in which to fatten, grow, and propagate its poison, which under such circumstances, it does to an unlimited extent."[28] Only human lassitude, not natural law, stood in the way of a salubrious South.

Southern sanitary reformers could draw upon European authorities for documented evidence when they claimed that hygienic improvements would advance the general health of the population. But if lawmakers were to be goaded into action, public-health expenditures would have to be for measures indubitably effective against yellow fever, the one disease that aroused the sensibilities of the electorate. Yet the 1840s and 1850s were not years of theoretical consensus about yellow fever prophylaxis. The growth in awareness of the South's unhealthy condition during this period was paralleled by an increasing tendency on the part of southern physicians to question the etiology of yellow fever and offer new explanations for it. An understanding of the course of yellow fever etiology in the South during the antebellum period is a necessary prerequisite for grasping the prophylactic options open to southerners aiming to obliterate their region's epidemiological stigma.

28. E. H. Barton, "Report on the Meteorology, Mortality, and Sanitary Condition of New Orleans, for the Years 1854 and 1855," *Transactions of the American Medical Association*, IX (1856), 728; "What We Have to Do about Epidemics," *Virginia Medical and Surgical Journal*, V (1855), 422–23.

MARGARET H. WARNER

The most important issue in theoretical considerations of yellow fever was its mode of production and dissemination and the ever-present concomitant question of how both could be prevented.[29] Until around 1840, nearly all southern physicians believed that yellow fever was a non-contagious disease. Many had been educated in Philadelphia under Benjamin Rush and his successors, or else trained under preceptors who themselves had been Philadelphia students. Rush, who experienced the devastating epidemics in Philadelphia in the two decades surrounding the turn of the century, was convinced by his observations of yellow fever that it was not contagious, and that it arose spontaneously from nonimported causes. He further believed that yellow fever was merely an aggravated form of the autumnal fevers that regularly plagued Philadelphia.[30]

Impressive evidence was marshaled against contagionism: when thousands fled from a city infected with yellow fever, the disease did not in large measure follow the refugees. The fact that cases which occurred among the emigrants rarely spread farther than the victim demonstrated conclusively that yellow fever could not be communicated from one person to another by contact. This was the accepted meaning of contagion, modeled on smallpox and syphilis transmission, and it was clearly inapplicable to yellow fever. Therefore, the disease could only arise from local causes. Importation, according to this argument, was impossible, for if it traveled at all, the disease must be conveyed (but was not) by human carriers.[31]

From the 1790s to the 1840s southern physicians, informed by Rush's work, shared a widespread conviction that yellow fever was non-contagious and quarantine hence futile, but this was not the case with the populace as a whole. Lacking the greater knowledge of yellow fever's peculiar behavior available to the medical profession, lay southerners found abundant evidence for the communicability of yellow

29. The yellow fever virus is spread from person to person by way of the *Aedes aegypti* mosquito, a fact that was not conclusively demonstrated until the experiments of Walter Reed and coworkers in 1900.

30. Creole physicians of Louisiana, many of them French-trained, also credited Nicholas Chervin, a prominent French anticontagionist, as a major influence on their ideas. See the comments of Dr. Beugnot in C. H. Stone, "Report on the Origin of Yellow Fever in the Town of Woodville, Miss., in the Summer of 1844. Read with Prefatory Remarks, before the Louisiana Medico-Chirurgical Society . . . ," *New-Orleans Medical Journal*, I (1844–45), 525.

31. William P. Hort, "An Essay on the Subject of Quarantine Laws; Read before the Physico-Medical Society of New-Orleans, at the Sitting of Feb. 15th, 1845," *New-Orleans Medical Journal*, II (1845–46), 3.

fever from infected persons and things. Quarantine followed a less steady course and was alternately praised and damned by politicians and newspaper editors in the South, depending upon whether it had appeared efficacious or worthless in the most recent epidemic or had been ignored altogether with the subsequent entry of yellow fever. While physicians might scoff at the possibility of yellow fever being personally contagious, few lay southerners approached the disease's victims without fear. The belief that yellow fever could be spread from one person to the next remained strong in the public mind, regardless of the physicians' pronouncements to the contrary.[32]

Some facts about yellow fever were accepted as common wisdom by the 1840s. The local causes that purportedly generated, or at least nurtured, yellow fever were widely believed to be related to heat, filth, and moisture. In the United States, yellow fever was a disease of late summer and autumn and appeared to be correlated with the degree of nearness to its year-round home, the West Indies. The more frequently a city's summer climate approximated that of the Caribbean, the more likely it was that yellow fever would occur there. Physicians described the "yellow fever zone" as a region with Charleston on its northern edge and Mexico and the West Indies at its heart. Occasionally, after a particularly warm summer, the zone might extend farther northward, some theorists argued; one explanation for the disappearance of yellow fever from the Northeast, based on this idea, was that the zone's northern boundary had apparently moved southward from its location earlier in the century.[33]

Yellow fever's limitation to cities and towns was a subject of speculation for physicians. Some, such as one professor at the Savannah Medical College, considered the miserable overcrowding of poor city dwellers to be the central condition for the development of yellow fever. The professor explained that the 1854 epidemic originated under the influence of excessive heat, "acting upon masses of human beings crowded together in cities and towns, in badly ventilated apartments, filthy in their habits, and breathing an atmosphere tainted by poisonous ex-

32. See, for example, Duffy, *Matas History*, I, 382–409, and II, 160–97.
33. These ideas were often assumed by the authors of yellow fever literature. The lecture notebooks of medical students are particularly good sources for the accepted knowledge about yellow fever. See, for example, Samuel Favel King, Notes on Lectures at the Medical College of South Carolina, Dr. [Thomas] Simons on Practice, 1837, Waring Historical Library, Medical University of South Carolina, Charleston; and Titus Munson Coan, Lectures of Dr. Alonzo Clark, 1859–60, Lectures Delivered at the College of Physicians and Surgeons, New York, New York Historical Society, New York.

halations from accumulations of putrid offal, with which their domicils abound."[34] Others argued that it was the presence of abundant animal, as opposed to vegetable, decay that distinguished cities. The miasmata of cities, resulting from dead animals, the by-products of slaughtering and rendering establishments, and piles of unremoved human excrement, seemed, according to one thesis written by a New Orleans medical student at Transylvania in 1826, "to differ from marsh miasmata in some essential quality; this I have very little doubt is owing to the decomposition of animal matter peculiar to cities added to that of vegetable, the peculiarity of season producing a vitiated atmosphere to a high degree." A third etiological factor peculiar to the urban environment, which was sharply condemned by the report of a Louisiana committee charged with studying the 1853 epidemic in New Orleans, was the upturning of soil during construction, which led to the exposure of putrefying matter and the emanation of dangerous miasmata.[35]

Whereas an earlier generation had been content to accept malarious influences without question, from the 1830s onward medical researchers both within and outside of the South attempted to discern in more detail the source of danger inherent in the miasmatic atmosphere. This questioning posture applied both to malaria of marshy, vegetable origin and to that indicted in the causation of yellow fever. As one Charleston physician noted in 1849, "The precise nature and composition of the noxious exhalations called technically miasma or malaria have never been discovered by the most skilful chemists," although attempts to isolate this data had been sincere.[36] Some sought to locate organic matter in foul air, and thus attribute the danger to floating microorganisms; others expected to find some poisonous chemical agent, such as hydrogen sulfide, that would explain the

34. P. M. Kollock, "Notes on the Epidemic Fever of 1854," *Southern Medical and Surgical Journal*, XI (1855), 469–70.

35. Luther Preston, "Aetiology of Bilious Fevers in Hot Climates" (M.D. thesis, Transylvania University, 1826), Special Collections and Archives, Frances Carrick Thomas Library, Transylvania University, Lexington, Ky.; A. D. Crossman *et al.*, "Report of the Sanitary Commission of New Orleans on the Origin and Spread of the Epidemic," in *Report of the Sanitary Commission on the Epidemic Yellow Fever of 1853* (New Orleans, 1854), 493–503.

36. Johnston, "Yellow Fever in Charleston," 155. Another approach, followed by William K. Bowling of the University of Nashville, fingered heat and moisture alone as the culprits. A student's admiring summary of his ideas is Joel Y. Bell, "Malaria" (M.D. thesis, University of Nashville, 1857), Special Collections, Vanderbilt University Medical Center Library, Nashville.

deadliness of malaria. Researchers generally looked for a specific component of the air whose presence was consistent with an overabundance of heat, moisture, and rotting substances. For example, John K. Mitchell of Cincinnati published the theory that malaria consisted of different varieties of fungal spores that respectively caused yellow fever, intermittent fever, and cholera. Nott, on the other hand, argued for the infectious qualities of tiny insects or animalcules that floated in the miasmatic mists.[37]

This recognition of the inadequacies of the older theory and search for a specific agent in the miasmata that caused yellow fever paralleled the belief that yellow fever was a disease sui generis, characterized by distinctive signs and symptoms that separated it from the periodic fevers. Those physicians, such as Rush and his followers, who believed that yellow fever was a particularly malignant version of intermittent fever had no difficulty ascribing the exacerbation to poor hygienic conditions or the poverty of the victim. But by the 1840s most southern physicians familiar with yellow fever had come to believe that it was a distinct nosological entity. Conscious of straying from his master's teachings, one Savannah physician described his anxiety over coming to see yellow fever as a disease in itself. "Among the opinions held by my distinguished preceptor [William R. Waring of Savannah] was this identical one, that Yellow fever was but a higher grade of Bilious fever," he recalled. "*He* had imbibed this from *his* preceptor, the celebrated Rush; it descended in a straight line to me, and many years rolled by before I dared to question its accuracy; and I did not do so, until repeated observations had given me data on which to base my belief." During the 1850s lists contrasting the phenomena of yellow and bilious fevers appeared frequently in the medical literature.[38] The association of yellow fever with cities only, its apparent antagonism with malarial diseases and ability to make them temporarily disappear, and the fact that physicians observed many cases of fatal bilious fever

37. J. K. Mitchell, *On the Cryptogamous Origin of Malarious and Epidemic Fevers* (Philadelphia, 1849); Josiah C. Nott, "Yellow Fever Contrasted with Bilious Fever—Reasons for Believing It a Disease Sui Generis—Its Mode of Propagation—Remote Cause—Probably Insect or Animalcular Origin, &c.," *New Orleans Medical and Surgical Journal*, IV (1847–48), 563–601.

38. Richard D. Arnold, "An Essay upon the Relation of Bilious and Yellow Fever—Prepared at the Request of, and Read before, the Medical Society of the State of Georgia, at Its Session Held at Macon on the 9th April, 1856," *Southern Medical and Surgical Journal*, XII (1856), 517. In addition to Arnold, "An Essay," and Nott, "Yellow Fever Contrasted," see, for example, W. J. Tuck, "An Essay on Yellow Fever," *New Orleans Medical and Surgical Journal*, XI (1854–55), 175–91.

that never resembled yellow fever even at the point of death, lent credence to their separate identities. This decision that yellow fever was a specific disease, with a specific cause of some sort, spurred the search for its etiological agent.[39]

The essential problem in the exploration of the etiology of yellow fever was to separate the cause or causes that were necessary for the development of the disease from those that only contributed to its virulence or spread. For this, cases of towns only occasionally visited by yellow fever proved the most revealing. "Where the disease is of annual occurrence, it must be difficult if not impossible to point to the sources of its origins," the committee of physicians who investigated the 1855 epidemic in Norfolk began.

> It is only where its visits are rare, with long intervals of healthy seasons, that we can hope, by contrasting all the conditions and circumstances of epidemic and healthy years, to discover the mysterious cause which gives rise to this terrible scourge. We ought, in the sickly years, to be able to find some local causes which had not previously existed, some unwonted meteorological conditions, some foreign and imported elements, or a combination of circumstances to furnish an explanation of the occurrence of so extraordinary an epidemic.[40]

This sort of analysis gave unpredictable results. According to the account presented by a Memphis physician in 1851, yellow fever prevailed at Bay St. Louis, Mississippi, in the absence of heat, moisture, filth, or imported influence. He suggested that local electrical forces were at fault. In other cases, even though the town was small, and circumstances supposedly crystalline, disputes over the local or imported origin of an epidemic raged as fiercely as if the epidemic had occurred in New Orleans.[41] Not only did theorists who supported a

---

39. Some authors also argued that yellow fever was antagonistic to other diseases as well, noting that in the regions where yellow fever prevailed, pulmonary infections were much less troublesome. See, for example, William Huston Ford, "On the Antagonism of Yellow Fever to 'Catarrh,' Pneumonia, and Consumption," *New Orleans Journal of Medicine*, XXII (1869), 1–22.

40. William Selden *et al.* [a Committee of Physicians], "Report on the Origin of the Yellow Fever in Norfolk during the Summer of 1855," *Virginia Medical Journal*, IX (1857), 91.

41. A. P. Merrill, "An Essay on the Yellow Fever, As It Appeared at the Bay of St. Louis, in 1820," *New Orleans Medical and Surgical Journal*, VIII (1851–52), 1–9. The epidemic in Woodville, Mississippi, in 1844 was the cause of considerable controversy. See Stone, "Report on the Origin"; and Andrew Kirkpatrick, "An Account of the Yellow Fever which Prevailed in Woodville, Mississippi, in the Year 1844," *New-Orleans Medical Journal*, II (1845–46), 40–57.

particular theory need to show that in every case their pet cause coincided with the onset of an epidemic, they also had to explain the absence of yellow fever when all causes were apparently present. After one season without yellow fever, a New Orleans medical editor exclaimed, "What a quandary the yellow fever wizards must be in! We have heat and moisture, dead dogs, cats, chickens, etc., all over the streets, and plenty of hungry doctors; yet Yellow Jack will not come. . . . How does the present differ from some of the past, in regard to the *peculiar* conditions?"[42] By and large, however, studies of isolated epidemics pointed to the transportability of yellow fever.

During the 1840s southern physicians began to challenge the assumption that yellow fever always originated spontaneously in the towns where it appeared. Works by three southern physicians, Benjamin B. Strobel, John W. Monette, and Wesley M. Carpenter, formed the vanguard of the new tradition supporting the transmissibility of yellow fever. "Now what is meant by transmissibility, is simply this," explained Carpenter, who was professor of materia medica at the Medical College of Louisiana:

> Under certain circumstances of temperature, population, &c., the introduction of cases of the disease from abroad; or of the air of other cities, where the disease is prevailing, whether in boxes or the holds of vessels, will tend to generate such a condition in the place, as to give rise to new cases, and finally to an epidemic of the disease. The point which we desire to prove, is, that the disease is transmissible, and consequently importable; and the question as to whether this transmission is by contagion or infection, does not enter into the general problem at all.[43]

Like Carpenter, many authors who wrote on yellow fever in this period struggled to explain the phenomena they had personally observed or on which they had gathered testimony. Yellow fever appeared in upriver towns only when an epidemic was active in New Orleans, but

42. "Health of Our City," *New Orleans Medical News and Hospital Gazette*, IV (1857–58), 358.

43. W. M. Carpenter, *Sketches from the History of Yellow Fever: Showing Its Origin: Together with Facts and Circumstances Disproving Its Domestic Origin, and Demonstrating Its Transmissibility* (New Orleans, 1844), 6. See also John W. Monette, *Observations on the Epidemic Yellow Fever of Natchez, and of the South-West* (Louisville, 1842); and B. B. Strobel, *An Essay on the Subject of Yellow Fever, Intended to Prove Its Transmissibility* (Charleston, 1840). Philadelphia physician Alfred Stillé described this attitude toward yellow fever's transmission, prevalent among southern physicians as early as 1841, in a letter to George Cheyne Shattuck, December 30, 1841, in Shattuck Papers, Vol. 17, Massachusetts Historical Society, Boston.

most people who traveled from yellow fever centers, even those sick with the disease, did not carry it with them. Epidemics apparently had been generated by the arrival of persons, baggage, clothing, or ships from yellow fever areas, yet many such events were innocuous. To most southern physicians in the decade before the Civil War, the evidence indicated that at least in some instances yellow fever had been transported from one infected community to another.

Few southern medical authors adopted Carpenter's insouciant attitude toward the question of contagion. A common ambition of nineteenth-century yellow fever literature was the demonstration that yellow fever was either contagious, that is, transmitted by personal contact, or infectious, a term of varying definition. One infection theory postulated that the disease was communicable to a limited extent, such that in a close, ill-ventilated room, a companion would receive a sufficiently large dose of the aeriform poison to become diseased. Supporters of the more common anticontagionist view of infection denied that yellow fever could be transported by *people* at all. Instead material goods and trapped air transmitted the germ of yellow fever from a diseased community. Such theorists variously believed that the specific etiological agent, be it termed virus, materies morbus, animalcula, or fungus, could be transported by physical means and released into a new location, where it would reproduce under the proper conditions of filth, moisture, and heat. This idea was not inconsistent with the notion that yellow fever could develop spontaneously in, say, New Orleans or Mobile. Whatever the germ's nature, it might well be resident in some American cities and require only a particular match of meteorological and hygienic conditions to develop.[44]

One center of the debate over transmissibility of yellow fever in the 1840s was rural Louisiana and Mississippi. The editor of the *New Orleans Medical Journal* noted in 1843, "We find that a good many of our oldest and most respectable physicians have changed their original opinions in regard especially to the transportability of Yellow Fever."[45] Two physicians of Rodney, Mississippi, for example, published their conclusion that yellow fever had been imported into their town from New Orleans in that same year, revealing the self-conscious break with authority of these lower Mississippi Valley physicians. "It is a difficult

44. Bennet Dowler outlined the various meanings of contagion and infection in *Tableau of the Yellow Fever of 1853* (New Orleans, 1854), 45–46. Curiously, the term "contingent contagion," popularly used to describe the communication of cholera in a suitably foul atmosphere, is rare in these discussions of yellow fever.
45. "Quarantine," 83.

matter to combat old and received opinions," they wrote. "We are aware that the views we have expressed are counter to those of many, perhaps a majority of our professional brethren. These convictions, however, have been forced on us from observation and reflection, in opposition to early imbibed impressions, and views of those in whose opinions we were thoroughly indoctrinated."[46] In a discussion about a much contested 1844 epidemic in Woodville, Mississippi, by the Louisiana Medico-Chirurgical Society, both the local origin and transmission theories were presented, though all agreed that they were anticontagionists and opposed to the idea of personal contagion.[47] By 1854 A. P. Jones, a physician of Jefferson County, Mississippi, could report that while "the practitioners of this section, with one exception, have heretofore been non-contagionists—local origin men—now, with one exception, they are all the other way."[48]

Almost to a man the apologists for the newly received theory of yellow fever's transmissibility maintained that their conviction resulted from personal observation of the disease and its spread, and that experience was no doubt the major factor in the transformation of their ideas. But the broader southern ideological tradition of agrarianism, which developed great strength in the 1840s and 1850s, also infused and supported their etiological conclusions. Some southern agrarians regarded the urban evils of commerce and manufacturing as antithetical to the virtues they attributed to southern agricultural society. In a like fashion, the physicians and government officials of inland towns condemned New Orleans for callously ignoring, in the name of commerce and greed, the disastrous consequences of their prosperous trade with yellow fever ports in the West Indies and Mexico. Commerce in this case went beyond vaguely striking at cultural values to threaten their lives, and quarantine, which destroyed trade, was a powerful weapon in their defense.[49]

New Orleans remained a bulwark of anticontagionist thought

46. William G. Williams and James Andrews, "An Account of the Yellow Fever Which Prevailed at Rodney, Mississippi, during the Autumn of 1843," *New-Orleans Medical Journal*, I (1844), 40.

47. Stone, "Report on the Origin." Even a committee of the state legislature voted that yellow fever was transportable, but their quarantine recommendations did not succeed in the legislature at large (Gillson, *Louisiana State Board of Health*, 26).

48. A. P. Jones, "Yellow Fever in a Rural District," *New Orleans Medical News and Hospital Gazette*, I (1854–55), 207.

49. On the agrarian ideal, see Dorse Harland Hagler, "The Agrarian Theme in Southern History to 1860" (Ph.D. dissertation, University of Missouri at Columbia, 1968).

throughout this period. The majority of New Orleans physicians, including the most prominent men in the profession—Barton, Samuel Cartwright, Fenner, and William P. Hort—were convinced that yellow fever could and did spontaneously originate in New Orleans. The Jefferson County practitioner Jones regretted "the pertinacity with which some of the leading practitioners and ablest writers of New Orleans still adhere to the local origin doctrine." In the city, yellow fever often first appeared simultaneously in widely scattered locations, belying the notion of a chain of communication, and was always worst in the filthiest quarters of town. The well-publicized committee report on the disastrous 1853 epidemic in New Orleans argued persuasively that the city was replete with noxious exhalations, heat, and humidity, so that there was no need to postulate some obscure imported cause. Even in New Orleans, however, the profession had come to believe by the 1850s that while not personally contagious, yellow fever could be transported. "The fact of transportability as a property belonging to this disease, no one now disputes," concluded the 1853 committee. "If it were ever doubtful, the current events of the past summer [1853] must be admitted as finally settling it."[50] Yellow fever had not been imported into the city, where it was an indigenous resident, but it had certainly been the city's most significant export in 1853.

The idea of the portability of yellow fever became popular in the Atlantic Coast southern cities as well during the 1840s and 1850s. Two prominent Charleston physicians, Samuel Henry Dickson and P. C. Gaillard, argued for the contagiousness of yellow fever in an appropriately noxious atmosphere. Editors of two medical journals, J. Dickson Bruns of the *Charleston Medical and Surgical Review* and L. A. Dugas of the *Southern Medical and Surgical Journal*, wrote editorials promoting the concept that yellow fever could be imported. After some years of respite the East Coast cities of Savannah, Charleston, Augusta, and Norfolk were ravaged by severe epidemics of yellow fever in the mid-1850s. Like many of his colleagues, H. L. Byrd of the Savannah Medical College was converted by his observations of the 1854 epidemic. "When a medical student in Philadelphia," he explained, "I imbibed the notion, from some of my teachers, that yellow fever was strictly a non-contagious disease, and though I had seen that disease—to a limited extent—during one or two seasons, I continued to regard it as a non-contagious disease, until some two or three weeks after the appearance of the epidemic of the past season."[51]

50. Jones, "Yellow Fever," 208; Crossman *et al.*, "Report of the Sanitary Commission," in *Report of the Sanitary Commission*, 479.

51. S. H. Dickson, "Epidemics," *Charleston Medical Journal and Review*, X (1855), 609–

An influential proclamation of the transmissibility of yellow fever came from the committee appointed to investigate the Norfolk epidemic of 1855. Their conclusions, widely affirmed by the lay and medical communities of Norfolk, were that the epidemic had been initiated in some way by the arrival of the steamer *Ben Franklin* from St. Thomas, then suffering a yellow fever epidemic. Nothing else was distinctive about Norfolk that summer, and although the disease had occurred there before, its appearance could always be traced to ships transporting goods from the West Indies. The events of these 1850s epidemics affected areas beyond the South. "Many of this assembly are doubtless now, for the first time, led to the conviction that the scourge is an imported disease—a conviction imposed on their judgment by the pestilential ravages of 1856, 1857, and 1858," declared a New York physician addressing a northern sanitary conference in 1859. "Let Norfolk and Memphis, and Charleston and Savannah speak."[52]

By the 1850s, the majority of southern medical authors, who had believed that yellow fever always arose locally, admitted the possibility that yellow fever was transportable. This transformation is difficult to explain. While Erwin Ackerknecht has argued that the evidence for both contagionism and anticontagionism was so evenly divided that no physician could decide on the basis of the facts alone, and so was swayed by liberal (anticontagionist) or conservative (contagionist) political inclinations, this pattern was by no means so clear among southern physicians choosing from the profusion of etiological theories current in the 1850s.[53] Anti-urban, agrarian sentiment apparently correlates somewhat with a propensity to favor quarantine. But it would be a thorny task indeed to attempt to discover the political associations of southern physicians, label them liberal or conservative,

20; P. C. Gaillard, "On Some Points of Hygiene, and Their Connection with the Propagation of Yellow Fever and Cholera," *Charleston Medical Journal and Review,* IV (1849), 280–95; "Yellow Fever in Charleston," *Charleston Medical Journal and Review,* XI (1856), 845–50; "Yellow Fever at the South-West," *Southern Medical and Surgical Journal,* IX (1853), 705; H. L. Byrd, "Observations on Yellow Fever," *Charleston Medical Journal and Review,* X (1853), 329.

52. Selden *et al.*, "Yellow Fever in Norfolk"; Edward C. Bolton, "The Yellow Fever at Norfolk" (M.D. thesis, University of Pennsylvania, 1858), Special Collections, Van Pelt Library, University of Pennsylvania, Philadelphia; Richard G. Parker, "Yellow Fever in Portsmouth Virg: During the Summer & Fall of 1855" (M.D. thesis, University of Pennsylvania, 1858), Special Collections; John W. Francis, remarks of April 29, 1859, *Proceedings and Debates of the Third National Quarantine and Sanitary Convention* (New York, 1859), 141–42.

53. Erwin Ackerknecht, "Anticontagionism between 1821 and 1867," *Bulletin of the History of Medicine,* XXII (1948), 562–93.

and then to make a case that political or even broader philosophical orientation determined their choices of disease theory. A more useful approach is to realize that even if they all had similar access to the medical evidence relating to yellow fever, physicians at different locations in the South actually saw the phenomena of yellow fever differently. The Atlantic Coast cities so ravaged by yellow fever in the 1850s were like the interior towns of Mississippi and Louisiana in that yellow fever was not an annual visitor, and those seeking to identify the essential elements in the production of yellow fever could therefore contrast the characteristics of the epidemic and the healthy years. In most cases such evidence resulted in the judgment that yellow fever had been imported into the town. This opportunity of treating the rare occurrence of yellow fever as a sort of laboratory experiment, with nonepidemic years as the control, seems more than any other factor to have critically influenced many southern physicians' decisions to accept the transmissibility of yellow fever.[54]

The concept of the transportability of yellow fever was to have a decided impact on the shape of southern public health, but this influence was not fully realized until the last two decades of the nineteenth century, when research on other diseases had provided the germ theory of yellow fever with a solid (if analogical) basis. By maintaining that both germ and environment were key elements in the development of yellow fever, the theory allowed for reconciliation between the advocates of sanitation and the proponents of quarantine. It proclaimed that both were useful and worthy of pursuit. Yet it would be an oversimplification to see this theory as a comprehensive, unified doctrine, recognized as such at the time; rather, it is better considered a group of assumptions that physicians had come to share, but that did not preclude strong differences among those physicians about the implications or elaboration of those assumptions. Too many issues, such as the nature of the germ and its mode of transport, were still unresolved, and the appropriate significance to be assigned to germ or environment in the prevention of yellow fever had yet to be settled.

With transportability no longer seriously at issue by the mid-1850s,

54. During the 1860s the possibility that yellow fever could be transported came to be increasingly accepted in Europe as well. Here, too, it was the study of epidemics in places where yellow fever rarely came that changed physicians' perceptions of disease etiology. The southern writings explicated here apparently had little influence on European authors. See William Coleman, *Yellow Fever in the North: The Methods of Early Epidemiology* (Madison, 1987); and C. E. Gordon Smith and Mary E. Gibson, "Yellow Fever in South Wales, 1865," *Medical History*, XXX (1986), 322–40.

the necessity for and nature of quarantine became a central topic for debate. The fact that yellow fever could be imported did not refute the possibility that it could also develop spontaneously from local causes, the same causes that acted in the West Indies, where it was endemic and indisputably indigenous. Prominent physicians in New Orleans and Mobile, such as Fenner and George A. Ketchum, grudgingly admitted that to quarantine seriously filthy ships was perhaps a wise practice, but they were convinced that the major source of yellow fever was to be found at home, in the unsanitary condition of their cities. Quarantines were useless for the prevention of yellow fever not because they were founded on a faulty theory, but because it was foolish to try to exclude an already-established local inhabitant. Physicians in towns less frequently visited by yellow fever were more likely to believe that though hygiene might limit the course of an epidemic, the main line of defense against the disease had to be quarantine. Thus C. B. Guthrie of Memphis, who accepted the impropriety of quarantine for Mobile and New Orleans, concurrently believed that a quarantine system was necessary for the protection of communities outside of the semitropical region where yellow fever developed spontaneously.[55] The public-health controversies of the 1850s revolved around the question of whether quarantine was relevant at all to the protection of southern communities. And, if quarantine were to be imposed, whom or what should be subjected to it?

While the idea that yellow fever could be transported renewed interest in quarantine, it also inspired a newly critical attitude toward its function and operation. Those who believed that people carried yellow fever within their bodies continued to advocate human isolation. Others who thought the danger lay primarily in the emanations of people as transmitted to their clothing and belongings argued that a thorough cleansing of the patient and his material accompaniments was sufficient to limit the personal spread of yellow fever. The more dominant view demarcated human beings as noncarriers of yellow fever and focused instead on physical objects, such as ships, clothing, and baggage. This theory was approved, for example, at a series of quarantine and sanitary conventions held in Philadelphia, New York, and Boston from 1857 to 1860. By a vote of 85 to 6, the 1859 convention, composed almost entirely of physicians and businessmen from the Northeast,

55. George A. Ketchum, "Report on the Diseases of Mobile for 1854," *Transactions of the Medical Association of the State of Alabama*, 8th session (1855), 114; E. D. Fenner, *History of the Epidemic of Yellow Fever at New Orleans, La. in 1853* (New York, 1854), 74; C. B. Guthrie, remarks of April 28, 1859, in *Third National Sanitary Convention*, 25–29.

renounced the theory of personal contagion but approved the quarantine of material goods. Rejecting the old system of mere detention, this convention and many reform-minded southerners argued for the disinfection of ships, baggage, and passengers through the use of agents known to halt fermentation and extinguish foul putrefactive odors, such as chloride of lime, steam, or the gas evolved from burning sulphur.[56] A variety of conflicting quarantine programs were thus postulated to meet the indications of the new faith in yellow fever's portability.

Among southern physicians, who were more likely to believe in personal contagion than their northern colleagues, the quarantine of people as well as material objects was granted more currency. Some commentators depicted this inclination as a peculiarly southern attitude. For example, the editor of a Charleston medical journal criticized the northern bias of the 1859 Quarantine and Sanitary Convention in language that echoed the growing southern dissatisfaction with the national division of political power. "It is 'national' inasmuch as some of the selected members came from various States; while the greater number, designed to shape and model the whole performance, and collected from the larger Northern cities, New York, Philadelphia, Boston, and Baltimore, furnished the mass of nationality, and can always do it, when any measure is beneficial to them," he wrote. He believed that the members of the meeting, especially the few southern ones who were present, had been chosen so as to predetermine a vote against quarantine, by which he meant quarantine as it had been and he thought should be practiced—against people as well as objects. "The Nationality of the Convention, as far as South Carolina is concerned, is purely fictitious, and we repudiate all design to be governed by its present or future National decrees. . . . It is patent that the meeting of the Convention was planned to effect the destruction of all Quarantines."[57] He went on to support quarantines as preventive measures that were in the South's interest, however much they might damage the trade centers of the Northeast.

A Louisiana physician likewise distinguished southern epidemiological knowledge from the anticontagionist and antiquarantine views

56. The vote on the quarantine question was recorded and discussed in *Third National Sanitary Convention*, 220–224. This volume also contains discussions of the value of disinfectants and a prescription for the new system of quarantine.

57. "[Review of] Proceedings and Debates of the Third National Quarantine and Sanitary Convention," *Charleston Medical Journal and Review*, XV (1860), 215.

considered gospel in European medical circles: "Because it is now in Europe almost conventional, that, to converse of the utility of quarantine for yellow fever is ridiculous, is that a reason that we, who have been eye-witnesses of facts contrary to this opinion, should prefer believing what others say, rather than the testimony of our own senses?"[58] The South did not need to import foreign theories from the North or Europe to eradicate its peculiar disease; southern observations had convinced southern physicians of the transportability of yellow fever, and southerners would boldly support quarantines, both personal and material, if southern knowledge indicated their value.

Certainly the impact of yellow fever on the South during the 1840s and 1850s prompted an active search for a remedy to the damage inflicted on the South by the disease. Towns outside of New Orleans, such as Natchez, instituted quarantines against the city during epidemics, with much analyzed results. Some years the quarantines appeared effective; in others yellow fever appeared in quarantined as well as in similarly situated but unquarantined nearby towns. Quarantine was debated and rejected frequently by New Orleans medical societies during the 1840s, and an effort to convince the state legislature to enact quarantine legislation failed during these years. Quarantine's advocates grew stronger in the 1850s, however. By 1854 the quarantine officer at Charleston, an avowed anticontagionist, was under attack for his lax administrative practices. Norfolk established a rigid quarantine system following its 1855 epidemic.[59]

The most widely heralded result of the resurgence of the popularity of quarantine in the South was the creation of a board of health for Louisiana in 1855 whose officers were "to be *selected in reference to their known zeal in favor of a Quarantine system.*" The quarantine law prescribed that if the ship were particularly foul or if there had been pestilential fever on board, the captain of the vessel was to be com-

58. Comments of Dr. Beugnot, in Stone, "Report on the Origin," 525.

59. On Louisiana, see Hort, "Quarantine Laws"; and Duffy, *Matas History*, II, 174–77. William Hume called for a stricter enforcement of Charleston's quarantine in "Report to the City Council of Charleston, on a Resolution of Inquiry Relative to 'The Source and Origin of Yellow Fever, As It Has Occasionally Prevailed in Charleston, and the Means of Prevention or Exclusion, As May Seem Worthy of Adoption, in Order to Obviate Its Future Occurrence,'" *Charleston Medical Journal and Review*, IX (1854), 145–64. J. C. Simonds cited Hume's work with approval in his 1854 report advocating a quarantine for New Orleans (Simonds, "Report on Quarantine," in *Report of the Sanitary Commission*, 502–523). Simonds' work was influential in the establishment of the 1855 Louisiana quarantine.

pelled to "land the sick at the Quarantine ground, [and] to fumigate and cleanse all such vessels."[60] The Louisiana quarantine was administered in its first years by Dr. A. F. Axson, who believed that the effluvia emanating from the sick were a source of danger, as were the air and articles about them. He did not deny the indigenicity of yellow fever to New Orleans, but reasoned that if one cause of the disease could be eliminated, it would be all the better for the city.[61]

Many New Orleans physicians pronounced the new quarantine system a failure when yellow fever reappeared in 1857, 1858, and 1859. The experiment had been fairly tried, they declared, and had proved a decided mistake. Quarantine was not and could not be the answer to the city's unhealthy condition if sanitary imperatives went unheeded.[62] Even contagionists like Gaillard of Charleston stressed that the crucial element in an epidemic was not the imported spark but the receptivity of the urban environment, which could be rendered nonflammable by civic hygiene.[63] The repetition of yellow fever epidemics in the 1840s and 1850s brought strident demands that the South's cities be drained and cleaned. As ephemeral boards of health were created and then disappeared during these years in New Orleans, each new incarnation brought appeals from Fenner, Barton, and other physicians for the promotion of the sanitary agenda. Likewise, in Charleston, Knoxville, Mobile, Savannah, and Norfolk, public-health advocates called for improved urban sanitation.

The South's hygienic reformers met with some success. Charleston was judged to be notably better drained, paved, and cleaned by the 1850s; in New Orleans the street cleaning contract was wrested from a corrupt monopoly and brought under municipal control.[64] But such

60. "[Review of] 'An Act to Establish Quarantine for the Protection of the State': Approved March 15, 1855," *New Orleans Medical and Surgical Journal*, XII (1855–56), 129, 132.

61. A. F. Axson, "Reply of the President of the Board of Health to the 'Memorial to the Legislature' Published in the Preceding Number of the N. O. Med. and Surg. Journal," *New Orleans Medical and Surgical Journal*, XV (1858), 360–62.

62. A. Mercier, "To the Honorable, the Members of the Senate and House of Representatives of the State of Louisiana, Now in Assembly Convened, at Baton Rouge," *New Orleans Medical and Surgical Journal*, XV (1858), 221–52. Mercier claimed that 19 out of 20 New Orleans physicians supported his position.

63. Gaillard, "Some Points of Hygiene," 292.

64. On Charleston, see Simons, "Epidemic Yellow Fever," 364. Although admittedly praising his own efforts, Simons' evaluation of the improvement of Charleston was not singular. Duffy, *Sword of Pestilence*, 19–20, discusses the New Orleans street-cleaning contract.

positive results were not typical. The very repetition of the litany of sanitary deficiencies indicates the general lack of action on the issue. This failure is evident in an 1860 review of the *Annual Report of the State of Louisiana Board of Health*. The reviewer first quoted the report as saying, "Its [the Board's] labors then and subsequently have been unavailing to inspire our city fathers with a sense of their importance . . . and the utter destitution of the city in every essential of sanitary regulation necessary to health, or even to decency and self-respect." He then went on in his words to conclude: "Pretty strong language, and appropriate; yet calculated to have as little effect on political eyes and ears as a morning mist or a schoolboy's pop-gun. New Orleans is the filthiest hole in the land, except New York City (which, in point of filth, it can never hope to rival), but there is no use in talking about it. Our city fathers wade through the filth to reach their seats in the hall, and they thus become accustomed to it."[65] Similarly, reformers in Savannah, Charleston, and Mobile continued to chide their legislators for ignoring urban filth and held forth cleanliness as the path that would elevate the South's salubrity. But sanitarians, foiled by the lack of agreement concerning the precise relevance of filth to yellow fever, could not convince their parsimonious lawgivers that such measures would save the South.

The research that the awareness of the Old South's health crisis sparked led not to the consensus necessary to inform practice and arouse legislative action, the objective envisioned by the proselytizers of yellow fever studies, but rather to a multitude of contending theories that weakened the chances for effective public-health reform. Although yellow fever's transmissibility was widely accepted, the species of quarantine required was left undecided, as was the degree to which filth contributed to the origin and growth of yellow fever. Sanitarians who sought to gain legitimacy for their efforts by tying them to the imperative of preventing yellow fever failed to persuade legislators that sanitation could eradicate the disease. The squabbling among quarantine theorists about appropriate quarantine procedure undermined attempts to improve quarantines and opened avenues of vulnerability for critics who ridiculed quarantine as based on uncertain speculations. By the eve of the Civil War, southerners had been for the most part unsuccessful in combatting their region's epidemiological reputation and reality.

65. "[Review of] Annual Report of the Board of Health to the Legislature of Louisiana, January, 1860," *New Orleans Medical News and Hospital Gazette*, VI (1859–60), 927.

CHAPTER 12

SOUTHERN MADNESS: THE SHAPE OF MENTAL HEALTH CARE IN THE OLD SOUTH

Samuel B. Thielman

I n the late 1890s, Theophilus O. Powell, superintendent of the Georgia State Sanitarium, was asked to chronicle the history of southern asylums in his presidential address to the American Medico-Psychological Association, for (he was told) due credit had never been given mental health reform in the South. Although Powell discussed the development of southern asylums in his address, few people since have explored the question of how mental health care evolved in the South. The reasons for this neglect of the southern response to madness are not hard to understand. The majority of the leadership of the asylum superintendents' organization, the Association of Medical Superintendents of American Institutions for the Insane, were from northern institutions. The major American asylum journal in the nineteenth century, *The American Journal of Insanity,* was edited and published in Utica, New York, and dealt primarily with the problems of asylums in the Mid-Atlantic and New England states. And virtually all of the "showcase" American institutions (the Worcester State Hospital, the Pennsylvania Hospital for the Insane, and the Bloomingdale Asylum) were northern institutions.[1]

1. T[heophilus] O. Powell, "A Sketch of Psychiatry in the Southern States," *Proceedings of the American Medico-Psychological Association at the Fifty-Third Annual Meeting* (N.p., 1897), 74. The most notable treatment of southern asylums is in Gerald N. Grob, *Mental Institutions in America: Social Policy to 1875* (New York, 1973), 343–47, 359–68. This discussion accentuates the problems of southern asylums and generally underestimates the knowledgability of the physicians involved with these asylums. On the development of antebellum mental health care in individual southern states, see Margaret Callender McCulloch, "Founding the North Carolina Asylum for the Insane," *The North Carolina*

Nonetheless, the neglect of southern mental health care in histories of American psychiatry is unfortunate, for it has led to generalizations about the development of the care for the insane in the United States that ignore regional differences. This is not to say that southern and northern institutions were entirely different, for they were not. Individuals in both regions dealt with the problem of managing the insane in the community. Asylum physicians in both regions faced problems of limited public funding, of convincing funding bodies that the asylum should be funded, and of living up to the public expectation that insanity was "curable" when, by mid-century, it was quite clear to most asylum physicians that a substantial number of mentally disordered patients would not be "cured." What was different was the social matrix within which these problems were addressed and the external resources that those dealing with madness were able to bring to bear on these problems. One issue, however, was uniquely southern: how to deal socially with the problem of insanity among blacks. Insane blacks almost always presented economic dilemmas, for free blacks were often indigent, and slaves were an economic burden on their masters. This chapter is a preliminary effort to present characteristic aspects of the southern approach to madness and to try to view the development of mental health care in the Old South in the context of the broader development of care for the insane in the United States during the antebellum period. I have included in this study all of the slave states of antebellum America, including the border states of Delaware, Kentucky, Maryland, and Missouri, and the District of Columbia. I have included a discussion of community as well as asylum management of madness, since the mad were treated in both places.

Historical Review, XIII (1936), 185–201; Hortense S. Cochrane, "Early Treatment of the Mentally Ill in Georgia," *Georgia Historical Quarterly,* XXXII (1948), 104–18; E. Bruce Thompson, "Reforms in the Care of the Insane in Tennessee, 1830–1850," *Tennessee Historical Quarterly,* III (1944), 319–34; Barbara Bellows, " 'Insanity is the Disease of Civilization': The Founding of the South Carolina Lunatic Asylum," *South Carolina Historical Magazine,* LXXXII (1981), 263–72; Robert O. Mellown, "The Construction of the Alabama Insane Hospital, 1852–1861," *Alabama Review* (1985), 83–104; John S. Hughs, "Alabama's Families and Involuntary Commitment of the Insane, 1861–1900: New Solutions to Old Problems" (Typescript in Hughs's possession); Ronald F. White, "Custodial Care for the Insane at Eastern State Hospital in Lexington, Kentucky, 1824–1844," and "John Rowan Allen, M.D., and the Early Years of the Psychiatric Profession in Kentucky, 1844–1854," both in *Filson Club Quarterly* (in press). See also Samuel B. Thielman, "Madness and Medicine: Medical Therapeutics for Insanity in Antebellum America, with Special Reference to the Eastern Lunatic Asylum of Virginia and the South Carolina Lunatic Asylum" (Ph.D. dissertation, Duke University, 1986).

Although the sources describing the community management of madness are less accessible than those on asylum physicians, the community was, nonetheless, the place where the management of madness began. What records are available indicate clearly that families, friends, and general physicians all participated in community care of madness. Home remedy books often gave recommendations for treating mental disorders such as hysteria, hypochondriasis, and melancholia. They recommended physical and mental treatments consistent with a medical understanding of mental disorders. Though such books often differed substantially in theoretical outlook, their approach to the treatment of mental disorders, particularly hysteria and hypochondriasis, is fairly uniform. They almost always advocated medicinal remedies, but sometimes included suggestions for moral (or psychological) therapeutics as well. One southern manual by Dr. Tomlinson Fort, a student of Benjamin Rush and a prominent physician in Milledgeville, Georgia, suggested that the affected patient should change bad habits and that the treating person should take a compassionate attitude toward the mentally troubled patient.[2]

Families were not always as medically oriented in their management of patients as were the home remedy manuals. John M. Galt, superintendent at the Eastern Lunatic Asylum at Williamsburg, Virginia, described a woman there who had been kept in a closet by her relatives prior to being sent to the asylum. In 1831, one physician at the South Carolina Lunatic Asylum described a violent wandering man from Abbeville, South Carolina, who had been chained by his neighbors for several weeks prior to his admission to the asylum after he tried to burn down his house.[3]

2. I have surveyed the following domestic medicine books that were published in southern editions: William Buchan, *Domestic Medicine: or, A Treatise on the Prevention and Cure of Diseases, by Regimen and Simple Medicines* (Charleston, 1807); Tomlinson Fort, *A Dissertation on the Practice of Medicine Containing an Account of the Causes, Symptoms, and Treatment of Diseases and Adapted to the Use of Physicians and Families* (N.p., 1849); John C. Gunn, *Gunn's Domestic Medicine, or Poor Man's Friend, in the Hours of Affliction, Pain, and Sickness* (Louisville, Ky., 1849). See Fort, *A Dissertation*, 510, 523. On Fort, see Evelyn Ward Gray, *The Medical Profession in Georgia, 1733–1983* (Atlanta, 1983).

3. "She was confined [by relatives] in a sort of cupboard or closet fixed in one of the rooms, so that she could not possibly get out. Was taken out to get fresh air. . . . Dr. Mason saw her twice, charged 10 dollars, but [she] might as well not have been [charged]" (Galt Family Papers, I, MsV 120, Earl Gregg Swem Library, College of William and Mary, Williamsburg); South Carolina Lunatic Asylum Treatment Record, I, 305, South Carolina State Archives, Columbia, S.C. (hereinafter cited as Treatment Record). Life at the Eastern Lunatic Asylum is reflected in the extensive Galt Family Papers collection (hereinafter cited as GFP; the collection is divided into Parts I and II).

There existed intermediate places of confinement between the home and the asylum. Many patients were kept in jails and almshouses, but there were other intermediate arrangements as well. A particularly illuminating example is that of the management of a Miss Simmons in South Carolina. Because she developed melancholy, a family acquaintance removed her to the home of his sister. Despite the "gentle treatment" of his sister, Miss Simmons became increasingly disturbed, and her disorder became "madness." Friends then placed her at "the house of a lady who had been accustomed to the care of persons in [this] unfortunate state of mind." Because her melancholia seemed to result from disappointment and shame, the treating woman attempted to divert her mind by providing a change of air and arranging a visit to the sea, all to no avail. Miss Simmons was then transferred to the asylum for management.[4]

Community physicians became involved in managing the insane when families consulted them. A Maryland physician boasted to a correspondent that he had successfully treated hundreds of patients, many of whom had been seen by the "finest medical gentlemen" in Philadelphia and Baltimore, and that he treated certain patients both in the hospital and as private patients. The asylum records at the Eastern Lunatic Asylum at Williamsburg and the South Carolina Lunatic Asylum reveal many instances of involvement of community physicians in the treatment of patients who eventually made their way to the asylum.[5] The Eastern Lunatic Asylum records contain a patient's ac-

4. Treatment Record, I, 374. On these lay-run houses for the mad, see the condemnation of private houses for the mad in South Carolina Lunatic Asylum Annual Report, 1842, 10.

5. For evidence of community physician involvement in the care of the insane in antebellum Virginia, see the following correspondence in GFP, II: R. L. Barrett to John M. Galt II, ca. October 15, 1858, Box XIII, folder 155; Wm. S. Scott to John M. Galt II, July 16, 1858, Box XII, folder 152; Wm. N. Yarborough to John M. Galt II, March 28, 1862, Box XV, folder 188; C. M. Stigleman to John M. Galt II, October 25, 1859, Box XIV, folder 169; [I.] W. Taylor to John M. Galt II, June 16, 1859, Box XIV, folder 169; O. A. Crenshaw to John M. Galt II, October 26, 1859, Box XIV, folder 164; B. R. F. to John M. Galt II, October 29, 1858, Box XII, folder 144; Robertson Cook to John M. Galt II, August 24, 1857, Box XII, folder 143; A. W. Fontaine to John M. Galt II, June 24, 1856, Box XI, folder 134; C. C. Buckner to John M. Galt II, June 18, 1856, Box XI, folder 134; G. [Wellford] to John M. Galt II, January 21, 1855, Box XI, folder 126; [J.] R. Harrison to John M. Galt II, September 12, 1849, Box IX, folder 111; Jas. Haller to John M. Galt II, October 28, 1858, Box XIII, folder 156; Charles Kemper to John M. Galt II, May 27, 1847, Box VI, folder 97; S. Edwards to John M. Galt II, July 20, 1847, Box IX, folder 100; Thomas D. Brown to John M. Galt II, October 11, 1844, Box IX, folder 112. See also Christian Boerstler to Andrew McCalla, May 5, 1826, John Moore McCalla Papers, Manuscript Collection, William R. Perkins Library, Duke University, Durham.

count of his involvement with his community physician:

> [The night I was taken with insanity, my brother] sent for the Doctor and as soon as I saw him I asked him if I might feel his head and after I told him what I thought of it he felt my pulse and ordered a cold cloth to be put to it which I think done a great deal of good. . . . the next day the Doctor gave me a dose of calomel and at night a dose of opium which he continued for about a week and did not allow me to eat anything but a little butter milk & bread but at last I got up and went to the table and told them I would have something to eat if it killed me so I took some bread & coffee.[6]

One of the more elaborate unpublished accounts of medical management in the community is the letter of a Dr. Lowry to the superintendent of the South Carolina Lunatic Asylum. In it he described a man he treated who suffered from outbursts of rage and the way he treated the man medically:

> At his worst times he appeared to abhor himself, and detest the whole human race with the bitterest . . . hatred and abhorrence. An observer might very readily have supposed that he was possessed of some evil spirit. When he felt these conditions coming on he would retire from company that he respected or such as held a restraint on him and vent his [desecrations] and bitter anathemas to the trees and woods. . . . He would then for a little be perfectly satisfied with himself and . . . [a short time after the incident would come to] detest and despise himself for what he had done—and be strongly induced to commit suicide to hide himself from himself or to get quit of the anguish of his own mind. All this time [if engaged in conversation] he would converse as rationally and soberly as any person whatever— but you could see vengeance and horror seethe from his soul through his countenance in torrents.[7]

Lowry treated him with purgatives, but obtained no improvement, so he advised the patient's friends to send him to the asylum.

Community physicians addressed these complex problems not only with physical remedies, but with nonmedicinal strategies as well. Christian Boerstler of Maryland wrote to an inquirer in 1826 that "the Moral treatment is all important [in treating furious mania]—and the benevolent plan of kindness and friendly attention has never failed with me." A physician in South Carolina treating a woman of "unstable mental constitutions" sent her on a trip to the mountains of North

6. Thomas I. Hancock to John M. Galt II, November 26, 1844, GFP, II, Box VII, folder 88.
7. Treatment Record, I, 234–35.

and South Carolina. He obtained a temporary good result, though the woman later went to the asylum for treatment.[8]

Although community treatment in the South must have been similar to that elsewhere, there was at least one major regional difference, for the presence of mad slaves in the South created a set of problems unique to the region. Legislation concerning insane slaves was among the earliest legislation concerning insanity in the colonies. The Council Chamber of South Carolina amended the Poor Relief Act of 1712 in 1745 to provide public funds for the maintenance of insane slaves of impoverished masters. And slaves were cared for both in the community and at a number of southern asylums. Providing for a mad slave was important to a slaveholder if for no other reason than that an insane slave placed a heavy burden on the master's family.[9] One desperate slaveowner wrote John Galt:

> My cook . . . became on Friday last . . . a *raving maniac.* . . . [S]he was very violent, though not exhibiting any disposition to do injury except by heaping curses upon certain persons. She was bled, cold water applied to the head, an opiate administered and then held by men upon the bed until midnight when she became more quiet. . . . I keep my best negro man constantly with her—a most serious loss to my business. [Even] if she were to get well enough to go about her usual occupations or any other, my wife, who is a delicate person of weak nerves, would be in constant dread of a recurrence. . . . I am told that there is no provision for slaves at the Hospital . . . [but any arrangement that you want to make in order to accept her as a patient] I am willing to do rather than have my wife and family subjected to the hourly dread of a maniac.[10]

Although some families attempted to care for insane slaves themselves, they sometimes called in physicians. A case in point is that described by W. T. Wragg and reprinted from the *Southern Journal of Medicine and Pharmacy* in the *Boston Medical and Surgical Journal.* Wragg

8. Christian Boerstler to Andrew McCalla, May 5, 1826, John Moore McCalla Papers.

9. *A Sketch of the Early History of the Insane in South Carolina* (N.p., n.d. [Located in the South Caroliniana Library of the University of South Carolina, Columbia, S.C.]), 1. Concerning problems raised by slaves becoming insane, see the following letters in GFP, II: W. B. Matthews to John M. Galt II, December 28, 1860, Box XV, folder 179; [I.] H. [Wombwell] to John M. Galt II, December 7, 1854, Box X, folder 125; R. L. Barrett to John M. Galt II, ca. October 15, 1858, Box XIII, folder 155; Wm. S. Scott to John M. Galt II, July 16, 1858, Box XII, folder 152; Jn. M. Gregory to John M. Galt II, March 31, 1857, Box XII, folder 141; [D.] F. Harrison to John M. Galt II, December 1, 1856, Box XI, folder 139; E. C. Taylor to John M. Galt II, January 23, 1855, Box XI, folder 126.

10. [D.] F. Harrison to John M. Galt II, December 1, 1856, GFP, II, Box XI, folder 139.

described his psychological formulation of the disease of a young slave on a Charleston plantation who had become convinced that he had died. Wragg observed:

> [The slave's] imagination . . . was awakened. He became impressed with the idea that he was dead. . . . This idea produce[d] a deep impression, and accordingly the patient . . . [exhibited] the most extravagant language and conduct. From his false ground he drew . . . [logical] inferences which failed to be rational only because they started from unsound premises. He said that, being dead, his flesh would soon begin to rot and drop from his bones; . . . [he] earnestly demanded that his grave clothes should be prepared and put upon him, and that he be laid out in the usual form. . . . [H]is countenance and his every action took a serious, a sublime expression from the thought [that he was dead], and his whole deportment was such as could not fail to touch and awe all who saw him.[11]

Wragg treated him with antiphlogistic measures, and the patient eventually recovered.

Thus, although our knowledge of the details of community management of insanity is limited, community management was clearly an important component of the social response to madness in the South. Other than in the management of slaves, community treatment in the antebellum South was probably similar in many respects to that in the North. Differences in management were more striking in the asylum.[12]

In 1773 the asylum at Williamsburg became the first American institution devoted exclusively to the care of the insane. Between 1773 and 1860, fifteen southern institutions came into being, slightly less than one third of the total number of asylums in the United States (Figures 1, 2; Table 1).[13] If one considers population differences, the

11. W. T. Wragg, "Remarkable Case of Mental Alienation," *Boston Medical and Surgical Journal*, XXXIV (1846), 309.

12. On community management in the North, see Ellen Dwyer, *Homes for the Mad: Life Inside Two Nineteenth-Century Asylums* (New Brunswick, 1987), 86–97; and Nancy Tomes, *A Generous Confidence: Thomas Story Kirkbride and the Art of Asylum-Keeping, 1840–1883* (Cambridge, England, 1984), 103–107.

13. Counting asylums can be difficult because not all asylums that existed are listed in secondary source material, and some sources list hospitals as being in existence earlier than they apparently were. Thus, the figures given in the text represent best estimates of the numbers of asylums in the North and South. Asylums were listed only if they could be verified through reliable sources, so the figures tend to underestimate rather than overestimate the number of asylums. My primary sources were Grob, *Mental Institutions*; Samuel W. Hamilton, "The History of American Mental Hospitals," in J. K. Hall (ed.), *One Hundred Years of American Psychiatry* (New York, 1944), 73–166; and the list of attendees and their hospitals of origin in "Proceedings of the Association of Medical Superin-

FIGURE 1.

REGIONAL DISTRIBUTION OF THE POPULATION OF THE UNITED STATES, 1800–1860

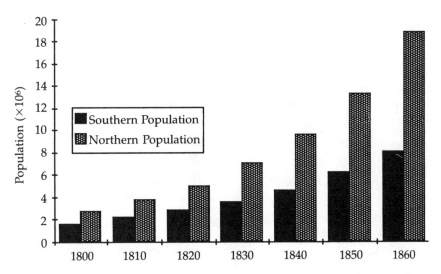

FIGURE 2.

REGIONAL DISTRIBUTION OF ASYLUMS IN THE UNITED STATES, 1800–1860

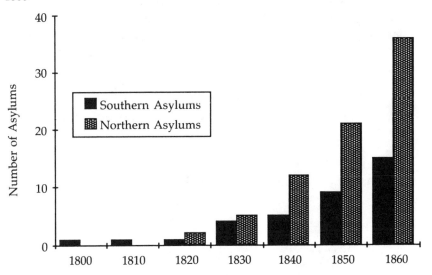

TABLE 1.
SOUTHERN ASYLUMS ESTABLISHED BEFORE 1860

Asylum	Location	Year Opened
Virginia Eastern Lunatic Asylum	Williamsburg	1773
Kentucky Eastern Lunatic Asylum	Lexington	1824
South Carolina Lunatic Asylum	Columbia	1828
Virginia Western Lunatic Asylum	Staunton	1828
Maryland Hospital for the Insane	Baltimore	1834
Mount Hope Institution	Baltimore	1840
Tennessee Hospital for the Insane	Nashville	1840
Milledgeville State Hospital	Milledgeville, Ga.	1842
Insane Asylum of Louisiana	Jackson	1848
Kentucky Western Lunatic Asylum	Hopkinsville	1854
Missouri State Lunatic Asylum No. 1	Fulton	1854
Mississippi State Lunatic Asylum	Whitfield	1855
Government Hospital for the Insane	Dist. of Columbia	1855
Insane Asylum of North Carolina	Raleigh	1856
St. Vincent's Institution for the Insane	St. Louis, Missouri	1858

proportion of asylums in the South was similar to that in the North.[14] There were, however, major differences in the way asylums were established in the North and South. One regional difference that influenced the development of asylums in the South, at least during the first three decades of the nineteenth century, was the lack there of sectarian religious reform. Quakers, of course, were a primary motivating force behind the establishment and maintenance of several northern asylums. The Friends' Asylum at Frankford, Pennsylvania, the Bloomingdale Asylum, and later the Pennsylvania Hospital for the Insane, all had been directly influenced by Quakers who had been motivated by piety and who modeled much of their treatment approach after that of the Quaker York Retreat in England. The Retreat's

tendents of American Institutions for the Insane," *American Journal of Insanity,* I–XV (1844–1860).

14. Population figures were derived from U.S. Bureau of the Census, *The Statistical History of the United States from Colonial Times to the Present* (Stamford, Conn., 1965).

great contribution to American asylums was its vision of the asylum as a therapeutic institution and its conviction that mental therapy and an appropriate physical regimen were the basic ingredients of asylum management.[15]

Direct Quaker influence on the establishment of southern asylums was, however, negligible, for outside of Piedmont North Carolina, there were few Quakers in the South. By the early nineteenth century, Quakers were a small minority, often persecuted for their abolitionist views, and they had little influence on the government or institutions of the Old South. The attitude adopted by the York Retreat, which viewed those deprived of reason more as children than as animals, and more as family members than patients, was reflected in Quaker asylums in the North in a way that it generally was not in the asylums of the South. As public asylums began to outnumber private asylums in the North, the Quaker attitude was diluted there also, but at least during the early years of the nineteenth century, the difference in attitude was a regionally noticeable one. This is not to say that the example of the York Retreat had no influence on the institutions of the South, for its humane and pragmatic approach to treatment was often admired, but the religious sect behind the Retreat had few sympathizers among southerners.[16]

What exactly *did* motivate those who sought to establish southern asylums is not always discernible. But when a rationale is evident, it is often more akin to the Enlightenment (and secular) philosophical approach of Philippe Pinel than to the religious thinking of the Tukes. One of the important motivations of those who established southern asylums seems to have been a belief in the primacy of reason and the consequent value of restoring reason to those who were mad. This

15. Tomes, *A Generous Confidence*, 47–49; Anne Digby, *Madness, Morality and Medicine: A Study of the York Retreat, 1796–1914* (Cambridge, England, 1985), 33–104. Other institutions had made provision for the insane, most notably the Pennsylvania Hospital (opened in 1752), the insane ward of the New York Hospital (opened in 1791), and the Maryland Hospital (opened in 1798), though the latter was plagued by severe financial problems (Grob, *Mental Institutions*, 15–39, 55–64; Albert Deutsch, *The Mentally Ill in America: A History of Their Care and Treatment from Colonial Times* [2nd ed.; New York, 1949], 59–61, 97–106).

16. See Edwin Scott Gaustad, *Historical Atlas of Religion in America* (Rev. ed.; New York, 1976), 22, 24–25, 94; Clement Eaton, *The Growth of Southern Civilization* (New York, 1961), 37, 77; Kenneth L. Carroll, "Quakerism in Caroline County, Maryland: Its Rise and Decline," *Bulletin of the Friends Historical Association*, XLVIII (1959), 83–102; Richard I. Zuber, "Conscientious Objectors in the Confederacy: The Quakers in North Carolina," *Quaker History*, LXVII (1978), 1–19; Digby, *Madness, Morality and Medicine*, 60.

notion, rooted in Enlightenment sensibilities, is clearly evident in the remarks made by the early advocates of the southern asylums. William Crafts, one of the two legislative sponsors of the South Carolina Lunatic Asylum, saw the public asylum as a means by which the state could help to restore reason to citizens who suffered from loss of reason.[17] In his oration at the laying of the asylum cornerstone in 1822, he argued that if the state had a responsibility to cultivate reason in its citizens through education, it had a similar responsibility to try to restore reason to the mad: "The beauty of reason is to propagate itself. The honor of States is to disseminate knowledge. . . . [D]oes not as strong an inducement exist to aid by public care and exertion, the *recovery* of reason, when it is lost, as to cultivate it when it exists[?]"[18]

A similar emphasis on the restoration of reason as a rationale for establishing a public asylum was apparent almost thirty years later when Dr. A. Lopez, an advocate for the establishment of an asylum in Alabama, told the state legislature of Alabama in 1850 that, "*Seven Hundred Human Beings* deprived of God's supremest gift to man [*i.e.*, reason], point out to you through us, the practical means by which that privation in a large population of cases, can be restored." For these reformers, reestablishing reason among the "unfortunate" members of society was an important motivating factor.[19]

A further distinguishing characteristic of southern asylums was their reliance, particularly during the first three decades of the nineteenth century, on lay superintendents. Of American asylums established prior to 1860, at least seven originally employed lay superintendents to administer the day-to-day affairs of the asylum. Two of these

17. The influence on asylum reformers of the concern with reason that occurred as part of the Enlightenment is discussed in George Rosen, "Irrationality and Madness in Seventeenth and Eighteenth Century Europe," in George Rosen, *Madness in Society: Chapters in the Historical Sociology of Mental Illness* (Chicago, 1968), 151–71; Andrew Scull, *Museums of Madness: The Social Organization of Insanity in Nineteenth-Century England* (New York, 1979), 43–44, 59–73; Andrew Scull, "Moral Treatment Reconsidered: Some Sociological Comments on an Episode in the History of British Psychiatry," and William F. Bynum, "Rationales for Therapy in British Psychiatry, 1780–1835," both in Andrew Scull (ed.), *Madhouses, Mad-Doctors, and Madmen: The Social History of Psychiatry in the Victorian Era* (Philadelphia, 1981), 105–18, 35–57. See also Bellows, " 'Insanity is the Disease of Civilization,' " 263–72; *Sketch*, 4; Henry M. Hurd, *The Institutional Care of the Insane in the United States and Canada* (4 vols.; Baltimore, 1916–17), III, 587–88.

18. William Crafts, *Oration on the Occasion of Laying the Corner Stone of the Lunatic Asylum, at Columbia, S.C., July 1822* (Charleston, S.C., 1822), 12–13.

19. Quoted in Katherine Vickery, *A History of Mental Health in Alabama* (N.p., n.d.), 27.

were in northern states (the Bloomingdale Asylum and the Friends' Asylum); five were in southern states. The use of lay superintendents was certainly not without precedent, for it represented a transplantation of the English madhouse system to American soil. Most of the southern asylums that employed lay superintendents had been established during the first three decades of the nineteenth century, when the practice of employing a physician superintendent was not standard in the United States. During the next three decades, however, the presence of a medical superintendent became a mark of excellence in the United States, and as a consequence, southern asylums with lay superintendents were at a disadvantage.[20]

The madhouse system that influenced the administrative structure of early southern asylums had grown up in the seventeenth and eighteenth centuries in England. There, with some important exceptions, madhouses served as custodial institutions, and the involvement of physicians in their daily operations was variable. English madhouses were administered sometimes by lay "keepers," sometimes by medical. Although lay keepers occasionally performed their jobs admirably, physician involvement at some level was seen as an integral part of proper asylum management in England.[21] Naturally enough, then, the Board of Governors of the earliest southern asylum, Williamsburg, retained a local physician, John de Sequerya, when it opened in 1773, and hired a layman, James Galt, to administrate the asylum as a keeper. Only in the 1840s did the asylum employ a physician, John M. Galt II, as superintendent. Likewise, the Kentucky Eastern Lunatic Asylum (established in 1824), the South Carolina Lunatic Asylum (1828), the Western Lunatic Asylum at Staunton (1828), and the Mount Hope Institution (1840) all originally had lay administrators and physician visitors. By the 1840s virtually all of these institutions had replaced

20. John M. Galt II, *The Treatment of Insanity* (1846; rpr. New York, 1973), 524, 544, 555; "Dr. William Stokes, of the Mount Hope Institution, Near Baltimore, Md., and the *American Journal of Insanity*," *American Journal of Insanity*, V (1848–49), 262–74.

21. William Lloyd Parry-Jones, *The Trade in Lunacy: A Study of Private Madhouses in England in the Eighteenth and Nineteenth Centuries* (London, 1972), 8–28, 74–75. William Pargeter, an influential English physician who wrote on insanity in the late eighteenth century, noted that madhouses kept by clergymen (and physicians) were usually superior to others (Parry-Jones, *The Trade in Lunacy*, 81). A woman treated in Miles' madhouse at Hoxton, England, complained in 1763 to a Select Committee of the House of Commons that she received no medical treatment and no medicines during her confinement there (Kathleen Jones, *Lunacy, Law, and Conscience, 1744–1845: The Social History of the Care of the Insane* [London, 1955], 35).

lay superintendents with physicians, the one exception being the Mount Hope Institution.[22]

Despite the presence of significant numbers of asylums in the Old South, southern asylum superintendents were not able to exert leadership nationally through the superintendents' organization, the Association of Medical Superintendents of American Institutions for the Insane (AMSAII). Such a situation would not, on the surface, seem to have been inevitable. The AMSAII was founded in 1844 through the efforts of Samuel B. Woodward, superintendent of the Worcester State Lunatic Hospital in Massachusetts, and Francis Stribling of the Virginia Western Lunatic Asylum. Although the organization grew out of the combined efforts of a northerner and a southerner, southern superintendents generally played a secondary role in the leadership of the organization. The most involved of the southern superintendents was Charles Nichols of the Government Hospital for the Insane in the District of Columbia, who served as President of the AMSAII for a number of years. But Nichols was born in Maine and had worked at the Utica and Bloomingdale asylums prior to taking the superintendency at the Government Hospital. Thus, he had more intimate ties to the leadership of the AMSAII than did most superintendents of southern asylums. Galt, who was superintendent at the Williamsburg asylum until 1862, attended all but one meeting of the association between 1844 and 1850, but attended no meetings of the association after 1850. Francis Stribling, a cofounder of the AMSAII, was always highly regarded in the association, but attended only four of the fifteen meetings held between 1844 and 1860. John Fonerden of the Maryland Hospital for the Insane and William Stokes of the Mount Hope Institution in Baltimore attended often, as did superintendents who joined the association somewhat later, such as William S. Chipley of the Lexington, Kentucky, asylum and William Cheatham of the Tennessee Hospital for the Insane in Nashville. Edward C. Fisher of the North Carolina asylum, who first came to the AMSAII meetings in 1854, had worked under Stribling at the Western Lunatic Asylum of Virginia and was well trained and influential; Thomas F. Green of Georgia attended meetings infrequently during this period but joined in the AMSAII discussions when he came.[23]

22. Norman Dain, *Disordered Minds: The First Century of the Eastern State Hospital in Williamsburg, Virginia, 1766–1866* (Williamsburg, 1971); Galt, *Treatment of Insanity,* 551–52, 555; *Sketch,* 10; Powell, "Psychiatry in the Southern States," 86.

23. Constance M. McGovern, *Masters of Madness: Social Origins of the American Psychiatric Profession* (Hanover, N.H., 1985), 2; Winfred Overholser, "The Founding and the

Part of the inability of southerners to exert national leadership may have been that, except for the Western Lunatic Asylum of Virginia, southern asylums were generally viewed as inferior to the best institutions in the North. The problem was not, however, that southern asylums had poorer physicians or that they were uninitiated into the humane techniques for managing the insane during the antebellum period. Southern physicians involved with asylums frequently acknowledged the value of moral therapy and humane treatment. Many even made visits to the North to learn more about humane approaches to treatment at the leading northern asylums. But most southern institutions were public, and in the South, as elsewhere, public institutions tended to receive indigent and chronic patients. Thus, even though asylum superintendents might have had the best of intentions, treatments were often limited by factors beyond their control.[24]

A case in point is that of John M. Galt II. Although Galt's father and grandfather had served as physicians at the Eastern asylum, and several of Galt's relatives had been lay keepers of the asylum, John Galt II, in his position as superintendent (a newly created post), was considerably more involved in patient treatment and asylum administration than other physicians in his family had been before him. He took the post of superintendent in 1841 at the age of twenty-two, having just received his medical degree from the University of Pennsylvania.

A bachelor throughout his life, Galt was able to divide his time between the asylum and personal study; consequently, he spent much of his personal time writing. He wrote about literature, philosophy, religion, medicine, and (especially) himself and kept many com-

---

Founders of the Association," in Hall (ed.), *One Hundred Years of American Psychiatry* (New York, 1944), 45–72. My estimate of the involvement of southerners in the AMSAII is based on a survey, "Proceedings of the Association of Medical Superintendents of American Institutions for the Insane," *American Journal of Insanity*, I–XV (1844–60).

24. On southerners' estimates of northern asylums, see South Carolina Lunatic Asylum Annual Report, 1842, 10; and South Carolina Lunatic Asylum Annual Report, 1850, 7; though in the South Carolina Lunatic Asylum Annual Report of 1853, the physician considered the Kirkbride plan of asylum construction to be inadequate for southern needs. On southern praise of moral therapy and humane treatment, see Maximilian Laborde's comments in South Carolina Lunatic Asylum Annual Report, 1842, 7; John M. Galt II, Medical Commonplace Book 1847, GFP, II, Box XV, folder 70; Vickery, *A History of Mental Health in Alabama*, 26; Insane Asylum of North Carolina Annual Report, 1858, 20–21; and White, "John Rowan Allen, M.D." On visits to northern asylums, see GFP, I, MsV 68, Commonplace Book, May 1842–July 1844; Powell, "Psychiatry in the Southern States," 86; South Carolina Lunatic Asylum, Minutes of the Board of Regents, November 9, 1828.

monplace books and a lengthy personal diary. Galt's writings reveal him as an introspective man concerned about discipline and order. His writing style (and presumably his interpersonal manner) was affected and sometimes condescending. He considered himself one of the literati and was particularly fond of poetry. The following diary entry, recorded during a trip to New England in the early 1840s, suggests something of his personal style:

> Went in the boat to New Haven; and from thence to Hartford in cars. A Bible in each room. First time in N. England. White servants were menial . . . in their behavior. A Bible in each room. [I took] Pleasure in [the] company of Mr. G's daughters. Younger said when she read [Keats's] Endymion, she threw the book down, so deeply did she feel the poetry. How this interview will linger in her heart's memory like the petals of a rose. Walked with her to Lecture on poetry. They allow no other amusement in the city.[25]

Whatever his personal idiosyncrasies, Galt attempted to investigate the treatment of mental disorders with great thoroughness. Galt made, by the standards of his day, careful written observations of the patients he treated to help him determine the best treatment approach for various types of insanity. He also read widely in an effort to determine the best way to manage the patients under his care at the asylum. His book, *Treatment of Insanity* (1846), is essentially a compilation of his notes on medical literature as it related to the treatment of mental disorders. He traveled North in the 1840s in an effort to broaden his knowledge about medicine and asylum management, touring the Pennsylvania Hospital, the Hartford Retreat, McLean Asylum, and the Maryland and St. Vincent's hospitals. Galt may be considered among the most careful and systematic practitioners of asylum medicine of the early nineteenth century.[26]

Early in his career, Galt began to realize that his patients were primarily the chronically mentally ill and would probably not improve, regardless of the therapy instituted. Prior to 1841, the year Galt took the superintendency of the asylum, the Virginia legislature had mandated that mad patients east of the Blue Ridge Mountains go to the Eastern Lunatic Asylum, and those west of them to the Western Lunatic Asylum. Because this arrangement gave the Western asylum a much larger population to serve than the Eastern, Stribling had the luxury of selecting higher-functioning cases, and Galt was forced to accept the "less desirable" patient residuum. In 1841, in an effort to redress the situation, the legislature required patients to apply to the asylum near-

25. GFP, I, MsV 68, Commonplace Book, May 1842–July 1844.
26. *Ibid.*

est home, but the situation did not improve since the great majority of the population of Virginia lived west of the Blue Ridge Mountains. Thus, the majority of patients at the asylum were the "incurable" insane. Not surprisingly, Galt's initial enthusiasm for the possibility of curing the insane waned as he began to realize the grim fact that the effectiveness of moral therapy was severely limited by the nature of the patient population he treated.[27]

Galt and the Eastern Lunatic Asylum were frequently the subject of controversy during Galt's superintendency. The most important on-going career difficulty facing Galt was the unfavorable comparison of the "cure rates" of the Eastern and Western asylums and the implicit comparison of the skill of Galt and Galt's counterpart at the Western Lunatic Asylum, Francis Stribling, by the state legislature. At one point Galt became so frustrated with his lack of recognition by the state legislature that he made the following entry in one of his commonplace books: "My reports before the Legislature are complete instances of 'casting pearls before swine.' For they have even ordered new editions of the report of the W[estern] A[sylum] and none of ours. . . . [T]he last of mine, was prepared with the utmost care . . . and diligence. Dr. Stribling's besides being written without any special care, . . . was short, and contained no new views whatever, indeed, he made the remark that 'a man after 20 years superintendence of an asylum could not be expected to have ought that is new.' "[28] Galt was never able to attain the degree of success at treatment he desired, not for any lack of study or knowledge, but because of the nature of the population he treated and (to a lesser degree) because of his lack of resources.

Similar to Galt's problems were those of James Davis, asylum physician at the South Carolina Lunatic Asylum from 1828 to 1836. Davis was born in Worcester County, Maryland, in 1774, but moved to South Carolina at the age of ten after the death of his father. His medical education apparently consisted primarily of an apprenticeship done with a Dr. George Ross from 1795 to 1797. He served in the state senate from 1804 to 1808 and was among the Commissioners who established the asylum in 1821.[29]

27. This account of Galt's problems in dealing with the chronically mentally ill is based on my own reading of the Galt Family Papers and the Eastern Lunatic Asylum annual reports, as well as the account in Dain, *Disordered Minds*, 105–27, 142–61.

28. GFP, II, Box V, folder 57, "Ideas on Insanity and Medicine."

29. Biographical information on James Davis is from the following sources: Joseph Ioor Waring, *A History of Medicine in South Carolina, 1670–1825* (N.p., 1964), 206–208; Senatorial Research Committee, *Biographical Directory of the Senate of the State of South Carolina, 1776–1964* (Columbia, S.C., 1964), 203; Vera Smith Pears, "Union Library Society Formed," Union (S.C.) *Daily Times*, October 16, 1969.

Davis, like others involved in the establishment of the Columbia asylum, wanted it to become the sort of therapeutic institution being established in the American North. Davis himself had, at least in the early phases of the establishment of the asylum, a strongly stated belief in the value of the "new" ways of managing the mentally disordered. In his annual report following the first year of operation of the asylum, Davis wrote:

> The old and barbarous practice of torture as a remedy is excluded in every shape; and when restraint and coercion become necessary for their own or others safety, and for the exhibition of medicine, they are imposed with the utmost lenity and mildness. In my immediate department, I have constant and special regard to moral influences upon the mind as well as to medicine upon the physical organs. . . . I endeavour to awaken [the patients'] acuity, to accustom them to cleanliness, and to order and propriety of conduct; [and] as far as possible to bring them to perceive and to feel, that they are yet members of the human family; that instead of being outcasts of society, they are objects of the sympathetic care, and the respectful regards of their fellow citizens.[30]

Davis continued by saying that he tried to arrange the patients' environment in such a way that they would not be confronted with anything that might stir up passionate or disagreeable emotions or painful associations. Instead, he tried to involve them in pleasant occupations and amusements that would encourage a rational mental life.

Though there is no reason to doubt the sincerity of Davis' desire to employ moral therapy in the asylum, his records of the treatment of individual patients do not indicate a great concern with the manipulation of their mental lives. This may be because moral therapy at the asylum was administered to all patients in a fairly uniform manner and therefore was not recorded in the treatment books. What *is* recorded suggests that medical treatment and the phenomenology and pathology of mental diseases were foremost in Davis' mind, and that moral therapy at the Columbia asylum served more as a rallying cry for state support of the institution than as a basis for the planning and implementation of asylum treatment.

Notably, the one southern institution that received some recognition for its therapeutic approach, the Western Lunatic Asylum of Virginia, eschewed black patients, and generally catered to a nonchronic, nonindigent population. In this respect it resembled the proprietary institutions of the North.[31]

30. Printed sheet inserted into Minutes of the Board of Regents, I.

31. Todd L. Savitt, *Medicine and Slavery: The Diseases and Health Care of Blacks in Antebellum Virginia* (Urbana, 1978), 263–66.

Prior to Reconstruction, the most common argument in favor of asylum segregation was moral therapy. One of the fundamental tenets of moral therapy was that patients should be separated from things that aroused disturbing associations, and that the asylum, where the patient could be free of disturbing family and home circumstances, was essential to restoring disordered mental process. Separation in the asylum, however, involved not only separation from problematic influences outside of the asylum, but from things within the asylum that might disturb as well. One of the things that seemed to disturb white patients (at least in the minds of some superintendents) was being placed in proximity to black patients. Writing for the AMSAII Committee on Asylums for Colored People in 1853, John M. Galt remarked: "The prominent disadvantage in the admission of lunatics of the two races into one asylum, is thought to be the prejudice existing in the United States as respects color. . . . [I]t is supposed that in the insane, the same feelings exist upon this point as with the sane, and hence from any admixture of races, a train of irritating circumstances would be likely to follow which must materially interfere with the comfort, the management, and the cure of both white and colored patients."[32]

Although Galt opposed separate asylums for blacks, favoring instead either segregation within the asylum or the judicious mixing of blacks and whites on the same ward, Galt's view was a minority one. Thomas Kirkbride, referring to Galt's ideas about asylum management, stated: "The idea of mixing up all colors and all classes, as is seen in one or two institutions of the United States, is not what is wanted in our hospitals for the insane, although it may be regarded by [Galt] as a desirable kind of liberty."[33]

Despite concerns about how black patients should be managed within the asylum, a number of southern asylums admitted blacks during the antebellum period. Not only the Eastern Lunatic Asylum, but the South Carolina Lunatic Asylum, the Maryland Asylum, and the Jackson (Mississippi) Asylum all admitted black patients.[34]

The issue of treatment for the "coloured insane" was as pertinent at the Eastern Lunatic Asylum as at any other American asylum for the insane. American medical theorists of the early nineteenth century frequently held that the treatment of disease should take the patient's

32. John M. Galt II, "Asylums for Colored Persons," *American Psychological Journal*, I (1853), 84.

33. "Proceedings of the Association of Medical Superintendents of American Institutions for the Insane," *American Journal of Insanity*, XII (1855), 43.

34. J. W. Babcock, *The Colored Insane: Read Before the National Conference of Charities and Corrections at New Haven, Conn., May, 1895* (N.p., [1895]), 6–23.

race into account. And one might expect a southern superintendent such as Galt to be a stringent advocate of separation of races during the treatment of insanity. In fact, the manner in which Galt felt race and servitude status affected treatment was considerably more complex. Galt, while no opponent of slavery, favored the admission of blacks, both slave and free, to the Eastern Asylum. Perhaps Galt was acting on humanitarian grounds in advocating a nondiscriminatory admission policy. However, the "cure rate" factor, which preoccupied Galt's relationship with Stribling and the Virginia legislature, may have been at work as well, for Galt was convinced that slave blacks not only had less insanity, but insanity more readily cured than that of whites.[35] Thus, in his annual report of 1848, Galt noted that since the legislature's act of 1846 allowing the admission of insane slaves, "those in charge of the asylum have had the privilege of ministering to the wants of all classes of persons laboring under . . . an insane mind, irrespective of color or social position." But he continued by observing,

> The proportionate number of slaves who become deranged, is less than that of free coloured persons, and less than that of the whites. . . . [Slaves] are removed from much of the mental excitement to which the free population of the Union is necessarily exposed in the daily routine of life. . . . When we look . . . to the number of slaves, with the view of making suitable provisions for the insane amongst them, the amount [of provision] required will be less than for the same number of free persons. . . . [Insanity] may be considered in general as less tenacious of its existence, and more readily yielding to remediate means [among slaves]. Moreover, we believed that these means are usually so applied, as either to result in the cure of the patient or to constitute the mode of management among them most suitable to the chronic insane.[36]

Further, Galt believed that black slaves were more likely to be

35. The issue of slave insanity has been dealt with in Savitt, *Medicine and Slavery,* 247–79. Savitt also deals with the general medical treatment of blacks on pp. 149–84. On race and science generally in America in the nineteenth century, see William Stanton, *The Leopard's Spots: Scientific Attitudes Toward Race in America, 1815–1859* (Chicago, 1960); and John S. Haller, Jr., *Outcasts from Evolution: Scientific Attitudes of Racial Inferiority, 1859–1900* (Urbana, 1971). On the controversy over insanity among slaves during the antebellum period, see Gerald N. Grob, "Edward Jarvis and the Federal Census: A Chapter in the History of Nineteenth-Century American Medicine," *Bulletin of the History of Medicine,* L (1976), 4–27; Albert Deutsch, "The First U.S. Census of the Insane (1840) and Its Use as Pro-Slavery Propaganda," *Bulletin of the History of Medicine,* XV (1944), 469–82. Galt's views on asylums and blacks are in "Asylums for Colored Persons," 73–88; his views on slavery are continued in [John M. Galt II], *A Voice from Virginia: Political Essays* (N.p., [1852]).

36. Eastern Lunatic Asylum of Virginia Annual Report, 1848, 18–20.

brought to the asylum early in their illness, thus increasing the like-lihood of cure. "The very fact that it is to the interest of his owner that a slave should recover from insanity, apart from feelings of kindness and a sense of duty induces him to send for a physician in the acute or incubative state of the disease," Galt wrote. Even if the slave did not entirely recover, he could be discharged from the asylum more readily than a free person, since his duties as a slave were structured for him by a master who would provide an environment for the slave similar to that provided for the chronically insane free persons by the asylum. Thus, while humanitarianism may have constituted *part* of Galt's motive in advocating a "liberal" admissions policy toward slaves, one suspects he had other motives as well.[37]

After the Civil War, however, a strong move toward strict segre-gation ensued. The Eastern Lunatic Asylum was transformed into an all-black asylum by the military governor of the state. The South Caro-lina Lunatic Asylum superintendent, Dr. Ensor, invoked the "natural antagonism of the races" when requesting money for provision for separate quarters for blacks in 1878. Although blacks were apparently not strictly segregated in Maryland after the war, in the 1890s, Dr. Richard Gundry, the superintendent, complained of the need for sepa-rate quarters for black patients since he found that they irritated whites.[38]

In conclusion, the South lacked the resources and social chemistry to provide national leadership in mental health care. While religious movements such as Quakerism and the Second Great Awakening cata-lyzed the asylum reform movement in the North, there was no analo-gous catalyst in the South. Nonetheless, antebellum southerners had among them individuals who were deeply concerned about providing mentally disordered patients a place to stay and humane management. Although organizational styles differed regionally and the South lacked the prominent proprietary institutions of the North, certain southerners conscientiously tried to care for mentally disordered people both at the community and the institutional level. Indeed, their experience, characterized by attempts to negotiate with frugal legisla-tures and to face realistically the problems of the chronically mentally ill, is in some respects quite similar to that of modern mental health policymakers who try to secure public assistance for troubled indi-viduals in a time of waning enthusiasm for government funding of mental health services.

37. *Ibid.*, 20.
38. Babcock, *The Colored Insane*, 7–11.

275

CHAPTER 13

UNLESS POWERFUL SICK: DOMESTIC MEDICINE IN THE OLD SOUTH

Elizabeth Barnaby Keeney

S outherners of the antebellum era employed a variety of techniques to maintain or restore health without the direct aid of professionals. Distrust of elites, uncertain access to physicians, the inefficacy of prevailing medical practices, and the relatively high cost of professional treatment all led many southerners to become their own physicians. Because the services of a physician were often expensive, inconvenient, or unavailable in the predominantly rural South, such lay medicine was widely used, either exclusively or as a first resort, with professional help being reserved for serious or stubborn cases. While southerners embraced do-it-yourself medicine with the same enthusiasm and for many of the same reasons as their northern and western contemporaries, they sometimes modified it, for example, to serve the peculiar health problems of the South and the institution of slavery. In doing so, southerners adapted traditional medicine for domestic use to fit their needs.[1]

The eschewal of professional medicine in favor of self-treatment or treatment by a friend or family member is as old as professional medicine itself. Folk medicine—the traditional use of homemade remedies—has been handed down from generation to generation as part of oral tradition; it is distinct rather than derived from professional therapeutics. In contrast, domestic medicine, as I will use the term, is medicine drawn from professional practice and generally disseminated

---

1. In this chapter, the "South" refers to the following states: Alabama, Arkansas, Florida, Georgia, Kentucky, Louisiana, Mississippi, North Carolina, South Carolina, Tennessee, Texas, and Virginia.

through published writings rather than oral transmission. By the early nineteenth century, Americans could choose from a wide selection of manuals. The flourishing publication not only of general manuals but of guides aimed at specific geographic regions, including the South, illustrates the popularity of domestic medicine in America. The thriving publication of specialized guides also suggests that domestic medicine is influenced by the culture of a region. The influence of such cultural variables as gender roles, the southern climate, and most especially the demands of slavery on domestic medicine offers the historian insight into both the medical and social history of the Old South.

Nineteenth-century American domestic manuals served several purposes. First, many of them offered extensive advice on the prevention of disease, focusing on hygiene, diet, and exercise. Second, they all described an array of diseases and disorders, their symptoms, and recommended treatment. Finally, they offered suggestions on when to call physicians and how to evaluate their services. Not surprisingly, the advice varied widely from manual to manual. The fragmentation of the antebellum medical community over therapeutic rationales is clearly reflected in these manuals, which greatly differed in the opinions they expressed on the prudence of heroic measures, such as bloodletting. The manuals represented various irregular medical sects and were tailored to regional differences as well, giving special emphasis to local problems. A close look at southern manuals and how they differed from those published in the North provides a good introduction to the practice of domestic medicine in the Old South.

At least eleven southern manuals appeared between 1807 and 1860, several running through multiple editions.[2] Although southerners were certainly not restricted to using manuals written for or by south-

---

2. Southern manuals I have identified include Simon B. Abbott, *The Southern Botanic* (Charleston, 1844); John W. Bright, *A Plain System of Medical Practice Adapted to the Use of Families* (Louisville, 1847); William Daily, *The Indian Doctor's Practice of Medicine or Daily's Family Physician* (Louisville, 1848); James Ewell, *The Planter's and Mariner's Medical Companion* (Philadelphia, 1807), thirteen editions; Tomlinson Fort, *A Dissertation on the Practice of Medicine* (Milledgeville, Ga., 1849); A. G. Goodlett, *Family Physician, or Every Man's Companion* (Nashville, 1838); J. C. Gunn, *Gunn's Domestic Medicine, or Poor Man's Friend* (Knoxville, Tenn., 1830), over one hundred "editions"; Samuel K. Jennings, *A Compendium of Medical Science, or Fifty Years Experience in the Art of Healing* (Tuscaloosa, Ala., 1847); Ralph Schenck, *The Family Physician: Treating of the Diseases Which Assail the Human System at Different Periods of Life* (Fincastle, Va., 1842); J. Hume Simons, *The Planter's Guide and Family Book of Medicine* (Charleston, 1848), two editions; and Isaac Wright, *Wright's Family Medicine, or System of Domestic Practice* (Madisonville, Tenn., 1833).

erners, many did elect to use them because they dealt with health problems southerners were especially likely to encounter and because they were apt to discuss the medical problems of blacks.[3] Some of the authors, including James Ewell, appealed to southern readers by claiming that they had gained special insight into southern diseases and constitutions through years of living and practicing medicine in the South: "On the important subject of domestic medicine, many books have been written, which though excellent in other respects, have greatly failed of usefulness to *Americans,* because they treat of diseases, which existing in very *foreign climates and constitutions* must widely differ from ours. The book now offered to the public has, therefore, the great advantage of having been written by a native American of long and successful practice in the Southern States, and who for years past has turned much of his attention to the composition of it."[4]

The earliest and one of the most popular of the manuals intended especially for a southern audience was *The Planter's and Mariner's Medical Companion,* written by a Savannah physician, James Ewell. The first of thirteen editions appeared in 1807. Even more popular and enduring was John C. Gunn's *Domestic Medicine, or Poor Man's Friend,* which went through one hundred printings between 1830 and 1870. The publishing success of these two manuals suggests that they were the most widely used, though other manuals were also available.[5]

The authors of the southern guides, like their peers elsewhere, generally were physicians.[6] James Ewell, for example, was trained through preceptorships under his uncle and another physician. In the

3. See, for example, Simons, *Planter's Guide,* 205–208; and Ewell, *Planter's and Mariner's Companion,* 34. See also Todd L. Savitt, *Medicine and Slavery: The Diseases and Health Care of Blacks in Antebellum Virginia* (Urbana, 1978), 11.

4. Ewell, *Planter's and Mariner's Companion,* vi–vii.

5. The popularity of nineteenth-century publications is difficult to assess, but one measure is the number of editions and printings. On the popularity of Gunn's work nationally, see Alex Berman, "The Impact of the Nineteenth Century Botanico-Medical Movement on American Pharmacy and Medicine" (Ph.D. dissertation, University of Wisconsin, 1954), 62; Madge E. Pickard and R. Carlyle Buley, *The Midwest Pioneer: His Ills, Cures & Doctors* (Crawfordsville, Ind., 1945), 93; and Charles E. Rosenberg, "Introduction to the New Edition" of *Gunn's Domestic Medicine* (1830; rpr. Knoxville, Tenn., 1986). Apparently, enough of the southern audience could read their manuals; southern literacy rates for whites reported in the U.S. Census of 1860 were lower than those for New England and the Mid-Atlantic and North Central regions, but higher than those of the West.

6. John B. Blake, "From Buchan to Fishbein: The Literature of Domestic Medicine," in Guenter B. Risse, Ronald L. Numbers, and Judith Walzer Leavitt (eds.), *Medicine Without Doctors: Home Health Care in American History* (New York, 1977), 11–30.

early years of the nineteenth century, Ewell practiced in Savannah, where he was a charter member of the Georgia Medical Society and ran a hospital for mariners. Following the publication of the first edition of his manual, he fell into disrepute among local physicians, who felt that his promotion of domestic medicine threatened their livelihoods. Ewell then left Savannah to practice in the District of Columbia and later in New Orleans.[7] John Gunn apparently studied medicine in New York before beginning practice first in Virginia and later in Tennessee. While the degree of Gunn's personal contact with medical leaders is uncertain, his writings reveal careful study of the works of Benjamin Rush, Phillip Syng Physic, and other authorities. Gunn's work reflects both a deep respect for the best of professional medicine and a belief that laypeople could often do just as good a job, or better, if properly guided.[8] Tomlinson Fort, author of *A Dissertation on the Practice of Medicine*, attended the University of Pennsylvania Medical School, where he studied under Benjamin Rush. He began his practice in 1810 in Milledgeville, Georgia, then the state capital. A founder and trustee of the Medical Academy (later the Medical College) of Georgia, as well as a Georgia and United States Representative, Fort had an extremely successful practice and was one of the leading figures of the town and the state. Fort's manual, written for physicians as well as laypeople, received favorable reviews in the South, but in national publications some reviewers attacked this attempt to inform the public, charging that medicine was too complex for the average reader.[9]

A comparison of the advice and perspectives given in northern and southern manuals reveals both similarities and differences in regional practices. On the surface, the similarities are most evident. Manuals written with other regions in mind, for example, George Capron and David B. Slack's *New England Popular Medicine* and Anthony A. Benezet's *The Family Physician*, were just as apt to stress prevention as their southern counterparts. The range of health problems they discussed and the remedies they recommended were also similar. But there were regional variations, especially in emphasis. Southern manuals, for example, included long sections on yellow fever and ague, two per-

7. Allan Westcott, "James Ewell," *Dictionary of American Biography*, VI, 229; Victor H. Bassett, "Plantation Medicine," *Journal of the Medical Association of Georgia*, XXXIX (1940), 116, 120.

8. Rosenberg, "Introduction." See also Ben H. McClarys, "Introducing a Classic: Gunn's Domestic Medicine," *Tennessee Historical Quarterly*, XLV (1986), 210–16.

9. William C. Roberts, "Tomlinson Fort of Milledgeville, Georgia: Physician and Statesman," *Journal of the History of Medicine and Allied Science*, XXIII (1968), 131–52.

sistent southern problems, while their northern counterparts treated both as infrequent problems. Northern manuals gave other disorders that flourished in the South but not the North the same curt attention given yaws by one northern writer: "Not one of the diseases of New England." And not surprisingly, southern manuals were more apt to discuss the special health problems of blacks.[10]

Comparing the specific remedies recommended in northern and southern manuals is hampered by the lack of uniformity even within those having a common regional focus. A look at the manuals of James Ewell and John Gunn and Isaac Wright's *Wright's Family Medicine* illustrates the variety. The advice these three southern manuals offered on the treatment of measles differed greatly. Ewell recommended keeping the bowels free by administering either castor oil or a cathartic mixture of glauber salts (sodium sulfate), lemon juice, sugar, and water. If the patient had a persistent fever, then bleeding, blistering the chest, and steam inhalation might also be tried. All cases called for rest, a light diet, and keeping warm. In contrast, Isaac Wright recommended prompt bleeding and the promotion of vomiting, together with warm baths, blisters, and doses of antimonial wine in dire cases.[11] Although Ewell and Gunn often recommended sharply contrasting remedies, they did agree about some things. Their recommendations for worms, for example, both focused on purges, and they each recognized the value of quinine in the control of malaria or intermittent fever.[12] While therapeutic recommendation may well have varied from North to South, the historical problem of contrasting the two is enormous because of the lack of regional conformity.

Despite their importance, manuals were by no means the only available source of medical information. Southerners recorded and shared their domestic remedies, advice, and experiences not only in domestic medical manuals but in popular journals and local newspapers. The number of periodical publications greatly increased during the ante-

10. George Capron and David B. Slack, *New England Popular Medicine* (Providence, 1846), esp. 603–604; Anthony A. Benezet, *The Family Physician; Comprising Rules for the Prevention and Cure of Diseases Calculated Particularly for the Inhabitants of the Western Country* (Cincinnati, 1826); see also Blake, "Buchan to Fishbein."

11. Ewell, *Planter's and Mariner's Companion*, 126–27; Wright, *Wright's Family Medicine*, 98–99.

12. Abbott, *Southern Botanic*, 136–42, 361–62; James Ewell, *The Medical Companion, or Family Physician* (Washington, D.C., 1827), 219, 585, 629; John C. Gunn, *Gunn's New Domestic Physician or Home Book of Health* (Cincinnati, 1861), 204–10, 553–55.

bellum period, and the South produced many of its own. Foremost among these were agricultural and planters' journals—*The Soil of the South, The Southern Agriculturist*, and *The Cultivator* to name but a few. Although none ran regular health columns, all frequently mentioned domestic medicine, as was common for agricultural periodicals nationally.[13] *De Bow's Review* also published pieces on health and had advertisements for home medicine chests and medicines in many issues. Literary journals occasionally reviewed and recommended medical works for lay audiences, and *The Southern Lady's Companion* ran articles on health and healing of special interest to women. No literate southerner with an interest in home treatment was at a loss for medical advice.

Reflected in these writings of the Old South was a broad base of concerns that fueled southern interest in domestic medicine. No theme emerges more strongly than the inconvenience and expense of getting a physician. A look at antebellum demographic characteristics reveals that southerners were indeed less apt to have easy access to a physician than many other Americans. Nationally the ratio of physicians to population rose dramatically between 1790 and 1850, and the number of physicians per capita in the South was close to the national average. But this trend was slow to affect many southerners because between 1830 and 1860, the percentage of southerners living in urban areas (populations greater than 2,500) remained less than half of the national average: it grew from less than 4 to 7 percent while the national average grew from 9 to 20 percent. As a result, southerners tended to live farther from physicians, whose economic interests made it desirable to live near large numbers of potential patients. Hence, professional help was often beyond reach.[14] As Paul Starr has recently observed, the cost of professional care included not only a fee for services rendered, but also a charge for the distance the physician had to travel to and from the patient. In antebellum Alabama, Georgia, and Mississippi, for ex-

13. A. L. Demaree, "The Farm Journals: Their Editors and Their Public, 1830–60," *Agricultural History*, XV (1941), 182. Also see Albert Lowther Demaree, *The American Agricultural Press, 1819–1860*, Columbia University Studies in the History of American Agriculture, VIII (New York, 1941), 146–48, 173–75.

14. U.S. Bureau of the Census, *Historical Statistics of the United States: Colonial Times to 1970* (Bicentennial ed.; Washington, D.C., 1975), Pt. 2, pp. 12, 24; J. D. B. De Bow, *The Seventh Census of the United States, 1850* (Washington, 1853), vi, lxxiv. See also James H. Cassedy, "Why Self Help? Americans Alone with their Diseases, 1800–1850," in Risse, Numbers, and Leavitt (eds.), *Medicine Without Doctors*, 31–48.

ample, physicians typically received travel fees of $1 per mile in the day and $2 per mile at night.[15] This fee may have varied from region to region, and from doctor to doctor, but its contribution to the cost of medical care, especially in a predominantly rural region like the South, was not insignificant. Other indirect costs—especially the lost work time spent summoning a physician—also contributed to the high cost of professional care compared to the cost of a domestic manual and medicines.[16]

Even those who had access to physicians and could afford to pay them did not always choose to seek professional assistance. Jacksonian Americans, including southerners, had little respect for elites or education.[17] Many southerners who used domestic medicine did so because they felt that they could do all a professional could, if not more. In 1842 for example, Bennet Barrow's Louisiana plantation was visited by epidemics of measles and scarlet fever. Barrow treated his slaves himself, bleeding and administering emetics at the first sign of illness. In contrast, local physicians were delaying treatment until the diagnosis was certain. Though local physicians lost many patients, Barrow's slaves all survived, which he attributed to his prompt treatment and personal attention. In another case a planter pulled all of his slaves through a local epidemic of "black tongue" by countering its debilitating effects with nourishing food, stimulants, and the healing power of nature. Area physicians, who used drugs that further weakened the system, were not as lucky.[18] Tales like these, which did little to bolster the reputation of physicians, encouraged southerners to rely on domestic healing.

Antebellum Americans had ample cause to be dissatisfied with the doctors and prevailing medical practices of the day. Mainstream, or

15. Bassett, "Plantation Medicine," 120; Howard L. Holley, A History of Medicine in Alabama (Birmingham, 1982), 37–38; Paul Starr, The Social Transformation of American Medicine: The Rise of a Sovereign Profession and the Making of a Vast Industry (New York, 1982), 67.
16. Starr, Social Transformation, 67–69.
17. On the connections between Jacksonian fervor and domestic medicine, see Martin Kaufman, Homeopathy in America: The Rise and Fall of a Medical Heresy (Baltimore, 1971), 21–22; Ronald L. Numbers, "Do-It-Yourself the Sectarian Way," in Risse, Numbers, and Leavitt (eds.), Medicine Without Doctors, 55; Holley, A History of Medicine in Alabama, 8.
18. Edwin Adams Davis, Plantation Life in the Florida Parishes of Louisiana, 1836–1846, as Reflected in the Diary of Bennet H. Barrow (New York, 1943), 42; Susan Dabney Smedes, Memorials of a Southern Planter (New York, 1965), 52–53. Black tongue has been identified by historians as pellagra; see, for example, Kenneth F. Kiple and Virginia Himmelsteib King, Another Dimension to the Black Diaspora: Diet, Disease, and Racism (Cambridge, England, 1981), 127–28.

allopathic, medicine often involved administering harsh drugs and letting large amounts of blood. Thousands of Americans reacted by turning to alternative medical sects, domestically or professionally, or by picking and choosing domestic applications from among the various systems. The most popular sects of antebellum America were Thomsonianism, which in its purest form was wholly domestic, and hydropathy and homeopathy, which had both professional and domestic adherents.[19]

Of the alternative sects the Thomsonians commanded far and away the largest number of domestic advocates in the South. Founded by Samuel Thomson, whose rallying cry, "Every man his own physician," inspired many antebellum Americans to adopt domestic botanic remedies, Thomsonianism swept the nation during the antebellum years, when manuals and certificates conferring the right to practice were sold throughout the nation. In 1835, Alva Curtis, one of the nation's leading botanics, claimed that twenty thousand Georgians were using Thomsonian remedies and that three thousand of the "family rights" that entitled one to use the system had been sold in the state. In the same year the governor of Mississippi claimed that Thomsonian "practitioners," both domestic and professional, treated one half of the people in his state.[20] Thomsonians in Tennessee and Kentucky made similar claims.[21] In South Carolina the sect was sufficiently popular that in 1838 the state legislature repealed licensure laws that prohibited Thomsonian practice.[22] Thomsonian journals, remedies, and books, including a southern domestic manual, were all readily available throughout the South through the mails or from agents authorized to sell them.[23] The domestic manual, written by Simon Abbott, generally adhered to orthodox Thomsonian practices and principles, advocating liberal use of cayenne and lobelia, a botanic emetic that was a warhorse of the Thomsonian arsenal nationally.[24] Also popular in the South was the Thomsonian remedy No. 6, Rheumatic drops, composed of "high wines, or fourth proof brandy, gum myrrh and

19. Numbers, "Do-It-Yourself," 49–72.

20. Berman, "Nineteenth Century Botanico-Medical Movement," 150–52.

21. William H. Pease and Jane H. Pease, *The Web of Progress: Private Values and Public Styles in Boston and Charleston, 1828–1843* (New York, 1985), 117–18.

22. W. Davenport, R. S. Dulin, and Benjamin Major, "Letter to the United States Thomsonian Botanic Convention," *Thomsonian Recorder*, II (1833), 52–53; "A Communication from Gallatin, Tennessee, dated October 1, 1833," *ibid.*, 53–54.

23. "List of Agents," *Thomsonian Recorder*, II (1833), unpaginated.

24. Abbott, *Southern Botanic*, 293–95.

cayenne."[25] Abbott, lamenting that "the benefits of Medicine as a trade will ever be confined to those who are able to pay for them; and of course, the far greater part of mankind will be every where deprived of them," felt that the Thomsonian system was especially appropriate for "the laboring class" because it eliminated the cost of a physician. Despite the cost of a manual and rights, many southerners, including John Walker, a Virginia planter, who bought his rights and some medications in June of 1834 for $23.87½ from agent Thomas Henley, concurred that Thomsonianism was a bargain. The fee, which was in line with the national average and was less than many slaveholders spent on professional care in a year, seemed to Walker to be a small price to pay to relieve his frustration with the inefficacy and harshness of allopathic medicine.[26]

Despite its immense popularity in the North and Midwest, homeopathy, which was based on the dual principle that a drug that induces a symptom in a healthy person will relieve it in an ill one and that drug potency increases as dosage decreases, never developed a large domestic following in the antebellum South. That homeopathic pharmacies, magazines, and societies were rare and short-lived in the South prior to 1860 indicates a lack of both professional and domestic interest.[27] The failure of homeopathy to become either professionally or domestically popular in the South is an issue still awaiting exploration. One possible explanation is the relatively urban appeal of the sect and the relatively rural nature of the South. While this argument certainly holds firmer for professional practice, the difficulty of obtaining supplies and advice may have discouraged domestic practice as well.[28]

Similarly, interest in the domestic applications of hydropathy, the medicinal use of water internally and externally, was greater in the

25. See, for example, P. C. Weston, "Management of a Southern Plantation," *De Bow's Review*, XVII (1857), 38–44, reprinted in James O. Breeden (ed.), *Advice Among Masters: The Ideal of Slave Management in the Old South* (Westport, Conn., 1980), 191; Berman, "Nineteenth Century Botanico-Medical Movement," 204.

26. Abbott, *Southern Botanic*, iii, 3; John Walker Diary, Southern Historical Collection, University of North Carolina at Chapel Hill. I thank John Harley Warner for this citation. See also Savitt, *Medicine and Slavery*, 169–70.

27. Thomas Lindsley Bradford, *Homeopathic Bibliography of the United States* (Philadelphia, 1892); Holley, *A History of Medicine in Alabama*, 247–48; Kaufman, *Homeopathy in America*, 28–47.

28. Elizabeth Barnaby Keeney, Susan Eyrich Lederer, and Edmond P. Minihan, "Sectarians and Scientists: Alternatives to Orthodox Medicine," in Ronald L. Numbers and Judith Walzer Leavitt (eds.), *Wisconsin Medicine: Historical Perspectives* (Madison, 1981), 48–53.

North. Southern water-cure establishments enjoyed success, though whether as vacation resorts or health retreats is often unclear. At least twenty-five water cures were established between 1850 and 1860 in southern states. Wealthy southerners often fled to water cures and other resorts to avoid disease, thereby spending the "sickly season" in healthful climes and vacationing at the same time.[29]

Avoiding disease, whether by flight or other means, was understandably a topic of great interest to antebellum southerners. Domestic manuals often included lengthy sections aimed at enabling readers "to protect themselves from ordinary diseases" through diet, exercise, and cleanliness.[30] Similarly, essays on the care of slaves, children, and pregnant women were full of tips aimed at preventing health problems. Female health, reputed in southern tradition to be frail, was nurtured with exercise, though always with the preservation of femininity in mind. Girls' schools established regular exercise periods, and many plantation women rode horseback and danced both to maintain their health and for recreation.[31]

Alas, preventive measures were not infallible, and southerners did succumb to sickness and injury. The abundance of remedies for simple ailments in the antebellum South reflects those health problems that concerned southerners most often. Southerners had, for example, a great variety of remedies for common injuries—cuts, burns, and insect bites—which is not surprising, considering their frequency and often minor nature.[32] Respiratory-tract problems also plagued southerners and gave rise to numerous remedies for coughs.[33] Because of their familiarity and ease of treatment, minor and common problems were those most apt to be treated domestically.

29. Catherine Clinton, *The Plantation Mistress: Women's World in the Old South* (New York, 1982), 147–50; Harry B. Weiss and Howard R. Kemble, *The Great American Water-Cure Craze: A History of Hydropathy in the United States* (Trenton, N.J., 1967); Marshall Scott Legan, "Hydropathy in America: A Nineteenth Century Panacea," *Bulletin of the History of Medicine*, XLV (1971), 267–80; Jane B. Donegan, *Hydropathic Highway to Health: Women and Water-Cure in Antebellum America* (Westport, Conn., 1986); Susan E. Cayleff, *Wash and Be Healed: The Water-Cure Movement and Women's Health* (Philadelphia, 1987).

30. See, for example, Abbott, *Southern Botanic*; and Wright, *Wright's Family Medicine*. Physicians also stressed prevention (see Charles E. Rosenberg, "The Practice of Medicine in New York a Century Ago," *Bulletin of the History of Medicine*, XLI [1967], 223–53).

31. Clinton, *Plantation Mistress*, 140–41.

32. For a sample, see *Soil of the South*, IV (1854), 57, 117, 276; *Soil of the South*, V (1855), 239, 382; *Soil of the South*, VI (1856), 103, 223.

33. George P. Rawick (ed.), *The American Slave: A Composite Autobiography* (19 vols.; Westport, Conn., 1972), vol. 12.1, p. 127. See also Savitt, *Medicine and Slavery*, 51–56, for the frequency of respiratory ailments.

The frequency of gastrointestinal problems is amply documented by the impressive array of recipes for home production of pills, cordials, and infusions that southern writers recommended. Remedies were rarely specific; what worked in small doses for simple diarrhea was used in heroic proportion for Asiatic cholera. Cholera, though only an occasional visitor during the antebellum period, inspired much fear. Following the outbreak of 1849–1850, recipes for domestic remedies swept planters' and popular journals, including *The Soil of the South* and *De Bow's Review*. Most revolved around brandy and were guaranteed by their contributors to work or to be "worth to any one at least five copies of *The Soil of the South*."[34] The inefficacy of cholera cures is painfully illustrated in one rice grower's daybook that lists five recipes for remedies. Presumably, when one failed he tried another until the patient recovered or succumbed.[35] Professionals were not much more successful. However, one of the reasons for so much interest in domestic cures for cholera may have been the continued professional use of heroic medicine, especially calomel, in the treatment of cholera—with markedly little therapeutic benefit.[36]

Lack of therapeutic effect was not confined to professional medicine. The practice of using domestic remedies first and turning to professional care as a backup when domestic attempts failed was widespread. For example, one slave recalled that his mistress only sought professional help for her family and slaves if her ministrations with oil, turpentine, and lobelia were ineffectual.[37] One planter, who relied heavily on domestic medicine, had so little faith in professionals that he considered sending for a physician to be giving up on the patient's recovery.[38] As a result, physicians complained about being called in too late to be of any use. But there was substantial agreement about the need for prompt professional care for some conditions, among them fractures. Isaac Wright in his *Wright's Family Medicine* recommended finding "an experienced operator" to set the bone immediately.[39] Si-

34. For typical statements, see Jno. M. C. Reed, "Cure for Cholera," *Soil of the South*, IV (1854), 231; E. J. Copell, "Recipe for Cholera," *Soil of the South*, III (1852), 411.

35. Albert Virgil House (ed.), *Plantation Management and Capitalism in Ante-Bellum Georgia: The Journal of Hugh Fraser Grant, Rice Grower* (New York, 1959), 279–80.

36. Charles E. Rosenberg, *The Cholera Years: The United States in 1832, 1849, and 1866* (Chicago, 1962), 151–53; Martha Carolyn Mitchell, "Health and the Medical Profession in the Old South, 1845–1860," *Journal of Southern History*, X (1944), 438–39.

37. Rawick (ed.), *American Slave*, vol. 7.2, p. 137.

38. Ralph Betts Flanders, *Plantation Slavery in Georgia* (Chapel Hill, 1933), 164.

39. Wright, *Wright's Family Medicine*, 237. See also Simons, *Planter's Guide*, 203–204.

mon Abbott, the Thomsonian, was one of the few who disagreed: "Any person of common sense knows how the bones ought to be when not displaced; And by exercising a little mechanical ingenuity, after the muscles are relaxed he will be able to return them to their proper situation." Even Abbott conceded, however, that "Surgical operations, and diseases which rarely occur, may require professional aid."[40] Emergencies did result in some domestic surgery, as in the case of one plantation mistress who recorded surgically removing a feather from her infant's throat.[41] Realizing that in some cases laypeople would have to perform surgery because no doctor was available, authors of some manuals provided instructions for operations. A. G. Goodlett assured his readers that "any man, unless he is an idiot or an absolute fool," can successfully amputate a limb.[42]

Southerners obtained drugs for domestic medicine either by manufacturing them at home or by buying them from physicians, from door-to-door peddlers, at stores, or by mail. Purchased drugs included both those that physicians also used—laudanum and quinine, to name two—and patent remedies, as is reflected in the advertisement of one Mobile merchant who offered to "families, physicians, and the public generally, in the city and the country" his "increasing assortment of Drugs, Chemicals, Family Medicines, fresh Garden and Flower Seed, Plants, Flowers, Herbs, Patent Medicines, Thomsonian and Eclectic Medicines, Leeches—all of which have been selected with the greatest care and are known to be fresh, excellent and genuine."[43]

A southern favorite among patent medicines was Swaim's Celebrated Panacea, a mixture of sarsaparilla, oil of wintergreen, and corrosive sublimate, which sold in 1853 for $1.50 per bottle or three bottles for $4.00. Swaim's claimed to be useful "for the cure of Incipient Consumption, Scrofula, General Debility, White Swelling Rheumatism, Diseases of the Liver and Skin, and all Diseases arising from Impurities of the Blood, and the effects of Mercury."[44] Advertisements like the following in southern publications stressed its effectiveness in treating the special health problems of blacks: "These diseases so frequently set

40. Abbott, *Southern Botanic*, 196, v.

41. Clinton, *Plantation Mistress*, 144.

42. Quoted in Blake, "From Buchan to Fishbein," 25.

43. Quoted in Weymouth T. Jordan, "Plantation Medicine in the Old South," *Alabama Review*, III (1950), 88.

44. *De Bow's Review*, XIV (1853), 634; and James Harvey Young, *The Toadstool Millionaires: A Social History of Patent Medicines in America before Federal Regulation* (Princeton, 1972), 58–66.

regular practice at defiance, and render their miserable victims both useless and expensive to their masters, that planters would study their own interest as well as that of humanity, by keeping always a supply of Swaim's Panacea, which appears to be the only thing which can be relied on in such cases."[45]

Many families and planters kept medicine chests. Indeed, James Ewell marketed chests designed to accompany his manual for $50 to $100.[46] In 1860, *De Bow's Review* recommended a $50 chest for sale in New Orleans. The contents, adequate for treating fifty to one hundred slaves, offer some insight into the favorite commercial remedies of antebellum southerners. Laudanum, paregoric, calomel, sugar of lead, mercurial ointment, and opium were all included in liberal proportions. The chest also contained two gallons of castor oil and six pounds of epsom salts, as well as quinine and specifics for worms and cholera. The case came with a graduated measure and a domestic manual. *De Bow's* suggested adding, among other things, ether, chloride of lime, a scale, and a mortar and pestle.[47] Those whose needs were less grandiose could purchase the items individually and in smaller quantities.

Somewhere on the border between folk and domestic medicine were the remedies many southerners made either by mixing basic ingredients or by preparing herbal remedies. Among the substances southerners commonly combined at home, alcohol, opiates, and red pepper featured prominently, as, for example, in Jno. M. C. Reed's "Cure for Cholera": "1 pint *good* brandy, 1 oz. laudanum, 1 oz. gum camphor, and ½ oz. cayenne."[48] Remedies made from native plants included infusions, for example, flaxseed tea, to be taken internally, and others to be applied externally, for example, a rinse of prickly ash bark, dogwood bark, walnut root, and water to be used for tetter and scald head.[49] Homemade remedies could be prepared as the need arose or stored for future use.

Domestic medicine knew no social bounds. Rich and poor, black and white, southerners all relied to some extent on home care. Within white families one adult, often a woman, assumed primary care for

45. *De Bow's Review*, XIV (1853), 634.
46. Mary Louise Marshall, "Plantation Medicine," *Bulletin of the Medical Library Association*, XXVI (1938), 125–26.
47. *De Bow's Review*, XXVIII (1860), 493–94.
48. Reed, "Cure for Cholera," 231.
49. "Recipe for Tetter and Scald Head," *Soil of the South*, V (1855), 78. Regional comparison of home remedies by a scholar with ethnobotanical expertise is needed to determine how southern remedies differ from those of other regions.

family health, nursing, dosing, and deciding when or whether to call a doctor. Slaves were sometimes allowed to nurse family members but also received care from owners, overseers, and fellow slaves. Providing medical care for slaves, whether few or many, was a very different experience from dosing one's own family. The most uniquely southern aspect of antebellum domestic medicine was its adaptation to fit the needs of slavery. Not only was the number of patients one person might treat expanded, but gender roles and authority structures were also challenged.

Although only about half of all slaveholders had more than twenty slaves, the plantation represents the extreme of the adaptation of domestic medicine to slavery. An example of one plantation's system of health care, though perhaps not typical or representative, serves to illuminate many issues. Plowden Charles Jennet Weston delegated much of the day-to-day running of his rice plantation, Hagley, in Georgetown County, South Carolina, to his overseer. Weston's model contract between overseer and owner, which spelled out duties and expectations, stressed that the most important consideration was always "the care and well being of the negroes." When a slave complained of ill health, the overseer was to determine whether the slave was sick or merely "shamming." Slaves who were "somewhat sick" were to be assigned lighter work than usual, and more serious cases were confined to the plantation sickhouse or "hospital" until they were able to return to work. Pregnant and postpartum women were to be treated with especial care and given reduced work. Those lying-in were attended to by the plantation midwife and then by a nurse for two weeks.

The hospital was kept by female slave nurses, who attended to simple nursing, cooking, and cleaning, with the further burden of keeping the patients from leaving. Choosing a nurse was a subject of much controversy. Some planters routinely appointed an older woman who was no longer fit for heavy work, but others argued that a young, intelligent nurse would give better service.[50] Weston's nurses administered medication only upon the orders of the attending physician. Weston limited the overseer's choice of medicines to "simple remedies such as flaxseed tea, mint water, No. 6, magnesia &c.," specifically forbidding the overseer to bleed slaves, unless so ordered by a physician, or to use "strong medicines, such as calomel or tarter emetic."

50. R. King, "On the Management of the Butler Estate and the Cultivation of the Sugar Cane," *The Southern Agriculturist*, I (1828), 527.

The overseer was assured that Weston "never grudges a Doctors bill," and was urged to call the physician when "serious" cases arose. In the event of both overseer and owner being absent, the nurse was to summon a physician for any ill slave. Weston himself was to be informed of serious illness or accident, death or epidemic.[51]

Because of the ease with which illness, particularly epidemics, spread in slave quarters, many planters stressed prevention even more than other southerners. On Weston's plantation this took the form of what he saw as generally good care and prompt treatment of illness. Others stressed the use of prophylactic measures. One South Carolina planter issued a dram of whiskey with assafetida (a foul smelling and tasting plant resin) each evening and during cotton-picking season in the morning as well. Rain-soaked slaves were similarly dosed. Assafetida bags were worn by children, and tonics and calomel were issued as prophylactics.[52] Maternal and infant death, a problem throughout the era for blacks and whites, was fought with special treatment, including modifications in the work loads of pregnant and nursing women and the provision of lying-in facilities and nurseries.[53] Preventing slave illness reduced loss of work time or even property and saved the owner from the bother, concern, and expense of providing treatment.[54]

Planters routinely isolated sick slaves to prevent the spread of infectious disease. "Hospitals" with separate rooms for males and females, as well as the lying-in facilities mentioned above, were common on large plantations.[55] Confining those who needed care facilitated the job of providing health care by allowing one person to supervise a number of patients. Unfortunately, isolation was not always sufficient to prevent the spread of infectious disease. The individuals caring for sick slaves—master, mistress, overseer, or fellow slave—were at high risk of contracting their patients' ills.

One ramification of the plantation practice involves authority. Slaves received medical care by order, not by choice, when they were

51. Weston, "Management," 191–92; George C. Rogers, Jr., *The History of Georgetown County, South Carolina* (Columbia, S.C., 1970), 257–59, and *passim*.

52. Joseph Ioor Waring, *A History of Medicine in South Carolina, 1825–1900* (Columbia, S.C., 1967), 6–7; Rawick (ed.), *American Slave*, vol. 6.1, p. 239, vol. 12.1, pp. 49, 127; Clinton, *Plantation Mistress*, 29–30, 187–88.

53. King, "On the Management of the Butler Estate," 527; Flanders, *Plantation Slavery*, 101–102.

54. Robert J. Draughton, "Houses of Negroes—Habits of Living &c," *Southern Cultivator*, VIII (1850), 66–67, reprinted in Breeden (ed.), *Advice Among Masters*, 168.

55. See Weston, "Management," 191.

treated by owners or their emissaries. Overseers, slave nurses, or midwives responsible for slave health worked within prescribed guidelines. Instructions to overseers—including Weston's—often described medical duties, including what book to follow, what medicines to use, and what doctor to call under what circumstances. An elementary knowledge of medicine was considered a necessary qualification for an overseer. One owner charged, "A great majority of the cases you should be yourself competent to manage, or you are unfit for the place you hold."[56] Overseers had the authority to treat slaves, but were by no means given a free reign.

In all but a few exceptional cases, slave nurses and midwives had still less medical autonomy than overseers. Even when midwives and nurses were charged with tending to the needs of patients, overseers and owners retained authority over diet, patient work load, medications, and other factors affecting health. The rule—as at Hagley—seems to have been that nurses were not to prescribe medication, though exceptions certainly existed. One owner had sufficient faith in his nurse to instruct his overseer that she was in charge of medical matters. When she felt that she could do no more, the overseer was to call the doctor. While the degree of autonomy of slave nurses and midwives varied widely, it is safe to conclude that even those who were operating under the strictest of supervision had a status greater than that of ordinary slaves. On those exceptional plantations where nurses were relatively autonomous, their word on medical matters sometimes superseded even the overseer's.[57]

The plantation system often gave white women, as well as black, increased responsibility. Planters' wives who became the primary providers of health care for plantations assumed tasks that subtly expanded the sphere of white antebellum women, though they remained traditionally feminine. Although Weston's overseer superintended health care, on many, perhaps most, plantations the owner, or more commonly his wife, assumed that responsibility. Many of the women found the duties tiring and unpleasant and complained in their letters and diaries about sick slaves and crying babies.[58] Yet,

56. "The Duties of an Overseer," *De Bow's Review,* XVIII (1855), 340; "Instructions by Alexander Telfair of Savannah, Ga. to the Overseer of His Plantation near Augusta, Dated June 11, 1832," in Ulrich B. Phillips (ed.), *Plantation and Frontier Documents, 1649–1863* (2 vols.; Cleveland, 1909), I, 127–28.

57. "Instructions by Alexander Telfair," 127–28.

58. Clinton, *Plantation Mistress,* 144–47; Sudie Duncan Sides, "Women and Slaves: An Interpretation Based on the Writings of Southern Women" (Ph.D. dissertation, University of North Carolina, 1969), 126–28.

though the work was often burdensome, some women found it peculiarly rewarding:

> I went on my usual round of visits today, first to the Negroes' hospital, then to see the young mothers who have recently been confined; afterwards to the children's ward, where they are kept during the day under the care of an old mammy, while their mothers are at work in the field. These and many other daily duties incumbent upon the mistress of a plantation leave one few spare hours. . . . I found the inmates of the hospital awaiting me with impatience and eagerness. . . . One of my greatest pleasures is in distributing the delicacies from our own tables to the invalids.[59]

Black or white, woman's traditional role as healer afforded her both special rights and increased burdens on the plantation.

The ministrations of the providers of plantation medicine—mistresses and masters, overseers, and slave nurses and midwives—are in a gray area on the boundary between professional and domestic medicine. On a large plantation like Weston's, the number of potential patients was far greater than anyone treating even an extended family would normally have seen. While this vastly broadened the experience a given practitioner might have, it also escalated the responsibility. In many cases the medical duties of those responsible for health care constituted a large part of their work. Yet their lack of training—admittedly a shortcoming of many antebellum professionals as well—and the widespread contemporary distinction between the plantation healers and professional physicians—clearly allies them more closely with domestic than with professional medical practitioners.

Like other southerners, those on plantations rarely used domestic medicine exclusively. Weston's instructions on when to call for the doctor exemplify the common plantation practice of using domestic medicine to handle any case possible and relying on professional medicine only as a backup. Instructions to overseers often reflected this mix of professional and domestic care, as well as the skill of the overseer, the availability of physicians in the locale, and the owner's preference for domestic or professional medicine; all of these factors were also reflected in the rules for deciding when to call the doctor.[60] Even owners who considered a knowledge of domestic medicine an important qualification for an overseer stressed that the overseer was to call for a physician whenever he felt it necessary.[61] The practice of resorting

59. Sides, "Women and Slaves," 122.

60. For two examples, see "The Duties of an Overseer," 340; St. George Cocke, "Plantation Medicine—Police," De Bow's Review, XIV (1853), 177–78.

61. "The Duties of an Overseer," 340; and Robert Collins, "Essays on the Treatment

to professional care as a last resort had its critics. Some doctors blamed "the almost universal practice on the part of owners and overseers, of tampering with their sick negroes for one, two or more days before applying for medical aid" for the high toll of epidemic diseases in slave quarters.[62] As an Alabama slave recounted, "Dey only had homemade medicines, an' dat is unless dey got sho'nuff powerful sick an' den dey would go to see a doctor."[63]

The larger the number of potential patients, the higher ran the cost of health care, especially the expense of hiring physicians, and many planters used domestic medicine to reduce the amount of costly professional care. One Mississippi planter bragged that despite the unhealthful climate in which he lived, his physician's bill for 150 slaves had averaged less than $50 per year because he provided domestic treatment when possible. The Mississippi planter's pride was justified; one Georgia plantation of about 250 slaves spent $550 in the early 1850s for a single year of professional medical care.[64]

Access to physicians was as much a problem for planters as it was for other rural southerners. Because several physicians practiced near Hadley, Weston was able to have his slaves treated professionally when the need arose without major inconvenience. Others were not as lucky, as one Georgia planter made clear in an 1849 letter to Tomlinson Fort, author of a domestic manual: "Having for many years past cultivated a plantation at some distance from the city, I have often sensibly felt the want of medical advice for my people, when medical attention could not be provided to meet the exigency of the moment."[65]

The adaptation of domestic medicine to fit the needs of slavery was obviously uniquely southern. Yet some attributes of domestic medicine were no different in the South than in the North. Although those on plantations often treated more patients than they might in even a large extended family, had different relationships with their patients, and in the case of women reaped different rewards and burdens, the

and Management of Slaves," *Southern Cultivator*, XII (1854), 205–206, reprinted in Breeden (ed.), *Advice Among Masters*, 23–24.

62. William Kauffman Scarborough, *The Overseer: Plantation Management in the Old South* (Baton Rouge, 1966), 85. See also Savitt, *Medicine and Slavery*, 165–66.

63. Rawick (ed.), *American Slave*, vol. 6.1, p. 69; vol. 6.2, p. 343; vol. 12.1, 75–76, 139, 164–165, 228.

64. Draughton, "House of Negroes," 168–70; Flanders, *Plantation Slavery*, 165.

65. Royce McCrary, "The Use of Home Medical Books in Ante-Bellum Georgia: A Letter by Macpherson Berrien," *Journal of the Medical Association of Georgia*, LXIV (1975), 137.

ELIZABETH BARNABY KEENEY

domestic remedies and the reasons southerners used them were similar to those of contemporaries elsewhere. Like northerners and westerners, southerners were dissatisfied with professional options and often found they could do as much or more themselves at a lower cost. Like pioneer westerners, rural southerners worried about access to physicians. And though domestic medicine was popular in the Old South, southerners, like their contemporaries, rarely used it to the exclusion of professional medicine. Adapting domestic medicine to their peculiar needs and environment, southerners blended unique regional factors with a typically American practice, creating a hybrid that was southern in particulars but national in character.

CHAPTER 14

BLACK MAGIC: FOLK BELIEFS OF THE SLAVE COMMUNITY

Elliott J. Gorn

Threatened with yet another beating by slave-breaker Edward Covey, Frederick Douglass hid out in the woods. There he met a fellow slave, a conjurer named Sandy, who gave him a magic root to prevent whippings. Although skeptical, repeated beatings in the past made Douglass willing to try anything. He returned home and was astonished that the root seemed to work for an entire day. When its magic powers failed, however, and Covey prepared to administer another whipping, Douglass resisted: "Whence came the daring spirit necessary to grapple with a man who eight-and-forty hours before, could, with his slightest word, have made me tremble like a leaf in a storm, I do not know; at any rate; I was resolved to fight, and what was better still, I actually was hard at it." I suggest that Douglass' "daring spirit" came from the sense of empowerment, however fleeting, engendered by the magic root.[1]

As this example illustrates, magic played an important part in the lives of Afro-American slaves. Douglass' experience with the supernatural at a moment of intense personal crisis was far from unusual, and Sandy the conjurer found his counterparts on countless farms and plantations. The following pages explore how black Americans shaped their supernatural traditions into an invaluable community resource.

To begin with, we must resist the tendency to dichotomize "primi-

The author wishes to thank Anna Yee, Alan Dundes, Peter Wood, William Ferris, Wayland Hand, Winthrop Jordan, Lawrence Levine, Leon Litwack, and Albert Raboteau for their ideas and encouragement.

1. Frederick Douglass, *The Life and Times of Frederick Douglass* (Rev. ed., 1892; rpr. Toronto, 1962), 136–40.

tive" superstition and "modern" science, for magical and scientific thinking are not as different as they first appear. Both are singularly empirical in that they match cause and effect through observation; both find pattern, regularity, and order where the untrained eye sees only random events; and both prescribe means of controlling the environment. The crucial difference, as the anthropologist Robin Horton observes, is that traditional cultures offer fewer alternatives to magic. Life's precariousness in prescientific societies makes the questioning of established patterns of thought seem especially dangerous. Moreover, the ever-present need to find meaning in events militates against belief in coincidence or randomness or absurdity, and the lack of alternatives to supernatural systems predisposes men to continued belief. On the other hand, scientists—especially theoretical scientists—are obliged to question their results constantly, to chip away at inconsistencies until new and better explanations emerge. They must not only match cause with effect and demonstrate how they are linked, but must also test hypotheses, discard them, and test new ones. Even as they reject theories, they remain ever confident that causes are logical and knowable. Unfortunately, individuals like young Frederick Douglass do not always have the luxury of scientific detachment. The relative sizes of scientific and magical realms vary from culture to culture, but both promise to fill the same fundamental human cravings for meaning, predictability, and control.[2]

Although we live in a "rational" age, folk beliefs or "superstitions" are still very much with us, even in the most technologically sophisticated societies and among highly educated and intelligent people. Baseball players, fishermen, graduate students confronting oral exams—all display superstitious behavior. So long as there is uncertainty in life that science and technology fail to control, there will be attempts to deal with it through the supernatural. The historical study of this cultural universal is important for precisely that reason. Folk beliefs reveal people's anxieties and their efforts to alleviate them. Studying folklore can help us understand a culture on its own terms.[3]

Recent research makes it clear that Afro-Americans developed a

2. Robin Horton, "African Traditional Thought and Western Science," *Africa*, XXXVII (1967), 50–71, 155–87. For a fine-tuning of Horton's thesis, which implies that an important distinction exists between applied and theoretical science, see S. J. Tambiah, "The Form and Meaning of Magical Acts: A Point of View," in Robin Horton and Ruth Finnegan (eds.), *Modes of Thought* (London, 1973), 199–229.

3. One of the best introductions to the study of folk beliefs is Gustav Jahoda, *The Psychology of Superstition* (Middlesex, England, 1971).

distinctive culture of their own, one that gave them a strong sense of group identity. A particularly rich folkloric tradition characterized black life, especially where slave populations were most concentrated. Not only did important African customs survive, but on the large plantations, black men and women possessed the necessary isolation from whites to fully develop their own distinctive ways. Indeed, black culture became a source of group esteem and therefore of psychic protection from the powerlessness of bondage.[4]

Afro-American culture afforded slaves relatively stable families based on their own patterns of marriage and kinship. Blacks refracted Christianity through a unique African perspective and created a sacred worldview compatible with their cultural assumptions and social needs. Slave preachers provided a corps of skillful leaders who counterposed black wisdom of the spiritual world to white domination of the secular sphere. In tales and songs, Afro-Americans not only forged their own aesthetic styles, they commented on racial relations, stripped away white pretentions, and taught each other crucial lessons in living. In all these ways and countless others, black culture offered compensation for material deprivations.[5]

An incredibly complex and varied body of magical practices forged

4. Among the most important works by historians on Afro-American culture are John W. Blassingame, *The Slave Community* (New York, 1972); Eugene Genovese, *Roll, Jordan, Roll* (New York, 1974), 217–32; Lawrence W. Levine, *Black Culture and Black Consciousness: Afro-American Folk Thought from Slavery to Freedom* (New York, 1977); Albert J. Raboteau, *Slave Religion* (New York, 1978); Herbert G. Gutman, *The Black Family in Slavery and Freedom, 1750–1925* (New York, 1976); Leon Litwack, *Been in the Storm So Long: The Aftermath of Slavery* (New York, 1979); Charles Joyner, *Down by the Riverside: A South Carolina Slave Community* (Urbana, 1984); Thomas L. Webber, *Deep Like the Rivers: Education in the Slave Quarter Community, 1831–1865* (New York, 1978); Robert Farris Thompson, *Flash of the Spirit: African and Afro-American Art and Philosophy* (New York, 1983).

5. These themes are treated at length in the works cited in note 4. The uses and pitfalls of slave sources are discussed in C. Vann Woodward, "History from Slave Sources," *American Historical Review,* LXX (April, 1974), 470–81; John Blassingame (ed.), "Introduction," *Slave Testimony* (Baton Rouge, 1977), xvii–lxv; Kenneth M. Stampp, "Rebels and Sambos: The Search for the Negro's Personality in Slavery," *Journal of Southern History,* XXXVII (August, 1971), 367–92; Norman R. Yetman, "Ex-Slave Interviews and the Historiography of Slavery," *American Quarterly,* XXXVI (Summer, 1984), 181–214; and David Thomas Bailey, "A Divided Prism: Two Sources on Black Testimony on Slavery," *Journal of Southern History,* XLVI (1980), 381–404. For instances where white interviewers clearly influenced their black informants, see George P. Rawick (ed.), *The American Slave: A Composite Autobiography* (Westport, Conn., 1972), vol. 9.3, p. 332; vol. 2.1, p. 69; vol. 3.4, p. 252; Georgia Writers' Project, *Drums and Shadows: Survival Studies Among the Georgia Coastal Negroes* (Athens, Ga., 1940), 84, 102. See also Zora Neale Hurston, *Mules and Men* (Bloomington, Ind., 1978), 18–19.

out of African, Anglo-American, and even Euro-Catholic traditions became a crucial part of black folk life. In all cultures, the chaos and uncertainty of life predispose the poor, the sick, and the socially marginal to heightened faith in superstitions. Folk beliefs, then, were encouraged by the material circumstances of bondage and by the slaves' lack of control over their daily lives. Blacks employed charms, amulets, potions, incantations, spells, and formulas to manipulate their surroundings, while dreams, signs, visions, prophesies, and fortune-telling gave them insight into the future. Perhaps more than any other part of Afro-American expressive culture, magical control of the environment held out the possibility of immediate, direct action, of change consciously willed and deliberately effected. Because much of their behavior was constricted, slaves often turned to their magical traditions to fashion an alternative reality, one that offered them a sense of order and control in their lives.[6]

The anthropologist Branislaw Malinowski commented on this association of magic and pragmatic control. Magic, he argued, concerns itself with concrete, specific, detailed problems, whereas religion addresses more fundamental issues, such as man's place in the universe, where he comes from and where he is going, the proper worship of spiritual forces, and obedience to the rulings of providence. Magic and religion may coexist, but they are functionally distinct.[7]

Malinowski drew this line too sharply, especially for slave magic and religion. Preachers also acted as folk healers; conjure potions sometimes relied on Trinitarian symbolism; hoodoo doctors invoked the

6. On folk beliefs and social class, see Jahoda, *Psychology of Superstition*, Chap. 9. Descendants of Anglo-Saxons and Celts were no less "superstitious" than Afro-Americans. See, for example, Tom Peete Cross, "Witchcraft in North Carolina," *Studies in Philology*, XVI (1919), 217–87; Wayland Hand (ed.), *Popular Beliefs and Superstitions*, vols. VI and VII of Newman Ivey White (gen. ed.), *The Frank C. Brown Collection of North Carolina Folklore* (Durham, 1961); Wayland Hand, *Magical Medicine* (Berkeley, 1980). On the English background of popular beliefs and superstitions, see Keith Thomas' magisterial *Religion and the Decline of Magic* (New York, 1971). Two indispensable works on Afro-American superstitions are Newbell Niles Puckett, *Folk Beliefs of the Southern Negro* (Chapel Hill, 1926); and Alan Dundes (ed.), *Mother Wit from the Laughing Barrel* (Englewood Cliffs, N.J., 1973), 357–427. For insightful discussions of antebellum black folk beliefs, see Levine, *Black Culture and Black Consciousness*, 55–80; Raboteau, *Slave Religion*, 80–86, 275–88; Joyner, *Down by the Riverside*, 141–63; and Blassingame, *Slave Community*, 45–49. Genovese, *Roll, Jordan, Roll*, 215–32, is especially helpful on the complex interaction of conjurers and masters.

7. Branislaw Malinowski, *A Scientific Theory of Culture and Other Essays* (Chapel Hill, 1944), 200.

Lord's name; and many slaves explained occult phenomena through Afro-Christian mythology. But Malinowski's point has validity if it is taken as a useful conceptual tool rather than a rigid dichotomy. God, Moses, and Christ were living presences, symbols of imminent deliverance, but they sometimes failed to intervene in daily life. Magical powers formed part of a continuum of spiritual forces pervading the material world. Like the lesser spirits of Africa, the supernatural was evidence of the unseen hierarchy mediating between human beings and the higher realms, a manifestation of a world far more spiritually animate than the modern one.[8]

For example, William Webb, a preacher on a Kentucky plantation, often led his fellow slaves in prayers for freedom and salvation, but he sometimes used magic to impress his congregants. The master on a nearby plantation had a reputation for cruelty, but Webb showed the man's slaves how to work roots to mollify his brutality. As preacher *and* conjurer, Webb exemplifies how magic and religion flowed into each other, yet remained functionally distinct. The former tended to serve immediate goals, offering practical solutions to daily problems, while the latter related to more basic moral and philosophical issues, and the ultimate questions of man's fate, sin, and salvation.[9]

All slaves had ready access to a range of highly adaptable folk beliefs. "You w'ite folks jest' go through de woods an' you don' know nuffin," Silvia King declared, counterposing black knowledge of the unseen world to white ignorance. Mothers prescribed traditional cures and preventatives, rarely respecting artificial distinctions between magical and natural healing. In less tractable cases, talented folk doctors—both male and female—drew on an extensive knowledge of local flora to create useful medicines. It was not just a matter of recognizing

8. See especially Levine, *Black Culture and Black Consciousness*, 55–80; Raboteau, *Slave Religion*, 275–88; Joyner, *Down by the Riverside*, Chap. 5; Thompson, *Flash of the Spirit*, Chap. 2. For examples of the living quality of the slaves' sacred world, see Ruth Bass, "Mojo," *Scribner's Magazine*, LXXXVI (1930), 83–90; Roland Steiner, "Braziel Robinson Possessed of Two Spirits," *Journal of American Folklore*, XIII (1900), 226–28; and Ruth Bass, "The Little Man," *Scribner's Magazine*, XCVII (1935), 120–23; all reprinted in Dundes (ed.), *Mother Wit*, 377–95. See also Elliott J. Gorn, "Black Spirits: The Ghostlore of Afro-American Slaves," *American Quarterly*, XXXVI (Fall, 1984), 549–65.

9. William Webb, *History of William Webb* (Detroit, 1873), 20–25. Slaves also believed that a turned-over washpot would miraculously absorb the sounds of their secret religious meetings, as they sang and prayed for freedom. See, for example, Rawick (ed.), *American Slave*, vol. 6, p. 68; vol. 10.6, p. 127; vol. 8.1, p. 120; vol. 15.2, p. 421; vol. 5.3, p. 44; vol. 19, pp. 24, 173.

natural cures and preventatives, but also of knowing the correct techniques for applying them. Slaves followed their African forebears' belief that proper administration was as important as the drug itself.[10]

A single slave's repertoire reveals some of the variety of black folk medicine. Janie Landrum, whose knowledge of healing was not at all unusual, described several of her remedies: lemon juice for foot corns; white sassafras-root tea for blindness; chinaberry roots, poke roots, and bluestone for scrofula; chicken gizzard linings for indigestion; roasted turnips or pine tar for frostbite; limewater or May rain as a general tonic. She also advised crossing pins over a wart and then hiding them, and making a cross with chimney soot to remove other blemishes; a penny on a string tied round one's neck staved off an upset stomach; placing an ax beside a sick person cut their pain, but moving their bed would surely bring death. All over the South, slaves practiced these and countless other folk cures for daily ills. If the efficacy of some remedies seems dubious, consider the alternatives— unwanted intimacy with masters or mistresses administering their own folk cures, or "professional" care, which was often primitive, alienating, and given grudgingly because of the cost. At least the slave healers offered their remedies amidst the warmth of kin and community.[11]

However, Afro-American folk beliefs went beyond simple health maintenance. Slaves made charms and amulets for a variety of domestic purposes, and they interpreted dreams, signs, and visions in order to glimpse the future. But the most powerful magic was practiced by specialists, sorcerers known variously as hoodoos, rootmen, voodoo priests, witch doctors, or, most commonly, conjurers. Slaves sought out these individuals when they wanted to accomplish especially difficult ends through magical means.[12] Conjurers borrowed their tech-

10. Rawick (ed.), *American Slave*, suppl. ser. 2, vol. 6.5, p. 2236; Puckett, *Folk Beliefs*, Chap. 5. For a compendium on Afro-American herbal medicine, see William Ed Grime, *Botany of the Black Americans* (St. Clair Shores, Mich., 1976). Also see Peter Wood, "People's Medicine in the Early South," *Southern Exposure*, VI (Summer, 1978), 50–53.

11. Rawick (ed.), *American Slave*, suppl. ser. 2, vol. 6.5, pp. 2263–71. The slave narratives still await systematic analysis of folk medicine. Also see Joyner, *Down by the Riverside*, 148–49.

12. Leonora Herron and Alice Bacon, "Conjuring and Conjure Doctors," *Southern Workman*, XXIV (1895), 117–18, 193–94, 209–11, reprinted in Dundes (ed.), *Mother Wit*, 359–68. Once again Puckett, *Folk Beliefs*, Chaps. 3, 4, contains a great deal of data, as do the first two decades of the *Journal of American Folklore*. For raw material on the subject, the most important source is Harry Middleton Hyatt's mammoth four-volume collection, *Hoodoo—Conjuration—Witchcraft—Rootwork* (Washington, D.C., 1970). See also Hand

niques and paraphernalia from black and white traditions, but the emphasis on sorcery—on supernatural services for hire, especially for harming and healing—was strongly African in origin. This essay focuses on conjuring as the most distinctive and the most powerful form of Afro-American magic.[13]

Conjurers' alleged skills ranged widely, and the black students who attended Hampton Institute in the 1870s compiled several examples:

> The power of snake-charming seems to be quite generally attributed to them. One is told of who claimed he could turn a horse to a cow, and kill a man or woman and bring them to life again by shaking up his little boxes. He could also whistle in the key-hole after the doors were locked, and make them fly open. Others are told of who "can trick, put snakes, lizards, terrapins, scorpions and different other things in you, fix you so you can't have any use of your limbs. They could put you in such a state that you would linger and pine away or so that you would go blind or crazy.

Some conjurers allegedly sacrificed healthy animals to heal sick ones, kept lovers from straying, and cured illnesses that stymied professional doctors. Even today, in the rural South, conjurers are said to influence the actions of policemen and control the outcomes of court trials, so that some blacks refer to the conjure charm as "de po man's lawyah."[14]

(ed.), *Popular Beliefs and Superstitions*. This chapter does not deal with voodoo as found in New Orleans because most plantation slaves did not have access to the elaborate rituals of this powerful hybrid of Afro-Caribbean religions. For more on voodoo, see George Washington Cable, "Creole Slave Songs," *Century Magazine*, XXXI (April, 1886), 807–27, reprinted in Bruce Jackson, *The Negro and His Folklore in Nineteenth Century Periodicals* (Austin, 1967), 211–42; Robert Tallant, *Voodoo in New Orleans* (New York, 1946); and especially Hurston, *Mules and Men*, Pt. 2, reprinted from *Journal of American Folklore*, XLVI (1931), 317–417, under the title "Hoodoo in America." For an Afro-Caribbean comparison, see Orlando Patterson, *The Sociology of Slavery* (London, 1967), Chap. 7.

13. Wayland Hand forcefully makes the point that African and British techniques blended, yet magic-for-hire was more distinctly African. See his "American Witchcraft and Conjuring: A Comparison," *Mannus: Deutsche Zeitschrift für Vor und Frühgeschichte*, XLVI (1978), 36–42. While the issue of origins is important, Afro-American folklore in general and magic in particular were so adaptable that questions of function and meaning hold more promise for future research, a point made throughout Levine, *Black Culture and Black Consciousness*. For a fine discussion of the implicit rules that structured conjurers' methods, materials, and results, see Michael Edward Bell, "Pattern, Structure and Logic in Afro-American Hoodoo Performances" (Ph.D. dissertation, Indiana University, 1980).

14. Herron and Bacon, "Conjuring and Conjure Doctors," 361; Norman E. Whitten, Jr., "Patterns of Malign Occultism Among Negroes in North Carolina," *Journal of American Folklore*, LXXV (1962), 311–25, reprinted in Dundes (ed.), *Mother Wit*, 408–409. See

No single source accounted for the root workers' powers. Some informants felt that magic was part of their African heritage, that hoodoo men were either Africans or descendants of African priests. Others took up the European concept of compact with the devil, but many professed Christians—preachers among them—contradicted this satanic view by contending that occult powers came from the Lord. Some resolved this conflict by claiming that good magic was from God, evil magic from the devil, though most slaves, like their African ancestors, rejected such a rigidly dichotomized Western morality. Still others argued for hereditary or physiological origins; the seventh son of a seventh son or one born with a caul possessed the power.[15] Some claimed that chewing a particular bone from a black cat was a powerful source of supernatural talent, but it was equally common for slaves to liken conjuring to a trade, handed down either to descendants or to apprentices. Gender proved no barrier to working magic, though more men than women seem to have been hoodoo doctors. Certainly, some whites patronized conjurers, and a few probably even practiced the root workers' arts, but as a general rule, racial barriers were observed; whites and blacks kept their magical trades largely to themselves.[16]

Conjurers had great influence in the slave community, commanding both fear and respect. Frederick Douglass described his friend Sandy as "famous among the slaves of the neighborhood. . . . He was a genuine African, and had inherited some of the so-called magical powers said to be possessed by the eastern nations." Henry Clay Bruce declared that slaves "believed and feared them almost beyond their masters." Two early students of this phenomenon concluded that "there was the most implicit faith in the conjure doctor's power. . . .

---

also Puckett, Folk Beliefs, 277–78; Bass, "Mojo," 380–87; Journal of American Folklore, IV (July-September, 1891), 267–69; Rawick (ed.), American Slave, suppl. ser. 2, vol. 2.1, pp. 17–18. Conjurers are also said to save businesses on the verge of bankruptcy.

15. For examples of African derived power, see W. E. B. Dubois, "The Religion of the American Negro," New World, IX (December, 1900), 618; Rawick (ed.), American Slave, vol. 12.1, p. 89. For examples of the concept of Satanic compact, see William Wells Brown, My Southern Home; or The South and Its People (Boston, 1880), Chap. 7; Rawick (ed.), American Slave, vol. 12.1, p. 245; vol. 3.4, pp. 244–45; vol. 4.2, p. 3; vol. 4.1, pp. 4–7. For Christian origins, see Douglass, Life and Times, 136–37; Puckett, Folk Beliefs, 204–205, 234, 526; Rawick (ed.), American Slave, suppl. ser. 2, vol. 2.1, pp. 16–22; suppl. ser. 2, vol. 7.6, pp. 2780–83. Herron and Bacon, "Conjuring and Conjure Doctors," 360, cite examples of all of the above origins of magical powers.

16. Rawick (ed.), American Slave, vol. 11, p. 331; vol. 12.1, p. 89; Blassingame, Slave Community, 45–48. I have found only one instance of a white man who allegedly had the power to conjure. See Rawick (ed.), American Slave, vol. 15.2, p. 121.

[T]he confidence in their abilities was unbounded." Even slave children, in their quest for heroes, played a game called "voodoo doctor."[17]

Some conjurers were legendary figures. "Doctor John," a free black who practiced in New Orleans before the Civil War, became a wealthy slaveholder with the fees paid to him by blacks and whites. Calling himself a Senegalese prince, he used his power to cure, to cause infirmity or death, to tell fortunes (slaves all over New Orleans worked as paid informants for him) and to make love potions. Similarly, William Wells Brown described a conjurer and fortune-teller named Dinkie. Though a slave, he worked only at the lightest tasks, only when he felt like doing them, and still avoided punishment. A full-blooded African, Dinkie proclaimed himself descended from a king in his native land: "Everybody treated him with respect. The whites throughout the neighborhood tipped their hats to the old one-eyed negro, while the policemen, or patrollers, permitted him to pass without a challenge. The negroes everywhere stood in mortal fear of 'Uncle Dinkie.' The blacks who saw him every day were always thrown upon their good behavior when in his presence." Like Doctor John, he harmed and cured, told fortunes and manipulated people supernaturally. Even Dinkie's superstitious owners came to him for aid and advice, and they too feared and respected him. "It was literally true," Brown concluded, "this man was his own master."[18]

How do we account for such beliefs? To begin with, faith in magic was received wisdom, inherited from Africa, then modified and reinforced by contact with Anglo-American, Euro-Catholic, and Creole superstitions. Fugitive slave Jacob Stroyer declared, "I held the idea that there were such things, for I thought the majority of the people believed it, and that they ought to know more than could one man." Moreover, conjurers cultivated the awe and respect of others. They shrouded their rituals in mystery and dressed or behaved in unusual ways. Many root workers lived on the margins of slave society as old, irascible, or physically deformed individuals; free blacks who existed

17. Douglass, *Life and Times*, 136–37; Henry Clay Bruce, *The New Man: Twenty-Nine Years A Slave* (1895; rpr. New York, 1969), 52; Herron and Bacon, "Conjuring and Conjure Doctors," 361; Rawick (ed.), *American Slave*, vol. 6, p. 49. See also Rawick (ed.), *American Slave*, suppl. ser. 2, vol. 3.1, p. 75.

18. Tallant, *Voodoo in New Orleans*, 33–35; Brown, *My Southern Home*, 10–11, 68–81. See also Rawick (ed.), *American Slave*, vol. 8.2, p. 61; suppl. ser. 2, vol. 3.2, p. 708; Eliza Dupuy, *Florence, or the Fatal Vow* (Cincinnati, 1852), 24–25; Blassingame, *Slave Community*, 45–48, 106.

apart from others; or recluses who voluntarily kept to themselves. As the folklorist Don Yoder observes, folk healers and sorcerers in diverse cultures often possess such ambivalent status. Charismatic outsiders, their powers both divide and reintegrate communities. Their acts may help unify people, but sorcerers and shamans frequently stand apart as eccentric, even fearsome individuals.[19]

Although theatrics reinforced fear of supernatural injury and hope of magical aid, most conjurers were not hypocrites. A few dissemblers notwithstanding, the majority genuinely believed in the origins and efficacy of their powers. Folklorist Newbell Niles Puckett personally knew many conjurers, and the conclusion he drew in the early twentieth century no doubt held true for the antebellum period. "Most of them I have seen," Puckett declared, "believe very firmly in the materials they prescribe and are willing to use charms prescribed for them."[20]

The pharmacopeia and rituals of Afro-American sorcery followed time-tested rules. In slave magic as in all other folklore, bits of old traditional materials were rearranged to produce something new. The hoodoo doctor put together a conjure bag (or "trick," "jack," "hand," "gris-gris," or "mojo," as they were called) from innumerable traditional items in countless familiar ways, but always with an eye to its symbolic power. Conjurers consistently followed the two universal rules of sympathetic magic, that like produces like (homeopathic magic), and that anything once in contact with someone's body continues to influence them (contagious magic). For example, placing peppers in a conjure bag to make a victim feel hot relied on the homeopathic principle; using fingernail clippings, hair, or even footprint tracks to direct magical power toward a specific individual was contagious magic.[21]

19. Jacob Stroyer, *My Life in the South* (Salem, 1890), 54; Herron and Bacon, "Conjuring and Conjure Doctors," 361; Bruce, *New Man*, 57; Puckett, *Folk Beliefs*, 201–203; Don Yoder, "Folk Medicine," in Richard M. Dorson, *Folklore and Folklife: An Introduction* (Chicago, 1972), 205. In Charles Chesnutt's fictional *The Conjure Woman* (Ann Arbor, 1969), originally published in 1899, free blacks were hoodoo doctors for slaves. It makes sense that free blacks would have turned to conjuring to supplement their meager incomes.

20. Puckett, *Folk Beliefs*, 211. For examples of fraudulent conjurers, see Rawick (ed.), *American Slave*, vol. 6, p. 47; vol. 12.1, p. 30. E. Fuller Torrey points out in his *The Mind Game: Witchdoctors and Psychiatry* (New York, 1972) that shamans frequently are aware that their cures have no inherent worth. But realizing that a patient's belief in their powers is often enough to effect real change, they knowingly prescribe bogus cures. These placebos are given with the assumption that anything which helps a patient is good. See also Jerome D. Frank, *Persuasion and Healing* (Baltimore, 1961), Chap. 3.

21. An excellent instance of both laws operating in a single sample came from Nannie

Other materials commonly found in conjure bags included grave-yard dirt (known as goopher dust), which was used to invoke spirits of the dead against the living; shroud ravelings, also used to bring illness and death; knotted string, used to symbolize impotence; insects, used to create infestations; and parts of loathsome reptiles and poisonous herbs, used to cause various afflictions. Often a multitude of items were merged into powerful symbolic combinations. "Aunt" Menthy, respected as the most gifted healer and feared as the most deadly conjurer on Mississippi's Bayou Pierre, described a potent death charm. She combined ash from scorched jaybird wing, squirrel jaw, and rattlesnake fang with goopher dust taken at sundown from the grave of an old and wicked person. She moistened this with the blood of a pig-eating sow, mixing it all with her left forefinger, Satan's "dog finger." She then placed the substance in a conjure bag, tied it up with shroud threads, named it for the intended victim, and buried it under his house. Although this example comes from the twentieth century, the constituent parts of Aunt Menthy's death charm and her techniques for combining them can be traced directly back to antebellum conjurers.[22]

The apparent effectiveness of magic constituted the single most important reason slaves believed in it. Sometimes conjurers prepared truly efficacious potions, sometimes sleight of hand matched means with ends, but faith comprised hoodoo's indispensable ingredient. In other words, conjuration functioned as a system of faith healing and faith harming that relied upon the suggestibility of the victim or client to achieve psychosomatic results. As one insightful former slave put it, "dem conjur-folks can't hurt you less'n you believes in 'em." That belief in magic can have physiological consequences is now widely accepted, and examples have been documented from diverse cultures.

Bradfield of Alabama. She claimed that a conjure doctor could take a person's garter or the top of his or her stocking, drape it in running water, and thus cause that person to be running for the rest of his or her life (Rawick [ed.], *American Slave*, vol. 6, p. 45). See also Jan Harold Brunvand, *The Study of American Folklore* (New York, 1968), 191–92; and Sir James Frazer, *The Golden Bough*, edited and abridged by Theodore H. Gaster (New York, 1959), 35–69.

22. I am especially indebted to Wayland Hand for compiling several examples in private correspondence. For innumerable other examples, Hyatt, *Hoodoo*, and Puckett, *Folk Beliefs*, are the best sources. As Hand pointed out, the "conjure bag," as opposed to the "witch bottle," was primarily part of Afro-American tradition (Hand, "American Witchcraft and Conjuring," 38). Aunt Menthy is described in Bass, "Mojo," 380–83. Her practice of naming the victim to her charm had Old World antecedents. In Africa, to name something was to have power over it (Horton, "African Traditional Thought and Western Science," 157).

Circular logic operated here: One had faith, faith produced the desired result, and faith was then further strengthened. And even when conjurers employed truly potent medicines or poisons, slaves attributed the effectiveness of these substances to the whole magic ritual surrounding their use; natural and supernatural powers reinforced each other.[23]

The sound practical advice that frequently accompanied magic also reinforced belief. A New Orleans conjurer who sold a man "French Love Powder" added the following counsel: "gib de 'oman ebbything she laks and lots uv hit—nebber cross her en make er mad no mattah how much she pesters you er flirts wid other men. Show her all de time dat she's de onliest 'oman you wants." In another example, a slave used a rabbit's foot to hoodoo the bloodhounds and run away from the plantation. He said a chant over the foot, took a bath, then began his journey by wading a long distance in a nearby creek. Obviously the bath and wading prevented the dogs from picking up his scent, but the former slave who told this story gave the rabbit's foot credit for success: "Dey didn't miss him till he clear gone and dat show what de rabbit foot done for him."[24]

---

23. Rawick (ed.), *American Slave*, vol. 13.3, p. 216; Puckett, *Folk Beliefs*, 301. Neurophysiologist Walter B. Cannon has identified a cross-cultural pattern of "voodoo death" in South American, African, New Zealand, Australian, Pacific Island and Caribbean cultures. Cannon asserts that persistent excessive activity of the sympatico-adrenal system, induced by fear of being hexed, stimulates adrenalin flow, but offers no target for terror or anger. Thus, witchcraft and sorcery victims go into shock similar to that sometimes experienced by slightly wounded soldiers or patients about to undergo surgery. A cycle of blood-vessel constriction and falling blood pressure exacerbated by lack of food and water may lead to death. Anthropologist David Lester argues for a more purely psychological explanation of witchcraft and sorcery deaths. Simply put, a hexed individual believes he is helpless in the face of magic, may feel responsible for being cursed, senses that he is cut off from his community, and because of his depressed psychological state, becomes susceptible to illnesses his body might otherwise resist. Barbara W. Lex accepts the idea of suggestion, but argues that it results not in lowered resistance, but in changes in the autonomic nervous system. Lex finds that witchcraft or sorcery beliefs activate stages of "autonomic tuning" that lead to various symptoms. The sorcerer manipulates the nervous system to create imbalances or restore balance in its subsystems. See Walter B. Cannon, "Voodoo Death," *American Anthropologist*, XLIV (1942), 169–81; Barbara Lex, "Voodoo Death: New Thoughts on an Old Explanation," *American Anthropologist*, LXXVI (December, 1974), 818–23; and David Lester, "Voodoo Death: Some New Thoughts on an Old Phenomenon," *American Anthropologist*, LXXIV (June, 1972), 386–90. See also *Health Services and Mental Health Administration Reports*, LXXXVI (April, 1971), 294.

24. Herron and Bacon, "Conjuring and Conjure Doctors," 362; Newbell Niles Puckett, "Race Pride and Folklore," *Opportunity: A Journal of Negro Life*, IV (1926), 82–84,

Already predisposed to belief in magic because of its apparent efficacy, slaves readily accepted conjurers' good-faith explanations of their failures. Perhaps the client did not follow the hoodoo doctor's instructions precisely, or a more powerful root worker cast a counterspell, or the patient did not have enough confidence in the magic. Just as the failure of one diagnosis does not destroy our faith in medicine, so a slave might lose faith in a particular conjurer, but not in conjuration.[25]

Equally important, the day-to-day practice of hoodoo gained justification from larger assumptions in Afro-American culture. Like their African ancestors of diverse cultures, slaves accepted the world's pervasive spirituality. Although West African belief systems varied widely, all tended to emphasize man's relationship to God and to the spiritual forces enveloping the world, forces tapped by charismatic shamans. The transfer of these beliefs to North America was somewhat fragmented—no equivalent of powerful and internally coherent religions such as the Caribbean's Vodun, Obeah, or Myalism emerged on these shores. But conjuring was one of several religious motifs—others included spirit possession, ecstatic trances, belief in witches, hag riding, and visitations from the dead—that became integrated into the slaves' worldview.[26]

Particular "Africanisms" pervaded the conjurer's art, especially ideas concerning the spirits of the dead. "Goopher" or graveyard dust was the most common substance used by hoodoo doctors. The word was derived from the Kikongo "kufwa," meaning "to die." Among the Bakongo of West Africa (a people from whom many American slaves

---

reprinted in Dundes (ed.), *Mother Wit*, 7; Rawick (ed.), *American Slave*, vol. 5.3, pp. 143–44.

25. Bruce, *New Man*, 53; Puckett, *Folk Beliefs*, 211–12. For an example of the persistence of belief after repeated failure, see Rawick (ed.), *American Slave*, vol. 7, pp. 245–49.

26. Joyner, *Down by the Riverside*, Chap. 5; Thompson, *Flash of the Spirit*, Chaps. 1, 2; Levine, *Black Culture and Black Consciousness*, 55–80; Raboteau, *Slave Religion*, 275–88. For a sampling of work on African and African-derived New World belief systems, see Roger Bastide, *African Civilizations in the New World*, trans. Peter Green (London, 1967); John S. Mbiti, *African Religions and Philosophy* (New York, 1969); George Eaton Simpson, "The Shango Cult in Nigeria and Trinidad," *American Anthropologist*, LXIV (1962), 1204–19; Harold Courlander, *The Drum and the Hoe: Life and Lore of the Haitian People* (Berkeley, 1960), Chaps. 2–7; Elsa V. Goveia, *Slave Society in the British Leeward Islands at the End of the Eighteenth Century* (New Haven, 1965), 245–49; Wade Davis, *The Serpent and the Rainbow* (New York, 1985); Alfred Metraux, *Voodoo in Haiti*, trans. Hugo Charteris (New York, 1959); Edward Brathwaite, *The Development of Creole Society in Jamaica, 1770–1820* (London, 1971), Chap. 15.

descended), ancestral spirits exerted a powerful influence on the world. Indeed, for the Bakongo, the world was divided into the land of the living and that of the dead. Water separated these two realms, but humans could contact spirits through charms called "minkisi" and thereby tap the medicinal powers god created. In much of West Africa, a person's grave was thought to be infused with his spirit, which continued to interact with the material world. Shamans in Africa and conjurers in America knew how to tap this spiritual essence to accomplish specific ends.[27]

Indeed, the use of goopher dust was part of a larger African-derived set of spirit beliefs, as revealed in Afro-American and Afro-Caribbean burial practices. Cemeteries in the United States, in Latin America, and in West and Central Africa often exhibited striking resemblances to each other, for in all, graves were places of communication with the dead. In America, relatives left personal objects on the graves of loved ones to placate or admonish their spirits and prevent them from wandering. Laying the dead east-to-west paralleled the African belief that the cosmos was oriented along the path of the sun; seashells, mirrors, and other shiny objects on top of grave sites symbolized the traditional African idea that rivers and seas separated the living from the souls of the dead. More than merely a collection of "survivals," these customs reflected African-derived spirit beliefs upon which conjurers implicitly drew.[28]

Although conjuring was rooted in the fundamental assumptions Afro-Americans had about the world, magic was not merely an ancestral "survival." Folk beliefs were, above all, useful and shaped themselves to daily life in a fashion characteristic of African cultures. Slaves believed in magic because it fulfilled needs not satisfied in other ways. The conjurers' powers ensured good luck, kept people friendly, strengthened love, and warded off disease. As in all cultures, slave folk beliefs provided tried and true means of coping with those anxiety-producing rites of passage—birth, puberty, marriage, and death—that touch all our lives. Perhaps W. E. B. Dubois best summed up the usefulness of the magic arts when he wrote that the conjurer "early appeared on the plantation and found his function as the healer of the

27. Thompson, *Flash of the Spirit*, 74, 105, 132–45; Elizabeth A. Fenn, "Honoring the Ancestors: Kongo-American Graves in the American South," *Southern Exposure*, XII (September, 1985), 42–43.

28. Joyner, *Down by the Riverside*, 143–45; John Michael Vlach, *The Afro-American Tradition in Decorative Arts* (Cleveland, 1978), Chap. 9; Fenn, "Honoring the Ancestors," 43–47.

sick, the interpreter of the unknown, the comforter of the sorrowing, the supernatural avenger of the wrong and the one who rudely but picturesquely expressed the longing disappointment and resentment of a stolen and oppressed people."[29]

Magic, then, found infinitely varied applications within the slave community, but two large patterns stand out. One centered on questions of power between whites and blacks, while the other revolved around regulating relationships within the slave community.

As in so much of black folklore, supernatural stories offered psychic escape through vicarious experience, a means of emotionally surmounting the frustrations of an oppressive white social structure. Slaves identified with the heroes of magical legends, finding in their abilities and actions wish-fulfilling experiences. But more than simply offering temporary release from daily anxieties, magical legends taught lessons in living. They demonstrated and sanctioned the use of folk beliefs to ameliorate the hardships of bondage.

Slaves learned their lessons well and constantly tried to improve their lot by supernatural means. Conjuring constituted a pragmatic and realistic method, given a situation of extremely limited alternatives, that slaves could use to cope with their masters. Magic itself did not engender an inclination to judge the morality of slavery or a radical ideology of liberation. Despite its internal complexities and contradictions, Afro-Christianity was a much more powerful ideological resource. An indispensable practical device, conjuring was available to both the individual bondsman trying to avoid a whipping and the leader of a slave rebellion recruiting new conspirators.[30]

The possibility of family separations was always a source of anxiety in the quarters, but slaves told each other legends about powerful conjurers who kept neighbors and kin from being sold away from each other. One woman allegedly conjured a steamboat so that it could not carry off the loved ones. In another example, slaves hired a renowned conjurer who made up a "hand," then buried it under the master's doorstep at midnight. Miraculously, when the white man walked through his door he lost the desire to sell his slaves, all of whom were now convinced they had momentarily tipped the balance of power in their own favor. Even properly interpreted dreams could prevent catastrophe: "if you dream of your master or your mistress counting

29. Dubois, "Religion of the American Negro," 618.

30. The use of slave magic to control whites is the main theme of Elliott J. Gorn, "No White Man Could Whip Me: Folk Beliefs of the Slave Community" (M.A. thesis, Berkeley, 1975).

money, and if you don't want anybody on the place to be sold, don't tell your dream until after sun-up—no one will be sold."[31]

Slaves employed a variety of techniques to keep their owners in a good mood. Hare Quarls recalled slipping up to the master's doorstep and driving a notched stick a little farther into the ground each night: "By de time de last notch down in de ground, it make massa good to us." Others chewed roots or carried a rabbit's foot to secure plenty of rations, obtain a good row to hoe, or stave off trouble with the overseer.[32] Controlling whites also meant avoiding whippings. Some conjurers allegedly made the master's lash miss its mark on every stroke, and one legendary bondsman miraculously deflected punishment onto his owner's wife: "When his master 'mence to whip him, eve'y cut he give de man, his wife way off at home feel de cut. Sin' wor' please stop cut lick de man. When he got home his wife was wash down wid blood." Conjurers supplied a variety of charms, roots, and conjure bags to keep the lash off their clients' backs, and fugitive slave Louis Hughes declared this custom to be "generally and tenaciously held to by all."[33]

Moreover, the world was filled with signs portending the future. The twitching of an eye, a rabbit crossing one's path, a kildee bird hollering, all warned of danger, and once interpreted properly, countermeasures prevented an impending whipping. No doubt chance, hard work, or good behavior coincided with magic to stave off beatings, but conjuring allowed slaves to believe they manipulated whites. Root workers who helped mollify brutal masters were seen as heroic

31. "Folklore and Ethnology," *Southern Workman*, XXVI (February, 1897), 37, reprinted from a student paper submitted in 1878; Bruce, *New Man*, 56–57; Rawick (ed.), *American Slave*, vol. 10.6, p. 7; "Folklore and Ethnology," *Southern Workman*, XXIII (March, 1894), 46. For parallel conjure stories, see Chesnutt, *Conjure Woman*, 36–63, 132–61. In another incident, a fortune-teller gave a woman information concerning the well-being of her daughter who had been sold away (Rawick [ed.], *American Slave*, vol. 19, p. 234).

32. Rawick (ed.), *American Slave*, vol. 5.3, p. 223; vol. 16, p. 95; suppl. ser. 2, vol. 4.3, p. 1134; Webb, *History of William Webb*, 21–23; Lyle Saxon and Robert Tallant (eds.), *Gumbo Ya Ya*, comp. Louisiana Writers' Program (Boston, 1945), 243–44; Puckett, *Folk Beliefs*, 276. For a fictional rendering of conjure improving the master's disposition, see "Mars Jeem's Nightmare," in Chesnutt, *Conjure Woman*, 64–102. Chesnutt discussed the influence of his boyhood in "Superstitions and Folklore of the South," *Modern Culture*, XIII (1901), 231–35, reprinted in Dundes (ed.), *Mother Wit*, 369–76. These stories are not to be confused with actual folklore, but they are interesting recreations by a man who was raised within the living tradition.

33. Elsie Clews Parsons, *Folklore of the Sea Islands, South Carolina* (New York, 1923), 61–62, vol. XVI of *The Memoirs of the American Folklore Society*; Louis Hughes, *Thirty Years a Slave, from Bondage to Freedom; Autobiography* (1897; rpr. New York, 1969), 108.

guardians and protectors, individuals who "just went around keeping people from getting killed." Again, magical power might be "unreal," but so long as slaves believed in and attempted to exercise it, their role never became one of total submission in the face of absolute authority.[34]

A similar pattern emerged in slaves' efforts to flee bondage. Legends of old-timers who knew how to fly back to Africa when life became too oppressive, narratives of blacks who left the plantation without a trace, stories about those who kept their tools working while they escaped, all sanctioned the use of magic to set limits on exploitation. One former slave claimed that his uncle made himself invisible whenever he wanted some time off: "He could disappear lak duh win, jis walk off duh plantation an stay way fuh weeks at a time. One time he get cownuhed by duh putrolmun an he jis walk up to a tree, an he say 'I tink I go intuh dis tree.' Den he disapeah right in duh tree." The fantasy of escape was made real by countless techniques for running away. Slaves used a wide variety of materials to hoodoo the bloodhounds and fool the patrollers. Conjurers prepared charms that caused the dogs to lose their way, bark up the wrong tree, or fail to recognize the slave they pursued. Hoodoo doctors also advised rubbing one's feet with pepper, snuff, or turpentine, all of which probably altered the dogs' ability to track, though slaves interpreted these acts within a larger supernatural context.[35]

34. For more examples, see Rawick (ed.), *American Slave*, vol. 5.3, pp. 161, 294; vol. 9.3, p. 166; vol. 6, p. 59; suppl. ser. 2, vol. 3.2, pp. 578, 756, 848; suppl. ser. 2, vol. 7.6, p. 2470; suppl. ser. 2, vol. 4.3, p. 1134; vol. 13.4, p. 263; vol. 13.3, p. 345; Puckett, *Folk Beliefs*, 318, 413; Bruce, *New Man*, 53; Monroe F. Jamison, *Autobiography and Work of Bishop Monroe F. Jamison, D.D.* (Nashville, 1912), 34. See also Herron and Bacon, "Conjuring and Conjure Doctors," 361; Brown, *My Southern Home*, Chap. 7; Richard Steiner, "Observations on the Practice of Conjuring in Georgia," *Journal of American Folklore*, XVI (July-September, 1901), 177; Genovese, *Roll, Jordan, Roll*, 221; "Folklore and Ethnology," *Southern Workman*, XXIII (March, 1894), 46; "Folklore and Ethnology," *Southern Workman*, XXV (January, 1896), 16; Rawick (ed.), *American Slave*, vol. 19, p. 139; Henry Bibb, *Narrative of the Life of Henry Bibb* (New York, 1850), 72. For efforts to mollify the master that failed, see Rawick (ed.), *American Slave*, suppl. ser. 2, vol. 3.2, pp. 633, 673; suppl. ser. 2, vol. 5.4, p. 1624.

35. Georgia Writers' Project, *Drums and Shadows*, 7, 28, 34, 41, 44, 79, 81, 116, 151, 156; John Bennett, "Folk Tales from Old Charleston," *Yale Review*, XXXII (Summer, 1943), 724–27; Rawick (ed.), *American Slave*, vol. 19, pp. 194–95; William R. Bascom, "Acculturation Among the Gullah Negroes," *American Anthropologist*, XLVII (1941), reprinted in August Meier and Elliott Rudwick (eds.), *The Origins of Black Americans* (New York, 1969), 41, vol. I of *The Making of Black America: Essays in Negro Life and History*; "Folklore and Ethnology," *Southern Workman*, XXIII (March, 1894), 46; Puckett, *Folk Beliefs*, 318; Herron and Bacon,

Not only magic but divination played an important part in slaves' efforts to abscond. William Wells Brown added almost as an afterthought that he visited a fortune-teller on the eve of his escape from bondage:

> I should have stated that just before leaving St. Louis, I went to an old man named Frank, a slave, owned by Mr. Sarpee. This old man was very distinguished (not only among the slave population, but also the whites). . . . I am no believer in soothsaying; yet I am sometimes at a loss to know how Uncle Frank could tell so accurately what would occur in the future. Among the many things he told was one which was enough to pay me for all the trouble of hunting him up. It was that I should be free!

How Frank knew that Brown intended to escape—perhaps Brown's demeanor gave him away, or Frank may have collected intelligence from other slaves—was unimportant, but the impact of the experience was crucial. Brown disclaimed belief in soothsaying, but why, then, did he seek out Frank? Clearly, Brown visited a fortune-teller because he was filled with anxiety and desperate to know how his dangerous plan would work out. He therefore turned to a method traditionally sanctioned within his culture, one that slaves frequently employed to bring a sense of security to their lives. Brown's mind was poised between credulity and disbelief, but his need for support inclined him for the moment towards faith. The experience with Old Frank gave Brown the confidence that comes from believing the future is tolerably predictable, not chaotic and filled with danger. Knowledge of the unseen world, then, tipped the scales toward freedom.[36]

In other important ways the supernatural provided a crucial sense of control over one's fate. Slaves developed their own standards for what they considered acceptable conduct from whites and enforced them magically. As early as 1773, Louisiana slaves attempted to kill their master and overseer with a gris-gris made from an alligator's heart, following the African precedent that called for a crocodile's

---

"Conjuring and Conjure Doctors," 361; Rawick (ed.), *American Slave*, vol. 13.4, p. 43; vol. 6, p. 230; vol. 12.2, pp. 235, 241; vol. 9.3, pp. 94–95; vol. 17, p. 15; vol. 16, p. 24; vol. 5.3, p. 248; vol. 11, p. 332; vol. 4.1, p. 42; suppl. ser. 2, vol. 2.1, p. 160; suppl. ser. 2, vol. 6.5, p. 1993.

36. William Wells Brown, *Narrative of William Wells Brown, A Fugitive Slave* (Boston, 1847), 91–93. Anthony Burns had a similar confidence-instilling experience with a fortune-teller who predicted his eventual freedom (Charles E. Stevens, *Anthony Burns* [Boston, 1856], 168–69).

organ. In another example, an old slave actually murdered her master and his family. Whites interpreted the event as simple poisoning, but as she was led to the gallows, slaves whispered among themselves about the woman's reputation as a conjurer. How often actual poisonings occurred is impossible to say, but clearly whites believed that some hoodoo doctors killed their masters.[37]

Generally, however, such murderous intentions remained confined to fantasy, or more precisely, to folk legends. South Carolina slaves told of a man beaten so badly by his master that he went to a conjurer to gain redress. The next morning "de white man was jus' as happy as happy can be; but de more de sun goes down, he commence ter sleep. At de same time he call to his Negro, 'Tomorrow you go an' do such an' such a tas'. Givin' out his orders kyan hardly hol' up his head. As soon as de sun was down, he down too, he down yet." Again, the conjurer held the power to even the score.[38]

Another legend taught that under unusual circumstances, bodily harm could be visited with impunity on a deserving white. The hero of this narrative was a conjurer, who, rather than kill his tormentor, reversed their power relationship: "There was another fellow on a joinin' plantation. He was a witch doctor. Brought him over from Africa. He didn't like his master 'cause he was mean. So he make a little man out of mud. An' he stick thorns in its back. Sure 'nuff, his master got down with a misery in his back. An' de witch doctor let de thorn stay in de mudman until he thought his master had got 'nuff punishment. When he tuck it out, his master got better." That the legendary slave decided when the master received " 'nuff punishment" is crucial. The conjurer assumed complete control over the question of discipline; the slave became master and his owner the slave.[39]

37. Laura L. Porteus, "The Gri-Gri Case," *Louisiana Historical Quarterly*, XVII (January, 1934), 50; Rawick (ed.), *American Slave*, vol. 3.3, p. 158; vol. 6, pp. 169, 223. A few slaves claimed magic only worked on other blacks (Rawick [ed.], *American Slave*, vol. 11, pp. 250–51; vol. 7, p. 207; vol. 19, p. 100). On the other hand, Ezra Adams, in Rawick (ed.), *American Slave*, vol. 2.1, p. 8, declared "De white chillun has been nursed by colored women and they has told them stories 'bout hants and sich lak. So de white chillun has growed up believin' some of dat stuff 'til dey natchally pass it on from generation to generation." For more examples of suspected poisonings of whites by conjurers, see Bertram Wyatt-Brown, *Southern Honor: Ethics and Behavior in the Old South* (New York, 1982), 424–25; and Peter H. Wood, *Black Majority: Negroes in Colonial South Carolina, From 1670 through the Stono Rebellion* (New York, 1974), 289–92.

38. Parsons, *Folklore of the Sea Islands*, 61–62.

39. Rawick (ed.), *American Slave*, vol. 11.7, pp. 20–21.

Like so much of Afro-American folklore, conjuring operated in fur-
tive and subtle ways. Zora Neale Hurston collected a postbellum legend about a planter who brutally killed one of his servants for some
minor indiscretion. Over the course of years, a friend and conjurer,
Old Dave, took revenge. Rather than simply kill the white man, he
conjured into insanity one member of his family after another. The
master's wife, daughter, and son mocked, attacked, and shot at him,
finally driving him from his own estate and stripping away all that he
cherished. The legend is significant because it cut to the very heart of
the southern value structure, revealing an acute knowledge of white
weaknesses. The hierarchical family was the central metaphor for
southern society. Authority, wisdom, and justice descended from the
father at the pinnacle, who dispensed largess and received the loving
obedience of others. But the legend of Old Dave denied the legitimacy
of patriarchal authority for masters who abused their power. Home,
family, and above all paternal prerogatives were undermined as one by
one the master's own kin betrayed him. On the level of fantasy, Old
Dave took away the white man's reason for living, literally a fate worse
than death.[40]

There are even hints that conjuring provided a screen behind which
interracial sexual taboos were broken. In South Carolina a master be-
queathed a fortune to his mulatto mistress. His kinsmen unsuccessfully challenged the will, claiming the woman supernaturally de-
ranged his judgment. Even more significant, in several court cases
male conjurers allegedly used their magic arts to seduce white women.
It is impossible to know for sure who really seduced whom, but once
again we have at least hints that magic offered a way of breaking
through social repressions. To violate patriarchal prerogatives and
female sexual "purity" was to deny the validity of the white code of
honor, the very core of the masters' values.[41]

Finally, those who could tap the supernatural became important
figures in slave rebellions. As early as 1712, a free black conjurer in
New York gave several conspirators magic powder, guaranteed to
make them invulnerable during their insurrection. Over a century
later, George Boxley rallied slaves to a rebellion, telling them that a
holy talking bird miraculously called them to the cause. In 1822, Denmark Vesey combined a Christian ideology of freedom with the prac-

40. Hurston, *Mules and Men*, 240–42. The ideology of southern paternalism is the
central theme of Genovese, *Roll, Jordan, Roll*.
41. Wyatt-Brown, *Southern Honor*, 313–16.

ticality of conjuring to create an extraordinarily powerful uprising. Vesey's lieutenant, "Gullah Jack," a renowned African conjurer, persuaded slaves to join the insurrection by promising supernatural protection; he then intimidated them into remaining loyal with threats of magical retribution. Less than a decade later, Nat Turner forged a militant Christian justification for freedom with interpretations of traditional dreams, signs, and portents. And on the eve of the Civil War, conspirators in Natchez, Mississippi, consulted a fortune-teller to gain insight into their dangerous future. Thus, if the supernatural did not engender an ideology of revolution, it did protect and legitimize those otherwise disposed to rebellious action. Magic bridged the sacred and secular worlds, reifying broad social goals and giving security, direction, and sanction to those embarking on a dangerous and radical course. In extreme cases then, the supernatural became a special esoteric power available to those bold enough to seize it.[42]

In all of these ways, the magical practices of slaves revealed continual strivings for autonomy and an unwillingness to accept white domination of their collective fate. Through traditional legends, slaves vented their submerged anger and gained a semblance of control over those who oppressed them. Manipulating the supernatural facilitated physical and psychological resistance to bondage and afforded slaves a genuine sense of selfhood. If magic failed to engender a critique of the

42. Kenneth Scott, "The Slave Insurrection in New York in 1712," *New York Historical Society Quarterly*, XLV (January, 1961), 47; Ulrich B. Phillips, *American Negro Slavery* (Baton Rouge, 1966), 476; Lionel H. Kennedy and Thomas Parker, *Official Report of the Trials of Sundry Negroes, Charged with an Attempt to Raise an Insurrection in the State of South Carolina* (Charleston, 1822), excerpted in Robert S. Starobin (ed.), *Denmark Vesey: The Slave Conspiracy of 1822* (Englewood Cliffs, N.J., 1972), 41–45. See also Vincent Harding, "Religion and Resistance Among Antebellum Negroes, 1800–1860," in Meier and Rudwick, *The Origins of Black Americans*, 186; Marion L. Starkey, *Striving to Make it My Home: The Story of Americans from Africa* (New York, 1964), 157, 187–88; Thomas R. Gray, reporter, "The Confessions of Nat Turner" (1831), reprinted in John Henrik Clarke (ed.), *William Styron's Nat Turner: Ten Black Writers Respond* (Boston, 1968), 99–105; Lemuel P. Connors, "Transcript of Slave Trials (1861)," Department of Archives and Manuscripts, Louisiana State University Library, Baton Rouge, 1, 8. Harriet Tubman, like Nat Turner, had visions, dreams, and revelations. See Harding, "Religion and Resistance," 192–93. All of this calls into question John Dollard's assertion that "magic accepts the status quo; it takes the place of political activity, agitation, organization, solidarity, or any real moves to change status" (Dollard, *Caste and Class in a Southern Town* [New York, 1937], 263). For an international perspective, see also Eugene Genovese, *From Rebellion to Revolution: Afro-American Slave Revolts in the Making of the Modern World* (Baton Rouge, 1979); and Michael Adas, *Prophets of Rebellion: Millenarian Protest Movements Against the European Colonial Order* (Chapel Hill, 1979), 92–164.

ELLIOTT J. GORN

social system, if folk beliefs could not alter the brute fact of servitude, they nevertheless were an antidote to feelings of powerlessness. Invoking the supernatural helped bondsmen and bondswomen survive with dignity.

Folk beliefs gave slaves a crucial sense of control over their masters, but blacks turned to the supernatural even more frequently in their dealings with each other.[43] As in many other cultures, magic offered a means of regulating behavior and enforcing communal norms. On the simplest level, this might involve discovering a thief. Conjurers used the old English technique of spinning a Bible or a pair of scissors, which pointed to the criminal. Still more effective, they made suspects drink graveyard dust dissolved in water, then questioned them about their role in the crime. If the thief lied, many assumed, the drink would kill him. No doubt belief in supernatural detection gave pause to those who contemplated antisocial behavior.[44]

Slaves also called upon conjurers to bring them good luck in gambling, help them collect debts, keep neighbors friendly, protect property, and prevent malicious magic. In interpersonal relationships, the

43. Responding to Stanley Elkins' thesis that slavery rendered its victims powerless and therefore psychically damaged, historians Genovese, Levine, Raboteau, Joyner, and Blassingame have asserted that cultural resources like conjuring were alternative repositories of authority and group self-worth. While I agree that folk beliefs offered a crucial measure of autonomy for psychic survival, the issue of direct supernatural control of whites has obscured the larger question of magic within the black community. Slaves conjured each other more than they conjured masters, but in either case, they exercised autonomous power. See Stanley M. Elkins, *Slavery: A Problem in American Institutional and Intellectual Life* (Chicago, 1959), Chap. 3.

44. See Stroyer, *My Life in the South*, 57–59. For English parallels to these customs, see Thomas, *Religion and the Decline of Magic*, 212–22. There were stories about clever masters who exploited their slaves' superstitiousness in similar ways: "One Mississippi slaveowner used a loaded cane to detect thieves. This 'jack' was supposed to rise up and work harm when the guilty man appeared, in case the slave did not confess of his own accord. Usually the threat was sufficient and the guilty slave confessed." On the basis of such stories, Puckett argued that masters disciplined their slaves by manipulating the slaves' fear of the supernatural (Puckett, *Folk Beliefs*, 281, 146). I have found very little evidence to back this claim, and Puckett offers nothing more of substance. Slaves carefully protected their magical lore, keeping this esoteric material as private as possible. For the few examples I have discovered, all of which involve the master detecting a thief, see Rawick (ed.), *American Slave*, vol. 7, p. 79; vol. 7, p. 113; vol. 3.3, p. 15; Kenneth M. Stampp, *The Peculiar Institution* (New York, 1956), 374; and Thaddeus Norris, "Negro Superstitions," *Lippincott's Magazine*, VI (July, 1870), 90–95, reprinted in Bruce Jackson, *The Negro and His Folklore*, 139–41. Gladys Marie Fry makes the argument for ghostlore as a form of social control, though her evidence is also questionable (Fry, *Night Riders in Black Folk History* [Knoxville, 1975]). For a critique of Fry, see Gorn, "Black Spirits."

316

conjurers rekindled old love affairs, broke up relationships, improved clients' sexual performance, and kept lovers faithful. Like all folk beliefs, slave superstitions offered a semblance of control over those ungovernable forces threatening peace, happiness, and security.[45]

Taken together, such magical practices added up to much more than a collection of useful tools for daily living. Afro-Americans' need for a sense of mastery was particularly acute because bondage, by definition, attempted to negate their individual and collective wills. The ideal slave was totally dependent, totally subjected to his owner's whims. Conjuring helped blacks psychically resist planter hegemony by offering them resources for acting in their own behalf and thereby rejecting white pretensions. The very existence of powerful slaves accomplishing useful ends through means that masters neither comprehended nor controlled was a living denial of black helplessness in the face of white omnipotence. Magic preserved a measure of autonomy that bondage otherwise threatened to strip away.

There was, however, a darker side to conjuring. Often the supernatural made the world seem less under control, not more. The power that hoodoo doctors wielded facilitated vendettas among slaves, and masters occasionally complained that their chattels' belief in magic caused serious health problems. Many bondsmen deeply feared being conjured into sickness or even death by their enemies. They related stories of friends or family members blinded, crippled, even driven insane. Some victims became so high-strung that they could not sit still, while others pined away and died. Countless reports by former slaves described men and women reduced to animality, barking like dogs, crowing like cocks, or crawling on hands and knees. Symbolically, these were especially grievous cases because they overturned human domination of the animal kingdom and equated individuals with mere beasts. Conjurers were commonly alleged to know how to make loathsome creatures live inside a person. They ground up charred lizards, frogs, snakes, spiders, maggots, or other vermin, put the powder in contact with intended victims, and before long, the vile beings were living inside them, growing, multiplying and eating their vitals. Such afflictions were not only potentially fatal, they symbolically rendered victims slaves to the disgusting creatures inside

45. Rawick (ed.), *American Slave*, vol. 13.3, p. 223; vol. 7, p. 228; *National Police Gazette*, II (March 27, 1847), 227; Puckett, *Folk Beliefs*, 245–46, 264–70, 283–84. For a modern example of the association of conjuring with organized crime, see George J. McCall, "Symbiosis: the Case of Hoodoo and the Numbers Rackets," *Social Problems*, X (Spring, 1963), 361–71, reprinted in Dundes (ed.), *Mother Wit*, 419–27.

them. One physician concluded that nearly all blacks were "kept in constant dread and terror by the conjurers."[46]

The reasons root workers inflicted these horrible maladies on others often seem remarkably trifling. A thoughtless word, some breach of neighborly etiquette, petty jealousies, envy of material goods, stealing someone's lover—all were cause for frightful curses leading to illness and death.[47] Susan Snow of Mississippi recalled being conjured by a man she treated with kindness. "It's a good thing you was good to me," the old conjurer told her, " 'cause if you hadn't, you'd be dead an' in your grave now." July Ann Halfner's neighbor accused her of stealing a blanket. She denied the charge, and her neighbor was very friendly, even as she prepared to afflict July with a painful illness. Some former slaves reported cases of conjuring in which there was no motive at all. "Yuh nebuh can tell who is a witch and who is workin' 'gainst yuh," one declared.[48]

A distinctly misanthropic view of humankind pervaded blacks' supernatural beliefs. A prominent theme in Afro-American folklore was that if one person suffered, another probably caused it. Declared one former Georgia slave, "T'ain't no need talkin'; folks can do anythin' to you they wants to. They can run you crazy or they can kill you. Don't you one time believe that every pore pusson they has in the 'sylum is just natchelly crazy. Some was run crazy on account of people not likin' 'em, some 'cause they was gettin' 'long a little too good. Every time a pusson jumps in the river don't think he was just tryin' to kill hisself;

46. See, for example, Genovese, *Roll, Jordan, Roll*, 209–32; Puckett, *Folk Beliefs*, 274–76; Herron and Bacon, "Conjuring and Conjure Doctors"; Rawick (ed.), *American Slave*, vol. 4.2, pp. 63–65; vol. 12.2, pp. 45, 123; vol. 13.4, pp. 358–59; suppl. ser. 1, vol. 4.2, pp. 580–91; vol. 13.4, pp. 261–88. On masters complaining about conjurers, see Stampp, *Peculiar Institution*, 374–75, and James O. Breeden (ed.), *Advice Among Masters: The Ideal of Slave Management in the Old South* (Westport, Conn., 1980), 170–71. Perhaps conjuring one's fellow slaves was a substitute outlet for aggression that could not be directed against whites. Although this argument may have merit, I believe that the violence associated with conjuring grew more out of specific grievances than out of free-floating anger.

47. See, for example, Herron and Bacon, "Conjuring and Conjure Doctors," 361; Rawick (ed.), *American Slave*, suppl. ser. 1, vol. 8.3, pp. 904–905; vol. 13.3, pp. 14–15; vol. 4.2, pp. 63–65; suppl. ser. 1, vol. 4.2, pp. 355–56, 426; vol. 13.3, p. 32; vol. 12.2, p. 45; vol. 13.4, pp. 259–62. Some could conjure by simply pointing a finger at an intended victim; others could put "bad mouth" on an enemy. See, for examples, Rawick (ed.), *American Slave*, suppl. ser. 2, vol. 4.3, p. 1329; suppl. ser. 2, vol. 6.5, pp. 2205–2206.

48. Rawick (ed.), *American Slave*, suppl. ser. 1, vol. 10.5, p. 2013; suppl. ser. 1, vol. 8.3, pp. 904–905; suppl. ser. 2, vol. 4.3, p. 1428; suppl. ser. 1, vol. 4.2, p. 591. See also Rawick (ed.), *American Slave*, suppl. ser. 2, vol. 9.8, p. 3864; suppl. ser. 1, vol. 3, pp. 138–39.

most times he just didn't know what he was doin'." Of course, pain, illness, and insanity are rendered doubly unbearable when we have no explanation for their origin. Belief in conjuring at least offered meaning: One suffered not because of chance or blind fate, but because a particular person acted out of malice. Anticipating supernatural assaults, many slaves took prophylactic measures. Conjurers sold charms to ward off the evil magic of others, and if a dime worn round one's neck turned black, it was a sure sign of being tricked. All too often, however, such counter-charms failed to constrain violent human impulses.[49]

The expectation of malice found encouragement in white southern life and thought. As Dickson Bruce observes, the antebellum South never had the North's optimistic faith in personal and social perfectibility. Implicitly, southerners took violence, selfish passions, and evil to be the lot of humankind. Even southern evangelicals anticipated more backsliding and expected less morally rigid behavior than their northern counterparts. Afro-Americans shared in and contributed to this regional outlook. More important, as victims of slavery—a social system embodying a pessimistic view of human nature because it assumed that masses of men were incapable of freedom and equality—blacks knew firsthand that benevolence was not to be fully trusted, that violence potentially lurked in all relationships. Hardship, suffering, and brutality were part of life in bondage, and they often struck suddenly and without apparent meaning. Narratives about malevolent conjuring drew upon and reinforced such assumptions.[50]

The belief in human finitude was part of a deeply personalistic worldview. Not institutions, technologies, nor ideologies, but men were responsible for daily occurrences. This outlook was also reinforced by the specific social circumstances Afro-Americans found in the New World. Like many other premodern labor systems, North

49. Rawick (ed.), *American Slave*, vol. 13.4, p. 279; Levine, *Black Culture and Black Consciousness*, Chap. 2. The slave narratives are full of anticonjure measures. See, for example, Rawick (ed.), *American Slave*, suppl. ser. 2, vol. 4.3, p. 1329; suppl. ser. 2, vol. 7.6, p. 2491; suppl. ser. 2, vol. 3.2, p. 896; suppl. ser. 2, vol. 4.3, pp. 1256–58; Puckett, *Folk Beliefs*, 287–300.

50. Dickson Bruce, *Violence and Culture in the Ante-Bellum South* (Austin, 1979). For a brilliant analysis of this pessimistic view in narrative folklore, see Levine, *Black Culture and Black Consciousness*, esp. Chap. 2. As Levine argues, this pessimism was counterbalanced by traditions emphasizing change and transcendence, especially in Afro-Christianity. A similarly misanthropic view was expressed in Afro-American ghostlore (see Gorn, "Black Spirits").

ELLIOTT J. GORN

American slavery was highly paternalistic; authority had a human visage, not an institutional one. Bondsmen were accustomed to regarding good and evil as the fruits of face-to-face contacts with particular individuals. "Massa" made the decisions about working hours, rations, whippings, and holidays for "his people." The southern social system encouraged slaves to expect pain and seek protection from above. Charismatic conjurers who harmed or protected individuals against evil were an Afro-American inversion of southern paternalism, a mirror reflection of the personalistic nature of slave society. Here blacks as well as whites could be great in their largess or terrifying in their power. It is not surprising, then, that masters and conjurers sometimes vied for influence over particular slaves.[51]

By encouraging a personalistic, often mistrustful worldview, southern white culture merely reinforced a tendency blacks inherited from Africa. Anthropologists have long known that African witchcraft and sorcery accusations grew out of community crises. Robin Horton observes that life in small, traditional African communities contained powerful sources of emotional stress. Circumscribed role choices and limited opportunities created deep personal frustrations, even serious problems in social adjustment. More important, petty fights and arguments easily radiated to all areas of life because members of small communities were forced to interact in a wide variety of daily activities. Close dependence on kin and neighbors often spread these disputes beyond the original antagonists to a large portion of the community, and once hostilities were kindled or social norms violated, individuals had little mobility to escape the sources of stress. There were, of course, tremendous differences between African peoples, and their supernatural beliefs varied considerably. Diversity notwithstanding,

51. The concept of paternalism is at the heart of Genovese, *Roll, Jordan, Roll,* esp. Book I and 209–32. A Louisiana physician complained in 1851:

> On almost every large plantation there is one or more negroes, who are ambitious of being considered in the character of conjurers—in order to gain influence and to make the others fear and obey them. The influence that these pretended conjurers exercise over their fellow servants would not be credited by persons unacquainted with the superstitious mind of the negro. . . . These impostors, like all other impostors, take advantage of circumstances to swell their importance and to inculcate a belief in their miraculous powers to bring good or evil upon those they like or dislike. It may be thought that the old superstition about conjuration has passed away with the old stock of native Africans; but it is too deeply radicated in the negro intellect to pass away; intelligent negroes believe in it, who are ashamed to acknowledge it.

In the war between slaveholders and conjurers, the doctor suggested good food, clothing, shelter, and the master's expressed concern for his slaves' well-being as prophylactics (Breeden [ed.], *Advice Among Masters,* 170–71).

320

African cultures historically ascribed personal or community problems to witchcraft and sorcery.[52]

Such magical beliefs, Horton observes, spoke in a personalistic idiom in contrast to modern science, which relies on an impersonal one. Traditional societies acknowledged "natural" causes of disease, but because they were so thickly communal, because so much of daily reality was constructed around tight interpersonal relationships, they gravitated toward human acts, thoughts, and motives to explain phenomena. To put the matter in a crude but useful way, scientific thinking perceives the world mechanistically; traditional patterns of thought seek explanations in the realm of human interactions.[53]

For this reason, African traditional healing more than Western medicine acknowledged the role of emotional stress in causing or exacerbating physical ailments. When disease persistently failed to respond to herbal or "natural" treatments, both doctor and patient began to suspect supernatural sources. At this point, Horton tells us, a diviner would be called in who generally cited human hatreds, misdeeds, or jealousies as the cause of illness. Good health, Africans believed, could not be restored until all sources of tension were discovered and rectified, and these healers therefore explored conflicts in their clients' social relationships. Diviners' findings often led to accusations of witchcraft or sorcery against their patients' enemies. Exposing the source of interpersonal tensions led the way to confessions, adjudication of wrongs, healing, and the restoration of community equilibrium.[54]

Although Afro-American slave communities were very different from traditional African societies, they shared important similarities that encouraged the retention of Old World belief systems. All were susceptible to the same sorts of nagging personal conflicts because all were essentially tightly bonded, closed social systems that offered limited role choice and mobility. As recent studies demonstrate, Afro-American culture was intensely communal. The plantation kept small

52. Horton, "African Traditional Thought and Western Science," 50–60. Horton reviews the anthropological literature.

53. *Ibid.*, esp. 64–65.

54. *Ibid.*, 53–56, 60. Africans, like Afro-Americans, recognized distinctions between "natural" disease subject to medical intervention and magically induced disease, which often led to death. Whereas the role of diviner was subsumed under that of conjurer among Afro-Americans, both African and American black cultures viewed the "medicine man" in the dual role of one who heals and one who inflicts disease. See Eva Gillies, "Causal Criteria in African Classifications of Disease," in J. B. Loudon (ed.), *Social Anthropology and Medicine* (London, 1976), 358–95.

numbers of slaves living cheek-by-jowl in rigidly confined space. Even the tiny slave quarters—usually "shotgun" houses, similar in layout to African homes—placed individuals in close and intimate contact. In America, as in Africa, such tight communality fostered cultural solidarity, but could also inflame interpersonal tensions.[55]

Thus, African belief in the human origins of disease, inherited faith in sorcery and witchcraft, a powerful communal ethos, the expectation that people act out of selfish impulses, and a deeply personalistic worldview all provided a foundation for faith in conjuring. These assumptions unleashed a fearsome power, sometimes setting slave against slave. But they also allowed Afro-American magic to develop into an extraordinarily useful community resource. A closer look at conjuring reveals that supernatural illness was part of a complex system for expressing grievances, seeking redress, and obtaining justice.

Since face-to-face relationships demanded constant interaction among slaves, etiquette and proper manners became vital to community cohesion. "Good manners will carry you where money won't," Gus Bradshaw was taught as a child, and he echoed the sentiments of many former slaves who thought that observing rules of decorum was essential to peaceful and stable relationships. Sometimes, however, manners failed to hold conflicts in check. If common courtesy bestowed honor, breaches of etiquette and personal slights denied it, so affronts were readily transformed into ugly crises. Yet because slaves were valuable property, masters restrained them from fighting each other. When one slave insulted or injured another, or committed some breach of community standards, the aggrieved party might be unable or unwilling to retaliate openly. Here, as in so many other facets of slave life, subtlety and indirection were essential. Conjuring became a hidden channel through which hostilities could flow. Largely deprived of direct aggression as an outlet for gnawing grievances, American blacks, like their African ancestors, turned to the supernatural.[56]

55. The communal quality of Afro-American culture is a central theme of Levine, *Black Culture and Black Consciousness*; Genovese, *Roll, Jordan, Roll*; and Vlach, *The Afro-American Tradition in Decorative Arts*. On black architecture, see George W. McDaniel, *Hearth and Home: Preserving a People's Culture* (Philadelphia, 1982).

56. Rawick (ed.), *American Slave*, suppl. ser. 2, vol. 5.4, p. 1504; suppl. ser. 2, vol. 2.1, p. 392. On slave violence, see Edward Ayers, *Vengeance and Justice: Crime and Punishment in the Nineteenth Century American South* (New York, 1984), 133. On conjure violence, see Herron and Bacon, "Conjuring and Conjure Doctors," 360; Puckett, *Folk Beliefs*, 167; Rawick (ed.), *American Slave*, suppl. ser. 1, vol. 7.2, p. 772. For other examples of malign magic, see Rawick (ed.), *American Slave*, vol. 3.3, pp. 78–79, 106–107; vol. 12.2, pp. 154–64; vol. 13.4, pp. 271–81.

Conjurers acted as neutral intermediaries—sorcerers—who accepted fees and provided services to others. Their powers were accessible to all, and slaves who felt injured could seek revenge by paying them to bring illness, insanity, or even death to their enemies. A former slave from Georgia recalled, "My aunt's son had took a girl away from another man who was going with her too. As soon as this man heard they was going to marry, he started studying some way to stop it. So he went to a root worker." The victim died.[57] Thus, slaves invoked magic to punish offenders and reestablish proper social relations; conjuring provided an outlet for the daily stresses of close communal contact, stresses that otherwise might have remained bottled up until they exploded. Because their talents were so useful, hoodoo doctors received great respect. Slaves feared conjurers, but unlike witches in Western cultures, they were never considered social pariahs worthy of persecution or death.[58]

The ability to injure supernaturally was a formidable weapon, and it invited abuses. But conjuring as a system contained internal restraints that limited the danger. Conjurers not only inflicted illness, they also cured it. Indeed, only a conjurer could remove magically induced disease; medical doctors, it was believed, were powerless to cure tricked victims. Once it became obvious to Francis Kimbrough, for example, that a jealous rival had conjured her, she abandoned regular cures and sent for a hoodoo doctor who healed her afflicted arm.[59]

Two other factors restrained potential abuses. First, slaves had to pay conjurers for their services, and bondsmen did not easily part with their small stock of material possessions. More important, having an

57. Rawick (ed.), *American Slave*, vol. 13.4, p. 278. Another ex-slave claimed that her niece "married a man that had been goin' 'round with a old woman who wasn't nothin.'" The scorned woman resorted to conjure (Rawick [ed.], *American Slave*, vol. 13.4, p. 348). Patsy Moses described a Knoxville conjurer who held ceremonies at night, where blacks "come ter git him ter work de evil charms on dey enemies" (Rawick [ed.], *American Slave*, suppl. ser. 2, vol. 7.6, pp. 2784–86). See also Rawick (ed.), *American Slave*, suppl. ser. 2, vol. 6.5, pp. 2205–2206.

58. See, for example, Rawick (ed.), *American Slave*, vol. 12.2, pp. 158–64. Whitten, "Patterns of Malign Occultism," 142, found during the 1960s that despite the injuries their magic inflicted, conjurers were generally considered to be good people performing useful work who had community prestige. Although individuals with evil intentions might hire hoodoo doctors, magical power itself was seen as value neutral.

59. Rawick (ed.), *American Slave*, vol. 13.3, pp. 14–15. For examples like Kimbrough's, see also Rawick (ed.), *American Slave*, vol. 13.4, p. 251; vol. 12.2, pp. 158–64; vol. 3.3, pp. 106–107; vol. 12.2, pp. 156–57. Dr. Ambrose McCoy of Penson, Tennessee, expressed consternation at being able neither to understand nor to cure conjured victims (see "Voodooism in the South," *Louisville Medical News* [December 18, 1884], 380–81).

enemy conjured involved considerable personal risk because the victim could have another hoodoo doctor "turn the trick," that is, send the illness back to the perpetrator. Once released, it was assumed that ill-fortune would not disappear, but must fasten on someone; if a conjure bag was discovered, setting it on fire burned your enemy, and throwing it in water drowned him. "Ma" Stevens, a former slave from Georgia, recalled a neighbor who always acted friendly, concealing deep jealousies. The neighbor conjured Ma, but as a hoodoo doctor herself, she knew how to make a "Hell Fire Gun." When Ma fired it, she caught three enemies working magic against her, all of whom eventually died. Similarly, another conjure woman perished in agony while her neighbors whispered "she was reapin' what she sowed." Narratives like these that warned slaves of the potential dangers of conjuring usually assured that magic was not invoked for light or transient causes.[60]

Whereas slaves who had their fellows conjured vented aggression and sought justice, many victims were atoning for their sins. Those who violated communal norms, for example, coveted someone else's loved one, spoke rudely, failed to show proper respect for another slave, or committed countless other social transgressions, were probably quite suggestible. Guilt and anxiety made them expect to be conjured, so practically any unusual event could trigger the belief that someone had indeed "fixed" them. In reality, the guilty slave might not have been conjured at all, and if he or she was, the magical charm hidden under the doorstep might be no more harmful than needles and human hair wrapped in red flannel. But the notion that someone conjured them, along with their unconscious belief that they deserved it, induced psychosomatic symptoms. In this way, disease became a self-fulfilling prophecy, and the nature, duration, and severity of the malady were determined partly by the victim's own sense of guilt.[61]

Illness, then, could be a form of self-chastisement for wrongdoing, and a return to health signaled successful atonement. Charles C. Jones,

60. Puckett, *Folk Beliefs*, 296–98; Rawick (ed.), *American Slave*, vol. 2.2, pp. 218–19; vol. 12.2, pp. 156–64; vol. 3.3, pp. 78–79, 106–107; suppl. ser. 1, vol. 4.2, pp. 588–89; vol. 13.4, pp. 270–72, 348–49; Herron and Bacon, "Conjuring and Conjure Doctors," 366–67; Whitten, "Patterns of Malign Occultism," 408.

61. On the idea of guilt and atonement, consider the following: A Reverend Dennis was sick for a year, but until he went to a hoodoo doctor—at his wife's insistence—he failed to recover. The doctor told him he had a snake in his leg, which got there because of some whiskey the Reverend drank, whiskey offered by his girlfriend. The entire situation—wife, girlfriend, and a whiskey-drinking preacher—seems ripe for the playing out of powerful feelings of guilt through supernatural illness (Rawick [ed.], *American Slave*, vol. 12.2, pp. 156–57).

a South Carolina planter, described his slaves' conjure beliefs with precisely this concept of making amends for offenses. Former slave Rosanna Frazier also made the connection between guilt and illness clear. One day she heard a mysterious voice say, " 'Rose, you done somethin' you ain't ought.' " The very next morning she was conjured into blindness. Speaking rudely to an elder, refusing to dance with someone, eliciting others' envy, all were given as reasons for being cursed. If suffering relieved the sense of guilt, then willingness to turn the trick signaled that one had atoned sufficiently, that now wrongdoing could be projected onto one's enemy. Thus, a woman conjurer who had her own malicious magic turned back on her died screaming, "Take 'em off of me, I ain't done nothin' to 'em. Tell 'em I didn't hurt 'em, don't let 'em kill me."[62]

As a system of faith healing and harming, conjuring offered slaves an important indigenous source of control over their social relationships. All cultures require general agreement on acceptable norms of conduct. Whenever possible, these are enforced by socialization, persuasion, and consensus. But fear is also an essential ingredient for regulating behavior. Some societies fall back on police forces, jails, or stockades to maintain their boundaries between acceptable and deviant conduct. Others turn to gossip, ridicule, and the supernatural. Among Afro-Americans, when the communal norms imbibed in church, taught by parents, and reinforced through folklore were violated, the conjurer held the power to reestablish equilibrium. Like any system of justice, conjuring could prove divisive. Magic sometimes caused needless anxiety and injured the innocent. But in the long run, it was an important stabilizing force, a means through which slaves themselves could handle violations of their own communal standards.

Finally, legends about magic were as important as magical practice itself. Slaves did not have to be conjured to know about sorcery. They were constantly reminded through countless narratives, many of which exaggerated the powers of conjurers to terrifying proportions, that people who violated standards of decent interpersonal behavior risked supernatural retribution. Susan Smith declared that she was always polite to everyone because she had heard stories about individuals who "sassed" others and paid for it supernaturally. She might

62. Charles C. Jones, *Negro Myths From the Georgia Coast* (Boston, 1888), 151–53; Rawick (ed.), *American Slave*, vol. 4.2, pp. 63–65; vol. 13.4, p. 272. Also see Rawick (ed.), *American Slave*, suppl. ser. 2, vol. 3.2, p. 674; suppl. ser. 2, vol. 10.9, p. 4147; Charles Chesnutt, "Superstitions and Folklore of the South," *Modern Culture*, XIII (1901), 231–35, reprinted in Dundes (ed.), *Mother Wit*, 374–75.

have had in mind the legend of children who harassed an old man by throwing rocks at him. He pointed at one who hit him in the face, threatening retribution. The child continued hurling stones, but the very next day he crumpled dead on the floor. From then on, no one bothered the old man.[63]

Such legends discouraged antisocial behavior by teaching slaves that those who acted rudely, encouraged jealousy, belittled others, trusted acquaintances too deeply, interfered between lovers, or committed other transgressions were subject to punishment. The following narrative, for example, must have served as a cautionary legend to all who heard it:

> Once a man named John tried to go with a girl but her step-pa, Willie, run him away from the house just like he might be a dog, so John made it up in his mind to conjure Willie. He went to the spring and planted somethin' in the mouth of it, and when Willie went there the next day to get a drink he got the stuff in the water. . . . In a few days somethin' started growin' in his throat. . . . Finally he got so bad off he claimed somethin' was chokin' him to death, and so his wife sont off and got a fortune teller. This fortune teller said it was a turtle in his throat. . . . It wasn't long after that 'fore Willie was dead. That turtle come up in his throat and choked him to death.

Here the stepfather—whose status as a nonrelative made his right to intervene in the situation tenuous to begin with—treated the girl's suitor with total contempt, thereby inviting magical retribution. Supernatural narratives, then, helped define and enforce the slave community's own norms of conduct.[64]

In all of these ways, whether conjuring helped Afro-Americans deal with the thousand nagging crises of daily life, gain a semblance of control over masters, feel that they understood the causes of human misery, or regulate social relations within their own communities, it offered black men and women the crucial awareness that they held some power over their own affairs, an awareness that bondage constantly threatened to strip away. Predicting the future, explaining the unknowable, controlling events, and providing symbolic meaning all made folk beliefs a vital part of Afro-American culture. Magic provided what human beings crave, a sense of mastery over the chaos of life.

63. Rawick (ed.), *American Slave*, suppl. ser. 2, vol. 9.8, pp. 3668–69; suppl. ser. 2, vol. 2.1, pp. 272–73.

64. Rawick (ed.), *American Slave*, vol. 13.4, p. 277. Certainly many of the narratives cited throughout this chapter as evidence of magical *practice* also served as magical *legends*—they described a core of events that became embellished into narratives.

CHAPTER 15

BLACK HEALTH ON THE PLANTATION: MASTERS, SLAVES, AND PHYSICIANS

Todd L. Savitt

S lavery was a fundamental element of southern life and society, one of several factors that made the region distinctive. Its presence created a special situation for two reasons: first, whites, responsible for slave medical care, in large part dictated the living and working conditions that promoted or destroyed blacks' health; second, some white southerners claimed (and many others believed) that blacks were medically different from whites and so in need of special treatment. This chapter will look at the three groups of southerners most directly involved in issues of black health and care—masters, physicians, and the slaves themselves—and show that matters of slave health contributed to the distinctiveness of southern society.[1]

This essay is extracted in large part from Todd L. Savitt, *Medicine and Slavery: The Diseases and Health Care of Blacks in Antebellum Virginia* (Urbana, 1978), 1–184. The author acknowledges the very helpful suggestions of James Breeden, Paul Escott, David Goldfield, Kenneth Kiple, Ronald Numbers, and James Harvey Young.

1. Except in the first section of this chapter, where I present a general overview of black-related diseases, the focus is on Virginia from the Revolution to the Civil War. Health conditions in the Old Dominion at that time were, in many respects, typical of those prevailing throughout the antebellum South. Residents suffered from malaria, parasitic worm diseases, and dysentery just as Mississippians and Georgians did. Yellow fever struck the state's major ports, though not so severely or so frequently as at Charleston, Mobile, or New Orleans. Virginia's position on the northern fringe of the slave South perhaps lessened the intensity and duration of warm-weather diseases, but not enough to render its diseases significantly different from those in the lower South.

During the time span under consideration, the black population and the health picture in Virginia were relatively stable. The slave trade had ended, there was little black immigration into the state, and tropical diseases brought from Africa and unable to survive in the new environment had all but disappeared.

I will first discuss how southern physicians used their own and others' observations of black medical differences to develop both a partial rationale for enslaving blacks in the American South and a special approach to their medical care and treatment. I will next describe the various ways in which the living and working conditions of plantation slaves, generally different from the conditions of agricultural workers in other regions of the country, affected black health. Finally, I will examine the various forms of black medical care that masters, physicians, and slaves themselves provided under this unique labor system known as "the peculiar institution."

"Scarcely any observant medical man, having charge of negro estates, fails to discover, by experience, important modifications in the diseases and appropriate treatment of the white and black race respectively."[2] Thus wrote the editor of a prominent Virginia medical journal in 1856, in an attempt to impress upon the state's physicians the importance of providing adequate health care to slaves. He could very well have been speaking to all southern doctors, many of whom believed that medical differences existed between blacks and whites. The issue was of both practical and political importance: it involved not only the health care of an entire racial group in the South, but also the partial justification for enslaving them.

Physicians who treated slave diseases had a pecuniary and professional concern with the subject. Their recorded opinions in medical, commercial, and agricultural journals, as well as in personal correspondence, attest to the seriousness with which they approached issues of black health. The politically minded physicians (all of whom practiced medicine) were also resolutely committed to explaining the southern position on slavery. In publications for the medical, commercial, and lay public, men like Josiah Clark Nott of Mobile and Samuel A. Cartwright of New Orleans used their knowledge of black medicine to rationalize the necessity and usefulness of slavery. These apologists for the peculiar institution, in order to prove that slavery was humane and economically viable in the South, argued that blacks had immunity to certain diseases that devastated whites. Slaveowners, they said, did not sacrifice blacks every time they sent them into the rice fields or canebrakes. Nor could physicians adequately treat blacks without knowledge of their anatomical and physiological peculiarities and disease proclivities. Blacks were medically different from and mentally inferior to whites, they asserted.

2. Editorial, *Monthly Stethoscope and Medical Reporter*, I (1856), 162–63.

In certain obvious physical ways Negroes did vary greatly from Caucasians. Old South writers particularly commented on facial features, hair, posture and gait, skin color, and odor. One school of American scientists spent much time and effort investigating cranium and brain size, as well as other characteristics, in part to discover whether blacks were inferior to whites. Physicians, slaveowners, and other interested persons also detected distinctions in the physical reactions of the two races both to diseases and to treatments. Their observations were often accurate, but at times they allowed racial prejudice to cloud their views. These observers remarked particularly about the relative immunity of blacks to southern fevers, especially intermittent fever (malaria) and yellow fever; blacks' susceptibility to intestinal and respiratory diseases; and their tolerance of heat and intolerance of cold. Black children, they noted, died more frequently of marasmus (wasting away), convulsions, "teething," and suffocation or overlaying than did whites.[3]

One of the most fascinating subjects of Old South medical authors was black resistance to malaria, the focus of constant comment during the antebellum period because blacks' liability to it appeared to vary from region to region, plantation to plantation, and individual to individual. In dispute was the degree of susceptibility and the virulence of the disease in blacks: Could slaves acquire some resistance to malaria by living in constant proximity to its supposed source? Were some slaves naturally immune? Did slaves have milder attacks of the disease than whites?

Modern science has answered many of the questions of immunity and prevention of malaria with which doctors and planters struggled in the antebellum period. Several factors contributed to the phenomenon of malarial immunity. Many blacks did possess an inherited immunity to one or another form of malaria. But Caucasians and Negroes without natural resistance to a particular type of plasmodium (the organism that causes malaria) could acquire malarial immunity or tolerance only by suffering repeated infections of the disease over several years, as was noted by the author of an article in the *New Orleans Medical News and Hospital Gazette* (1858–59). For this to occur, one of the four species of plasmodium—falciparum, vivax, malariae,

3. These and other diseases and conditions are discussed in an important book on black medical differences, Kenneth F. Kiple and Virginia Himmelsteib King, *Another Dimension to the Black Diaspora: Diet, Disease, and Racism* (Cambridge, England, 1981). On the life and thought of one southern medical thinker, see Reginald Horsman, *Josiah Nott of Mobile: Southerner, Physician, and Racial Theorist* (Baton Rouge, 1987).

and ovale—had to be present constantly in the endemic region, so that with each attack a person's supply of antibodies was strengthened against further parasitic invasions. Interruption of this process, such as removal to nonendemic areas for the summer (when exposure to the parasite was useful in building immunity) or for several years (during schooling or travel), prohibited the aggregation of sufficient antibodies to resist infection. In truly endemic areas, acquiring immunity this way was a risky affair: unprotected children struggled for their lives, adults suffered from relapses of infections contracted years before, and partially immune adults worked through mild cases. It is no wonder, then, that slaves sold from, say, Virginia, where one form of malaria was prevalent, to owners on a Louisiana bayou or South Carolina rice plantation, where a different species or strain of plasmodium was endemic, had a high incidence of the disease. Even adult slaves from Africa had to go through a "seasoning" period because the strains of malarial parasites in this country differed from those in their native lands.

Generally speaking, most malaria in the upper South and in inland piedmont areas was of the milder vivax type, whereas vivax coexisted with the more dangerous falciparum malaria in coastal and swampy inland portions of both the lower and upper South. Rare pockets of the malariae type (quartan fever) were scattered across the South. Ovale malaria appears not to have been present in the United States. Of course, epidemics of one type or another could strike any neighborhood and bring sickness and death even to those who had acquired resistance to the endemic variety. *Plasmodium falciparum* usually caused such epidemics, especially in the temperate regions of the South.[4]

The major reason for black immunity to vivax or falciparum malaria relates not to acquired resistance, but to selective genetic factors. At least three hereditary conditions prevalent among blacks in parts of modern Africa appear to give their bearers immunity to malaria. Recent medical research indicates that the red blood cells of persons lacking a specific factor called "Duffy antigen" are resistant to invasion of *Plasmodium vivax*. Approximately 90 percent of West Africans lack Duffy antigens, as do about 70 percent of Afro-Americans. This inherited, symptomless, hematologic condition is extremely rare in other racial groups. All evidence points to the conclusion that infection by

4. For a discussion of the southern disease environment from colonial times to the present, see Albert Cowdrey, *This Land, This South: An Environmental History* (Lexington, Ky., 1983).

Plasmodium vivax requires the presence of Duffy-positive red blood cells. Since most Negroes do not possess this factor, they are immune to vivax malaria. It can be safely assumed that the vast majority of American slaves and free blacks were therefore resistant to this form of the disease.

Some antebellum blacks had additional protection against malaria resulting from two abnormal genetic hemoglobin conditions, sickle-cell disease (a form of anemia) and sickle-cell trait (the symptomless carrier state of the sickling gene). People with either of these conditions had milder cases of, and decreased risk of mortality from, the most malignant form of malaria, falciparum. Many of those who had sickle-cell *disease* died from its consequences before or during adolescence; however, blacks who had sickle-cell *trait* lived entirely normal lives and could then transmit the gene for sickling to their offspring. Since people with the trait had one normal gene and one abnormal gene for sickling (in contrast to those with the disease, who had two of the abnormal genes), their offspring could inherit sickle-cell anemia only when each parent contributed a gene for sickling. Because the sickle-cell condition was not discovered until 1910, physicians in the antebellum South were unaware that this was one reason why some slaves on plantations appeared to be immune to malarial infections. One other genetic condition with a high incidence within the former slave-trading region probably affords some malarial resistance: deficiency of the enzyme glucose-6-phosphate dehydrogenase (G-6-PD deficiency).

It is impossible to provide an exact calculation of the prevalence of sickle-cell and G-6-PD deficiency gene among antebellum southern blacks. An estimate might be ventured, however, on the basis of known gene frequencies among present-day Afro-Americans and those Africans residing in former slave-trading areas. One leading medical authority on abnormal hemoglobins has estimated that at least 22 percent of the Africans first brought to this country possessed genes for sickling. Other medical scientists have determined that approximately 20 percent of West Africans have genes for G-6-PD deficiency. Overall, then, a conservative estimate would be that approximately 30 to 40 percent of newly arrived slaves had one or both of these genes. Recent evidence points to a higher-than-expected frequency of the G-6-PD gene in patients having sickle-cell disease, which might reduce this estimate by a few percentage points. Thus, a large proportion of blacks were immune to the severe effects of falciparum malaria and to the less virulent vivax malaria, facts which planters and physicians in the South could not help but notice and discuss openly.

As with malaria, planters and physicians speculated publicly on blacks' intolerance of cold climates but could never adequately prove their contentions. It was the confirmed opinion of many white southerners that blacks could not withstand cold weather to the same degree as whites because of their dark skin and equatorial origins. Their major concern was that blacks seemed to resist and tolerate respiratory infections less well than whites. Since the germ theory of disease was years in the future, these men and others explained their observations with a combination of then-current though not universally accepted medical, anthropological, and scientific logic—and occasionally with unfounded theories. Blacks, natives of a tropical climate, were physiologically ill-suited for the cold winter weather and cool spring and fall nights of the temperate zone. They breathed less air, dissipated a greater amount of "animal heat" through the skin, and eliminated larger quantities of carbon via liver and skin than whites. In addition, the exposure of blacks to the elements for much of the year placed a strain on heat production within the body. One medical extremist, Samuel A. Cartwright of New Orleans, even claimed that inefficient functioning of Negroes' lungs caused "defective atmospherization of the blood." Some noted that slaves often slept with their heads (rather than their feet) next to the fire and entirely covered by a blanket; this was seen as proof that they required warm, moist air to breathe and to survive in this climate. Blacks were, these men concluded, physiologically different from whites.

Even today there is some confusion among medical authorities regarding the susceptibility of blacks to severe pulmonary infections. Some claim a racial or genetic predisposition, while others deny it. Historically, blacks have shown a higher incidence and more severe manifestations of respiratory illness than have whites. Explanations for this phenomenon are numerous. First, Negroes did not experience bacterial pneumonias until the coming of the Caucasian. The entire newly exposed population was thus exquisitely sensitive to these infections and developed much more serious cases than whites, who had had frequent contact with the bacteria since childhood. Second, black African laborers who today move from moist tropical to temperate climates (e.g., to the gold mines of South Africa) contract pneumonia at a much higher rate than whites. Though the incidence of disease decreases with time, it always remains at a more elevated level than among Caucasians. The same phenomenon probably operated during slavery. At first the mortality rate from pneumonia among newly arrived slaves was probably inordinately high, but with time the figure decreased somewhat, though it remains higher than in Caucasians. Third, there appears to be a close relationship between resistance to pulmonary infection and exposure to cool, wet weather. Slaves, who worked outdoors in all seasons and often lived in drafty, damp cabins, were therefore more likely to suffer from respiratory diseases than their masters. Fourth, poor diet, a common slave problem, predisposes people to infections such as pneumonia and other respiratory problems.[5] Finally, overcrowding and unsanitary living conditions increased the incidence of respiratory diseases. Slaves living in small cottages or grouped together in a large community at the quarters, where intimate and frequent visiting was common, stood a greater chance of contracting airborne infections than did the more isolated whites. Undoubtedly, all these factors combined to increase the occurrence of respiratory illness among southern blacks.

The most serious nonfatal manifestation of cold intolerance was frostbite. At least one proslavery apologist claimed that the Negro race was more susceptible than whites to this condition: "Almost every one has seen negroes in Northern cities, who have lost their legs by frost at sea—a thing rarely witnessed among whites, and yet where a single negro has been thus exposed doubtless a thousand of the former have."[6] The condition was a serious one, especially for slaveowners who stood to lose the labor of valuable workers.

Blacks are in fact more susceptible to cold injury than whites. Studies conducted during and after the Korean War indicate that the adaptive response of blacks to cold exposure is poorer than that of whites in the following ways: blacks' metabolic rates increase more slowly and not as much as those of whites; their first shivers (one of the body's defensive responses to cold) occur at a lower skin temperature than for whites; and their incidence of frostbite is higher and their cases more severe than those of whites. Even after blacks have acclimated to cold (and they do so in a manner physiologically similar to whites), they are then only slightly less liable to sustain cold injury than they had been previously. Those antebellum observers who warned against overexposure of slaves to cold were essentially correct.

Racial differences in tolerance to heat also exist but may be modified under certain conditions. Again, antebellum observers agreed that blacks, having originated in an area known for its heat and humidity,

5. Kiple and King, *Another Dimension*, emphasize dietary considerations in their explanations of many slave health problems.
6. John H. Van Evrie, *Negroes and Negro "Slavery"* (New York, 1861), 25.

were ideally suited for labor in the damp, warm South. One northern physician, John H. Van Evrie, explained blacks' resistance to heat in both religious and physiological terms:

> God has adapted him, both in his physical and mental structure, to the tropics. . . . His head is protected from the rays of a vertical sun by a dense mat of wooly hair, wholly impervious to its fiercest heats, while his entire surface, studded with innumerable sebaceous glands, forming a complete excretory system, relieves him from all those climatic influences so fatal, under the same circumstances, to the sensitive and highly organized white man. Instead of seeking to shelter himself from the burning sun of the tropics, he courts it, enjoys it, delights in its fiercest heats.[7]

Modern medical investigators would not agree with Van Evrie's reasoning. But they have discovered that under normal living conditions, Negroes in Africa and the United States are better equipped to tolerate humid heat than Caucasians. However, both races possess the same capacity to acclimatize to hot, humid conditions. The physiological mechanisms by which the human body acclimatizes to heat can be readily observed and measured. Increased external temperature causes the body to perspire more, resulting in a greater evaporative heat loss, a decline in skin and rectal temperatures, and a drop in the heart rate from its initially more rapid pace. When whites and blacks are equally active in the same environment over a period of time, there is little difference in heat tolerance.

From this information it can be assumed that in the Old South slaves and free blacks possessed a higher *natural* tolerance to humid heat stress than did whites. In addition, blacks became quickly acclimatized to performance of their particular tasks under the prevailing climatic conditions of the region. This natural and acquired acclimatization enabled black laborers to withstand the damp heat of summer better than whites, who were unused to physical exertion under such severe conditions. White farm and general laborers, however, also must have adjusted to the heat and fared as well as blacks. One physiological difference between Caucasians and Negroes that might have affected work performance in the hot, humid South was the latter's inherent ability to discharge smaller amounts of sodium chloride and other vital body salts (electrolytes) into sweat and urine. Excessive loss of those salts leads to heat prostration and heatstroke. Thus conservation of needed electrolytes gave slaves an advantage over laboring whites, whose requirements for replacement of the substances were greater. In

7. Van Evrie, *Negroes and Negro "Slavery,"* 251, 256.

the case of heat tolerance, then, white observers were correct in noting a racial difference, but they tended to ignore the fact that many whites did become acclimatized to the hot, humid environment.

Whites detected, or thought they detected, distinctive variances in black susceptibility to several other medical conditions common in the antebellum South. Many believed that slave women developed prolapsed uteri at a higher rate than white women, though modern anatomists have shown that Negroes are actually less prone to this affliction than Caucasians. Observers also noted that slaves were frequent sufferers of typhoid fever, worms, and dysentery, though we now know that the reason for this high prevalence was environmental rather than racial or genetic. Blacks did, however, have a greater resistance to the yellow fever virus than whites.[8]

One disease that drew great attention because of its frequency and virulence was consumption (pulmonary tuberculosis), a leading cause of death in nineteenth-century America for members of both races. A particular form of the disease—characterized by extreme difficulty in breathing, unexplained abdominal pain around the navel, and rapidly progressing debility and emaciation, usually resulting in death—struck blacks so commonly that it came to be known as Negro consumption or *Struma Africana*. In all likelihood most of the cases that white southerners described as Negro consumption were miliary tuberculosis, the most serious and fatal form of the disease known, in which tubercles occur in many body organs simultaneously and overwhelm what natural defenses exist. The reason that rapidly fatal varieties of the disease (so-called galloping consumption) afflicted Negroes more frequently than Caucasians may be related to the fact that Caucasians (like Mongolians) had suffered from tuberculosis for many hundreds of years and had developed a strong immune response to the infection, whereas Africans (and American Indians and Eskimos) had been exposed to tuberculosis only since the coming of the white man and had not yet built up this same effective resistance. Others have discounted racial immunity as an explanation and have argued that, as a "virgin" population, blacks were highly susceptible to serious first attacks of tuberculosis. Additional factors such as malnourishment, preexisting illness, or general debility also contributed to the apparent black predisposition to tuberculosis.

8. For examples of the political use some white southerners made of the relative immunity of blacks to yellow fever and of blacks' ability to labor in humid heat, see Jo Ann Carrigan, "Yellow Fever: Scourge of the South," in Todd L. Savitt and James Harvey Young (eds.), *Southern Disease and Southern Distinctiveness* (Knoxville, Tenn., 1988).

Neonatal tetanus (also called *trismus nascentium*) was a common cause of death among newborn slaves throughout the South. Slave-owners and physicians, few of whom recognized that it was caused by the improper handling of the umbilical stump, often discussed it in their writings. It still kills large numbers of children in undeveloped countries. *Clostridium tetani*, the same bacterium that causes tetanus in older children and adults, infects newborns through unwashed and frequently touched umbilical stumps. In a typical antebellum case, related by Dr. Albert Snead of Richmond to his colleagues at a medical society meeting in 1853, an eight-day-old black child first refused her mother's breast and gave a few convulsive hand jerks. Soon the baby's entire muscular system was rigid, with her head bent back, fists and jaws clenched, and feet tightly flexed, as the bacterial toxin affected her central nervous system tissue. In this case death from suffocation owing to respiratory muscle paralysis did not intervene until the eighteenth day (though it usually occurred within seven to ten days).

One cause of death not considered a disease that seemed to occur almost exclusively among the slave population was "smothering," "overlaying," or "suffocation." Observers assumed that sleeping mothers simply rolled onto or pressed snugly against their infants, cutting off the air supply, or that angry, fearful parents intentionally destroyed their offspring rather than have them raised in slavery. Modern medical evidence strongly indicates that most of these deaths may be ascribed to a condition presently known as Sudden Infant Death Syndrome (SIDS) or "crib death," which, for reasons yet unexplained, affects blacks more frequently than whites.[9]

The diseases and conditions discussed above represent only some of the several that whites noted affected blacks and whites differently. Others are difficult to trace back to slavery times either through direct records or by implication through comparative West African medicine. Among those not mentioned, the most important is hypertension (high blood pressure). Others include polydactyly (six or more fingers per hand); umbilical hernia; cancers of the cervix, stomach, lungs, esophagus, and prostate; and toxemia of pregnancy. At the same time, Negroes are much less susceptible to hookworm disease, cystic fibrosis, and skin cancer than Caucasians.

Though blacks are not the only racial or ethnic group possessing increased immunity and susceptibility to specific diseases, they were

9. Recent historical discussions of SIDS include Kiple and King, *Another Dimension*, 107–10; and Michael P. Johnson, "Smothered Slave Infants: Were Slave Mothers at Fault?" *Journal of Southern History*, XLVII (1981), 493–520.

the only group whose medical differences mattered to white residents of the Old South. Reports of black medical "peculiarities" appeared regularly in periodicals and pamphlets, presumably to alert southern physicians to problems they might encounter in practice. Agricultural and medical journal articles and medical student dissertations also discussed racial differences in responses to medical treatments. Most writers agreed that blacks withstood the heroic, depletive therapies of the day (bleeding, purging, vomiting, blistering) less well than whites.

Despite many writings on the subject of black diseases and treatments, no comprehensive discussion existed in any standard textbook for student doctors or practitioners. Some articles on the subject of treatment provided vague information, such as "the Caucasian seems to yield more readily to remedies . . . than the African," or "it is much more difficult to form a just diagnosis or prognosis with the latter [African] than the former [white], consequently the treatment is often more dubious."[10] In 1855 an editor of the *Virginia Medical and Surgical Journal* suggested that a Virginian write a book on "the modifications of disease in the Negro constitution." The subject, he proclaimed, stood "invitingly open"; no medical student "fresh from Watson or Wood [textbooks of the day], with his new lancet and his armory of anti-phlogistics" had been properly trained to treat many of the diseases to which the black man was subject: "Has he been taught that the African constitution sinks before the heavy blows of the 'heroic school' and runs down under the action of purgatives; that when the books say blood letting and calomel, the black man needs nourishment and opium?"[11] Other southern medical writers put forth similar pleas for medical school courses and books on black medicine. Northern textbook authors and professors at northern medical schools, they asserted, could not and did not accurately or adequately discuss diseases afflicting blacks in the South.[12]

John Stainbach Wilson, a physician in Columbus, Georgia, who had spent years practicing medicine in southern Alabama, came closest to

10. E. M. Pendleton, "On the Susceptibility of the Caucasian and African Races to the Different Classes of Disease," *Southern Medical Reports*, I (1849), 336–37.

11. Editorial, "The Medical Society of Virginia," *Virginia Medical and Surgical Journal*, IV (1855), 256–58.

12. On the matter of southern medical nationalism, see James O. Breeden, "States-Rights Medicine in the Old South," *Bulletin of the New York Academy of Medicine*, LII (1976), 348–72; John Duffy, "Medical Practice in the Antebellum South," *Journal of Southern History*, XXV (1959), 53–72; and John Harley Warner, "A Southern Medical Reform: The Meaning of the Antebellum Argument for Southern Medical Education," *Bulletin of the History of Medicine*, LVII (1983), 364–81.

actually producing a textbook on black health. Its advertised title indicated the wide scope of the proposed contents: *The Plantation and Family Physician; A Work for Families Generally and for Southern Slaveowners Especially; Embracing the Peculiarities and Diseases, the Medical and Hygienic Management of Negroes, Together with the Causes, Symptoms, and Treatment of the Principal Diseases to Whites and Blacks.* But apparently the outbreak of hostilities in 1861 interrupted Wilson's plans. It was not until more than one hundred years later, in 1975, that a book entitled *Textbook of Black-Related Diseases* was finally published, written this time by black physicians.

For southern whites, black medical problems and health care had political as well as medical ramifications. Men like Cartwright, Nott, and Wilson, advocates of what historians have labeled "states-rights medicine," were writing for a sectional audience who wished to hear that blacks were distinct from whites. This was, after all, a part of the proslavery argument. Medical theory and practice were still in such a state of flux in the late eighteenth and early nineteenth centuries that there was little risk of any true scientific challenge to a medical system based on racial differences. Observers were correct in noting that blacks showed different susceptibilities and immunities to a few specific diseases and conditions. They capitalized on these conditions to illustrate the inferiority of blacks to whites, to rationalize the use of the "less fit" racial group as slaves, to justify subjecting Negro slaves to harsh working conditions in extreme dampness and heat in the malarious regions of the South, and to prove to their critics that they recognized the special medical weaknesses of blacks and took these failings into account when providing for their human chattel. But in terms of an overall theory of medical care predicated on racial inferiority, the issue was a false one. It is instructive to note here, for example, that no writer ventured beyond vague and cautious statements about bleeding or purging blacks less than whites. None presented an account of the amount of blood loss or the dose of medicine that was optimal for blacks. Remarks on the subject were always couched in terms that placed whites in a position of medical and physical superiority over blacks, perfect for southern sectional polemics and useless to the practitioner.

The state of slave health depended not only on disease immunities and susceptibilities, but also on living and working conditions. And in those matters, the South stood out from the rest of the nation. Nowhere else did one group exert such great control over most aspects of their workers' lives as did slaveowners and overseers over the daily

338

routines of their black slaves. How whites in the slave South provided for sanitation, housing, food, clothing, and children's and women's special needs, and how they worked and disciplined their human chattel, necessarily affected the health of their black work force.[13]

Most slaves lived on plantations or farms in a well-defined area known as the "quarters." Here was an ideal setting for the spread of disease, similar to the situation in antebellum villages and urban areas. What might have been considered a personal illness in the isolated, white, rural family dwelling became in a three- or ten- or thirty-home slave community a matter of public health and group concern.

At the slave quarters sneezing, coughing, or contact with improperly washed eating utensils and personal belongings promoted transmission of disease-causing microorganisms among family members. Poor ventilation, lack of sufficient windows for sunshine, and damp earthen floors merely added to the problem by aiding the growth of fungus and bacteria on food, clothing, floors, and utensils, as well as the development of worm and insect larvae. Improper personal hygiene (infrequent baths, hairbrushings, and haircuts; unwashed clothes; unclean beds) led to such nuisances as bedbugs, body lice (which also carried typhus germs), ringworm of skin and scalp, and pinworms. In a household cramped for space, these diseases became family, not individual, problems. And when two or more families shared homes and facilities, the problem of contagion was further aggravated.

Contacts outside the home also facilitated the dissemination of disease. Children who played together all day under the supervision of a few older women and then returned to their cabins in the evening spread their day's accumulation of germs to other family members. Even mere Sunday and evening socializing in an ill neighbor's cabin was enough to "seed" the unsuspecting with disease. Contaminated water, unwashed or poorly cooked food, soil infested with worm larvae, and disease-carrying farm animals and rodents also contributed their share to the unhealthfulness of the quarters.

The two major types of seasonal diseases—respiratory and intestinal—that afflicted southern blacks reflected living conditions within most slave communities. Respiratory illnesses prevailed during the cold months, when slaves were forced to spend much time indoors in

13. For examples of typical planters' writings on the management of slaves, see James O. Breeden (ed.), *Advice Among Masters: The Ideal of Slave Management in the Old South* (Westport, Conn., 1980).

intimate contact with their families and friends. Several important contagious diseases were spread through contact with respiratory system secretions: tuberculosis, diphtheria, colds and upper respiratory infections, influenza, pneumonia, and streptococcal infections (including sore throats and scarlet fever). The community life of the slave quarters also provided excellent surroundings for dissemination of several year-round diseases contracted through respiratory secretions. People today tend to regard these illnesses—whooping cough, measles, chicken pox, and mumps—as limited to the younger population, but adult slaves who had never experienced an outbreak of, say, measles in Africa or the United States were quite susceptible to infection and even death. Measles and whooping cough are still important causes of fatality in developing countries, as they were in the antebellum South.

As warm weather arrived and workers spent more time outdoors, intestinal diseases caused by poor outdoor sanitation and close contact with the earth became common. Respiratory diseases decreased in frequency and insects became important culprits in the spread of disease, particularly maladies of the digestive tract and various "fevers." What more could a mosquito or housefly wish than a large concentration of human beings, decaying leftover food scraps, scattered human feces, or a compost heap? Mosquitoes discharged yellow fever or malarial parasites while they drew fresh blood from their victims. Flies transported bacteria such as *Vibrio* (cholera), *Salmonella* (food poisoning and typhoid), and *Shigella* (bacillary dysentery); the virus that causes infectious hepatitis; and the protozoan *Entameba histolytica* (ameobic dysentery) from feces to food. Trichina worms, embedded in the muscles of hogs inhabiting yards often shared with bondsmen, were released into a slave's body when the meat was not completely cooked. Finally, there were the large parasitic worms, a concomitant of primitive sanitation.

Intestinal disorders were at least as common among antebellum Virginia's blacks as were respiratory diseases. The human alimentary tract is distinguished among all other body systems in that it receives daily large amounts of foreign material, usually in the form of food, which it must sort and assimilate into a usable form. In the Old South, where living conditions were generally unhygienic, seemingly good food and drink often concealed pathogenic organisms ranging from viruses to worm larvae. Hands entering mouths sometimes contained the germs that others had cast off in feces, urine, or contaminated food. It is not surprising to find that dysentery, typhoid fever, food poisoning, and worm diseases afflicted many southerners, especially those living in the poorest, most crowded circumstances, without sanitary facilities or time to prepare food properly. Slaves often fit into this category.

Though their major medical problems were communicable diseases, blacks, in the course of a day, also faced health challenges unrelated to contagion or parasites. Inadequate clothing and food, poor working conditions, harsh physical punishment, pregnancy, and certain bodily disorders also made slaves sick or uncomfortable, at times rendering them useless to their masters and burdensome to friends and family.

Though adequate clothing was important for slaves, it did not play as crucial a role in the maintenance of health as did housing. Of course clothing covered and protected the body from exposure to wind, sun, rain, snow, cold, and insects. It also limited the severity of many minor falls to cuts, scrapes, and bruises, and of some accidents to smaller areas of the body. But only a few disorders are spread by contact with infected clothing (smallpox, body lice, impetigo, typhus) or by contact of exposed skin with other objects (tetanus, yaws, hookworm, brucellosis).

Except in cases where slaves were truly underclothed in winter and therefore possibly had less resistance to respiratory ailments, the danger of contracting disease through inadequate or dirty wearing apparel was relatively small. Of the articles of clothing that masters provided their bondsmen, shoes were probably the most important in terms of health and disease. Not only did they provide warmth in the winter to feet and toes highly susceptible to frostbite, but they also protected slaves against hookworm penetration, scrapes, scratches, burns, and some puncture wounds that would otherwise have caused tetanus.

Did slaves receive a diet adequate to keep them healthy, laboring, and producing vigorous offspring? Opinions vary on this question, for diets differed from individual to individual, and our understanding of nutritional needs has changed often. Based on current dietary standards, the typical daily ration, one quart of whole ground, dry, bolted cornmeal, prepared from white corn (the South's favorite) and half a pound of cured, medium-fat ham with no bone or skin, could not have provided enough essential nutrients to sustain a moderately active, twenty-two-year-old male or female, much less a hard-working laborer or a pregnant or lactating woman. Field hands fed this diet alone (with water) would soon have become emaciated and sickly and would have shown symptoms of several nutrient deficiencies. It is highly unlikely that any slave could have survived very long on a diet consisting solely of pork and cornmeal.

Most masters provided supplements to the basic hogmeat and corn-meal, a practice most urgently recommended by agricultural writers throughout the South. Vegetables topped the list of required additional foods. Planters could, if they planned ahead, have a ready supply of at least one or two varieties throughout the year. These writers also suggested adding, when available, fish, fresh meat, molasses, milk, and buttermilk to slave diets.

Many agricultural authors and slavemasters indicated in their writings that blacks often raised vegetables, poultry, and even pigs on their own plots of land near the quarters. The assumption was that extra food from this source would supplement rations supplied by the master. Surprisingly, however, some of these same writers also pointed out that slaves usually sold what they raised to the master or at the marketplace, thereby defeating the major purpose of the plan. In all likelihood the slaves did not dispose of all their produce, but saved some for future needs. The fact that there were bondsmen who sold rather than kept food indicates that, other than those saving every available penny to purchase their freedom, some slaves received sufficient nutrition from their regular rations, supplemented by homegrown food, to feel quite comfortable relying on their masters for proper nutrition.

Kenneth F. Kiple and Virginia H. King, in their book *Another Dimension to the Black Diaspora*, assess the adequacy of a slave diet consisting primarily of pork and cornmeal supplemented occasionally with other foods.[14] Using recently discovered knowledge of human nutritional needs and nutrient actions and interactions in the body, they conclude that slaves received sufficient amounts of carbohydrates and calories but generally lacked some essential amino acids, vitamin C, riboflavin, niacin, thiamine, vitamin D, calcium, and iron. And slave children, who all too often began life with nutritional deficiencies owing to their mothers' poor pre- and postnatal diets, also lacked sufficient magnesium, calories, and protein in their diets. Not surprisingly, Kiple and King assert, slave adults and children suffered higher morbidity and mortality than whites because of lower resistance to infection and disrupted basic metabolic pathways. Among the most common resul-

14. Kiple and King, *Another Dimension*. See also Robert A. Margo and Richard H. Steckel, "The Heights of American Slaves: New Evidence on Slave Nutrition and Health," *Social Science History*, VI (1982), 516–38; Steckel, "A Peculiar Population: The Nutrition, Health, and Mortality of American Slaves from Childhood to Maturity," *Journal of Economic History*, XLVI (1986), 721–41.

tant black health problems were respiratory and intestinal diseases, skin and eye afflictions, "teething," tetanus, "fits and seizures," and rickets. Diet, controlled to a large degree by the master, greatly affected slave health.

In addition to providing food, clothing, and housing, slaveowners also directed working conditions, punishments, and care of women and children. Though warm weather helped the crops grow, it did not always have the same effect on the black laborers who tended them. Planters recording the effects of excessive heat on their field hands made it clear that even though blacks originated in tropical Africa, they were not immune to sunstroke. For instance, Hill Carter of Shirley Plantation wrote during the 1825 wheat harvest, "Hotest day ever felt—men gave out & some fainted."[15]

Slaveowners also recognized the potential hazards of overexertion and exposure. Some indulged their slaves by easing their tasks; others found this impossible, especially at certain times of the year. Hill Carter and no doubt many others worked their blacks in intense heat when it was necessary to harvest a crop. Charles Friend of Prince George County, Virginia, on the other hand, had second thoughts when the ditching operation to which he had assigned many slaves evolved into a messy and unhealthy job: "We have the ditchers knee deep in water and mud. If I had known how bad it was I should not have put them to work at it but hired labor to do it."[16]

Farm accidents also took their toll on slaves. Falls, overturned carts, runaway wagons, drownings, limbs caught in farm machines, kicks from animals, and cuts from axes or scythe blades were the commonest types. Occasionally slaves suffered more remarkable mishaps, as when a 260-pound Culpeper County field hand jumped eight feet from a hay loft onto a pile of hay in which a wooden pitchfork lay concealed. The point punctured the man's scrotum and passed into his abdominal cavity, but miraculously pierced no internal organs. Thanks to prompt surgical attention he was doing "light work" around the plantation about three weeks later.

The whip was an integral part of slave life in the Old South. Those bondsmen who had not experienced its sting firsthand were acquainted with persons, usually friends or relatives, who had. Whites held out the threat of whipping as a means of maintaining order. When

15. Shirley on the James Farm Journals, June 23, 1825, Library of Congress.
16. Quoted in Wyndham B. Blanton, *Medicine in Virginia in the Eighteenth Century* (Richmond, 1931), 161 (Blanton cites no source).

strong discipline was called for, so, very often, was the lash. Even the mildest and most God-fearing of masters permitted application of this painful instrument in extreme cases, though some insisted that the slave's skin not be cut or that a responsible witness be present when punishment was administered.

From a medical point of view, whipping inflicted cruel and often permanent injuries upon its victims. Laying stripes across the bare back or buttocks caused indescribable pain, especially when each stroke dug deeper into previously opened wounds. During the interval between lashes, victims anticipated the next in anguish, wishing for postponement or for all due speed, though neither alternative brought relief. In addition to multiple lacerations of the skin, whipping caused loss of blood, injury to muscles (and internal organs, if the lash reached that deep), and shock. (Rubbing salt into these wounds, often complained of as a further mode of torture, actually cleansed the injured, exposed tissues and helped ward off infection.) The paddle jarred every part of the body by the violence of the blow, and raised blisters from repeated strokes. In addition to the possibility of death (uncommon), there was the danger that muscle damage inflicted by these instruments might permanently incapacitate a slave or deform him for life. An Old Dominion slave who experienced the sting of the paddle recalled years later: "You be jes' as raw as a piece of beef an' hit eats you up. He loose you an' you go to house no work done dat day."[17] No work done that day or, in many cases, for several days. Ellick, a rebellious member of Charles Friend's White Hill Plantation slave force, was slapped one day "for not being at the stable in time this morning," and "soundly whipped" the next day for running away and for not submitting to a flogging earlier that morning. He spent the next week recovering in bed, only to receive another whipping upon his return to work. This time he ran off for two days before settling back into the plantation routine.

The daily routines of slave women and children were often upset by health conditions peculiar to these groups.[18] Female slaves probably

17. Interview of William Lee, n.d., in WPA Folklore File, Manuscript Room, Alderman Library, University of Virginia, Charlottesville.

18. On slave women's and children's health conditions, see also Kiple and King, *Another Dimension*; Richard H. Steckel, "A Dreadful Childhood: The Excess Mortality of American Slaves," *Social Science History,* X (1986), 427–65; J. Campbell, "Work, Pregnancy, and Infant Mortality Among Southern Slaves," *Journal of Interdisciplinary History,* XIV (1984), 793–812; Deborah Gray White, *Ar'n't I a Woman?: Female Slaves in the Plantation South* (New York, 1985), 79–87, 124–26.

lost more time from work for menstrual pain, discomfort, and disorders than for any other cause. Planters rarely named illnesses in their diaries or daybooks, but the frequency and regularity with which women of childbearing age appeared on sick lists indicates that menstrual conditions were a leading complaint. A Fauquier County, Virginia, physician considered the loss of four to eight workdays per month not unusual for slave women. Among the menstrual maladies that afflicted bondswomen most often were amenorrhea (lack of menstrual flow), abnormal bleeding between cycles (sometimes caused by benign and malignant tumors), and abnormal discharges (resulting from such conditions as gonorrhea, tumors, and prolapsed uterus).

Some servants took advantage of their masters by complaining falsely of female indispositions. One unnamed Virginian who owned numerous slaves complained to Frederick Law Olmsted about such malingering women:

> The women on a plantation will hardly earn their salt, after they come to the breeding age; they don't come to the field, and you go to the quarters and ask the old nurse what's the matter, and she says, "oh she's not well, master; she's not fit to work, sir"; and what can you do? You have to take her word for it that something or other is the matter with her, and you dare not set her to work; and so she lays up till she feels like taking the air again, and plays the lady at your expense. [19]

Masters found it difficult to separate the sick from the falsely ill; as a result, they often indulged their breeding-aged women rather than risk unknown complications. Thomas Jefferson, for instance, ordered his overseer not to coerce the female workers into exerting themselves because "women are destroyed by exposure to wet at certain periodical indispositions to which nature has subjected them." [20]

If whites treated women's gynecological complaints with a certain delicacy, they regarded pregnancy as almost holy. In addition to receiving time off from work and avoiding whippings, expectant women in Virginia were protected from execution in capital offenses until after parturition. [21] At least three cases arose between the Revolution and the Civil War in which slave women obtained execution postpone-

---

19. Frederick Law Olmsted, *A Journey in the Seaboard Slave States, with Remarks on Their Economy* (New York, 1856), 190.

20. Thomas Jefferson to Joel Yancey, January 17, 1819, in Edwin M. Betts (ed.), *Thomas Jefferson's Farm Book* (Princeton, 1953), 43.

21. There were, of course, exceptions to these statements. See, for example, Johnson, "Smothered Slave Infants," 511–20.

ments for this reason, though all were presumably put to death following delivery.

Children, like women, were exposed to certain unique disorders that caused illness or death. Though their labor did not usually account for much, young slaves' serious illnesses did mean lost time from work for mothers watching over them at home or distractedly worrying about them while performing daily tasks. Slave children suffered more frequently than their white counterparts from most illnesses, especially diarrhea, neonatal tetanus, convulsions, "teething" (not really a disease, but considered a cause of sickness and death prior to the twentieth century), diphtheria, respiratory diseases, and whooping cough, owing to poorer living conditions and diet. And their mortality rate far exceeded that of whites, especially in infancy.[22]

Worms occurred frequently in black children. The poor sanitary conditions at many slave quarters were conducive to the development of these parasites in the soil. Children playing in the dirt inevitably picked up worm larvae as they put fingers in mouths. Failure to use, or lack of, privy facilities only served to spread worm diseases to other residents of the quarters and to visiting slaves, who then carried these parasites to their own plantation quarters.

Some black children had overt sickle-cell disease with irregular hemolytic crises, severe joint pains, chronic leg ulcers, and abdominal pains. The medical records relating to antebellum Virginia do not provide any clear descriptions of the disease, probably because its symptoms resemble so many other conditions and because the sickness was not known until 1910. These children were often the "sickly" ones, useless for fieldwork or heavy household duties, expensive to maintain because of frequent infections, and, if female, often unable to bear children if they survived puberty. Their lot was a poor and painful one.

Slave children also developed diseases that no one could identify or treat. John Walker's young servants appeared one day with "head ach sweled faces & belly diseases"; Colonel John Ambler's evidenced swollen feet and faces, and bones cutting through the skin; and Landon Carter's had "swelling of the almonds of . . . [their] ears which burst inward and choaked . . . [them]." The white tutor at Nomini Hall, Philip Vickers Fithian, noticed that one slave mother on this estate in Westmoreland County, Virginia, had lost seven children successively, none of whom had even reached the age of ten: "The

22. Steckel, "A Dreadful Childhood," 427–29.

Negroes all seem much alarm'd."[23] Childhood was generally the least healthy period of a slave's life.

In many ways, then, the state of southern blacks' health depended on the kind of living and working conditions whites provided. These conditions varied widely from place to place and individual to individual, and became a subject of much comment in both northern and southern publications.

Bondage placed slaves in a different position with regard to health care. When taken ill they had a limited range of choices. Masters wished their slaves, legally an article of property, immediately to inform the person in charge about any sickness so the malady might be arrested before it worsened. But some blacks, as people, felt reluctant to submit to the often harsh prescriptions and remedies of eighteenth- and nineteenth-century white medical practice. They preferred self-treatment or reliance on cures recommended by friends and older relatives. They depended on Negro herb and root doctors or on influential conjurers among the local black population. This desire to treat oneself, or at least to have the freedom to choose one's mode of care, directly conflicted with the demands and wishes of white masters, whose trust in black medicine was usually slight and whose main concern was keeping the slave force intact.

To further compound the problem, unannounced illnesses did not entitle slaves to time off from work. To treat their own illnesses, slaves had to conceal them or pass them off to the master as less serious than they actually were. Masters who complained that blacks tended to report sickness only after the disease had progressed to a serious stage often discovered that slaves had treated illnesses at home first. The blacks' dilemma, then, was whether to delay reporting illnesses and treat those diseases at home, risking white reprisal, or to submit at once to the medicines of white America and, in a sense, surrender their bodies to their masters. The result was a dual system in which some slaves received treatment both from whites and blacks.

When illness afflicted a slave, whites responded in several ways. They almost always applied treatments derived from European experience. Most often the master, mistress, or overseer first attempted to

23. John Walker Diary, April 23, 1853, Southern Historical Collection, University of North Carolina at Chapel Hill; Jack P. Greene (ed.), *The Diary of Colonel Landon Carter of Sabine Hall, 1752–1778* (2 vols.; Charlottesville, 1965), I, 377 (March 31, 1770); Hunter Dickinson Farish (ed.), *Journal and Letters of Philip Vickers Fithian, 1773–1774: A Plantation Tutor of the Old Dominion* (Williamsburg, 1957), 182.

treat the ailment with home remedies. If the patient failed to respond to these home ministrations, the family physician was summoned. Some slaveowners distrusted "regular" doctors and called instead "irregular" practitioners: Thomsonians, homeopaths, empirics, and eclectics, for example. Masters who hired out their bondsmen to others for a period of time arranged for medical care when signing the hiring bond. Whatever the situation, white southerners often displayed concern for the health of blacks in bondage. The reasons were threefold: slaves represented a financial investment that required protection; many masters felt a true humanitarian commitment toward their slaves; and whites realized that certain illnesses could easily spread to their own families if not properly treated and contained.

Those responsible for the care of sick slaves made home treatment the first step in the restorative process. They knew that physicians, though they possessed great knowledge of the human body and the effects of certain medicines on it, were severely limited in the amount of good they could do. Because no one understood the etiology of most diseases, no one could effectively cure them. Astute nonmedical observers could make diagnoses as well as doctors and could even treat patients just as effectively. Physicians played their most crucial roles in executing certain surgical procedures, assisting mothers at childbirth, and instilling confidence in sick patients through an effective bedside manner. At other times, their excessive use of drugs, overready cups and leeches, and ever-present lancets produced positive harm by depleting the body of blood and nourishment and exhausting the already weakened patient with frequent purges, vomits, sweats, and diuretics. Laymen often merely followed the same course of treatment that they had observed their physicians using or that they had read about in one of the ubiquitous domestic medical guides. Anyone could practice blood-letting or dosing with a little experience. And a physician's services cost money, even when no treatment or cure resulted from the consultation.

Home care, of course, stemmed from people's natural instincts to relieve their own or their families' illnesses as quickly as possible. The unavailability of physicians, the inaccessibility of many farms to main highways, and the lack of good roads and speedy means of transportation reinforced such thinking among rural southerners. Even when a doctor was summoned, hours or even a day passed before his arrival, during which time something had to be done to ease the patient's discomfort. People learned to tolerate pain and to cope with death, but the mitigation of suffering was still a primary goal. To that end most

people stocked their cabinets with favorite remedies (or the ingredients required for their preparation) in order to be well equipped
when relief was demanded. On large plantations with many slaves this
was a necessity, as Catherine C. Hopley, tutor at Forest Rill near Tap-
pahannock, Essex County, Virginia, noted: "A capacious medicine
chest is an inseparable part of a Southern establishment; and I have
seen medicines enough dispensed to furnish good occupation for an
assistant, when colds or epidemics have prevailed."[24] Some physicians
made a living selling medicine chests and domestic health guides designed specifically for use on southern plantations. Self-sufficiency in
medical care was desirable on farms and even in urban households,
especially when financial considerations were important.

An additional feature of home medical care for slaves was the plantation hospital or infirmary. Its form varied from farm to farm, and it
existed primarily on the larger slaveholdings. It was quicker and more
efficient to place ailing slaves in one building, where care could be
tendered with a minimum amount of wasted movement and where all
medicines, special equipment, and other necessary stores could be
maintained. Of course, infectious diseases could spread quite rapidly
through a hospital and subject those with noncontagious conditions to
further sickness.

Armed with drugs from the plantation or home dispensary, one
person, usually white, had the responsibility of dosing and treating ill
slaves. The master, mistress, or overseer spent time each day with
those claiming bodily disorders and soon developed a certain facility in
handling both patients and drugs.[25] The approach was empirical—if a
particular medication or combination of drugs succeeded in arresting
symptoms, it became the standard treatment for that malady in that
household until a better one came along. Overseers and owners in-
scribed useful medical recipes into their diaries or journals and clipped
suggestions from newspapers, almanacs, and books.

An overseer's or owner's incompetence or negligence was the
slave's loss. New and inexperienced farm managers, unskilled in the
treatment of illness, necessarily used blacks as guinea pigs for their
"on-the-job" training. As a consequence of living on the wrong plantation at the wrong time, some slaves probably lost their lives or be-

24. Catherine C. Hopley, *Life in the South: From the Commencement of the War* (2 vols.;
London, 1863), I, 103.

25. On the healing roles of white women on the plantation, see Catherine Clinton,
The Plantation Mistress: Women's World in the Old South (New York, 1982), 28, 43, 187.

came invalids at the hands of new, poorly trained, or simply inhumane overseers or masters.

Despite the policy of many masters of delaying a call to the physician until late in the course of a slave's disease, there were times when owners desperately wished for the doctor's presence. More practitioners should have retained in their files the numerous hastily scrawled notes from frantic slaveowners begging for medical assistance or kept a record of each verbal summons to a sick slave at a distant farm or village household. For physicians did play important roles, both physiological and psychological, in the treatment of illness. Dr. Charles Brown of Charlottesville, Virginia, for instance, had a thriving country practice during the early nineteenth century. He handled many types of problems: James Old wanted him to determine whether his slave woman, then "in a strange way," was pregnant or not; Bezaleel Brown needed his opinion "if I must bleed her [Jane, who had pain in her side and suppression of urine] either large or small in quantity"; and Jemima Fretwell wished Brown to "cut of[f] the arm" of a four-month-old slave who had been "so very badly burnt" that "the [elbow] joint appears like it will drap of[f]."[26] Sometimes physicians made daily visits to dress slaves' wounds or to keep track of household epidemics. In emergencies some owners panicked and fretted away many hours after learning of their physician's temporary absence.

Between the household remedies and the standard treatments of the physicians stood "irregular" medicine. The impact of alternative movements on the medical care of blacks in at least one southern state, Virginia, was greater than historians have recognized. Most slaveowners there either treated with conventional medicines or called in regular doctors and rejected the new cults as quackery, but a sizable minority, difficult to estimate, became enthusiastic proponents of the system known as Thomsonianism. This movement, which had followers in areas of heavy slave concentrations (64 percent of the Tidewater counties and 66 percent of the Piedmont counties during the 1830s and 1840s), appealed to masters who were fed up with the ineffective and expensive treatments of their regular physicians. One Tidewater resident turned to Thomsonianism after experienced Norfolk physicians had unsuccessfully managed a household scarlet fever outbreak. All twenty cases, the happy slaveowner reported to the editors

26. For more examples of such notes, see Todd L. Savitt (ed.), "Patient Letters to an Early Nineteenth Century Virginia Physician," *Journal of the Florida Medical Association,* LXIX (1982), 688–94.

of a Thomsonian journal, had been cured. Another man, in Goochland County, stated that a local Thomsonian practitioner had cured his slave of a disease that one of the most respected regular physicians of the area had found intractable to the usual blister and salivation treatments. And a Prince Edward County Thomsonian doctor claimed to have cured a ten-year-old slave who had been suffering from rabies (a misdiagnosis, no doubt). With adherents to the sect so widely diffused throughout the state, the services or success stories of practitioners no doubt reached at least a portion of the slaveholding class and influenced its thinking.[27]

Beyond the master's and overseer's eyes, back in the slaves' cabins, some blacks took medical matters into their own hands. When under the surveillance of whites, slaves usually (but not always) accepted their treatments. Some even administered them in the name of the master. But others developed or retained from an ancient African heritage their own brand of care, complete with special remedies, medical practitioners, and rituals. The result was a dual system of health care, the two parts of which often conflicted with each other.

Masters did not appreciate slaves overusing the plantation infirmary, medicines, or the family doctor, but they preferred this to black self-care for several reasons. Their quarrel with slaves was the same as the physicians' with the masters: they waited too long before seeking medical assistance and often misdiagnosed illnesses. Owners permitted blacks a small amount of freedom in treating minor ailments at home, but lost their patience when sickness got out of hand. James L. Hubard, in charge of his father's lands during the latter's vacation at Alleghany Springs, Virginia, reported that Daphny had treated her own son with vermifuges (worm medicines) for several days before realizing that the boy was suffering not from worms but from dysentery. Hubard quickly altered the medication and summoned a doctor, blaming the entire affair on "the stupidity of Daphny." An enraged Landon Carter found a suckling child with measles at the slave quarters. "The mother," he wrote in his diary, "let nobody know of it until it was almost dead."[28]

Whites also accused slaves of negligence or incompetence in the care

27. The best treatment of Thomsonianism in a southern state is James O. Breeden, "Thomsonianism in Virginia," *Virginia Magazine of History and Biography,* LXXXII (1974), 150–80.

28. James L. Hubard to Robert T. Hubard, August 4, 1857, in Robert T. Hubard Papers, Manuscript Room, Alderman Library, University of Virginia, Charlottesville; Greene (ed.), *Carter Diary,* II, 812 (May 20, 1774).

of their fellow blacks. Dr. G. Lane Corbin of Warwick County, Virginia, for instance, promoted slaves' use of collodion, a syrupy dressing, because it required so little attention once applied: "This I consider of moment in regard to our slave population, whose negligence and inattention to such matters [as the proper dressing of wounds] must have attracted the notice of the most superficial observer."[29] Negroes frequently were charged with irresponsibility, ignorance, slovenliness, and indifference in the management of other blacks' illnesses. "They will never do right, left to themselves," declared one Franklin County planter.[30]

Furthermore, some whites argued, slaves did not even care for their own personal health properly. Recovery was retarded and even reversed, Dr. W. S. Morton of Cumberland County remarked, "by their [slaves'] own stupid perversity in refusing confinement to bed, and to follow other important directions when in a very dangerous condition."[31] Masters and physicians often confirmed this but were powerless to combat it. It was difficult for whites, unless they were present at all times, to force ailing blacks to take medicines or to remain constantly in bed. A most spectacular instance of death following defiance of medical orders occurred in Portsmouth when a black male patient of Dr. John W. Trugien, confined to bed with a stab wound of the heart, sustained a massive effusion of blood from that organ upon exerting himself by rising from his pallet.[32]

To offset the failures and harshness of white remedies or the negligence of masters, or perhaps to exert some control over their lives, some slaves treated their own diseases and disorders or turned to other trusted blacks for medical assistance, with or without the master's knowledge.[33] Black home remedies circulated secretly through the slave quarters and were passed down privately from generation to generation. Most of these cures were derived from local plants, though

29. G. Lane Corbin, "Collodion on Stumps of Amputated Limbs," *Stethoscope and Virginia Medical Gazette*, I (1851), 489.

30. L. G. Cabell to Bowker Preston, October 8, 1834, in John Hook Collection, Manuscript Room, Alderman Library, University of Virginia, Charlottesville.

31. W. S. Morton, "Causes of Mortality Amongst Negroes," *Monthly Stethoscope and Medical Reporter*, I (1856), 290.

32. John W. H. Trugien, "A Case of Wound of the Left Ventricle of the Heart.—Patient Survived Five Days;—with Remarks," *American Journal of the Medical Sciences*, n.s., XX (1850), 99–102.

33. See, for more information and references, Lawrence W. Levine, *Black Culture and Black Consciousness: Afro-American Folk Thought from Slavery to Freedom* (New York, 1977), 55–80.

some medicines contained ingredients that had magical value only. Occasionally whites would learn of a particularly effective medicine and adopt it, as when Dr. Richard S. Cauthorn announced in the *Monthly Stethoscope* (1857) that an old folk remedy (milk weed or silk weed, *Asclepias syriaca* in the United States Dispensatory) that had been used for years by blacks in the counties north of Richmond worked almost as well as quinine for agues and fevers.[34] Otherwise, most whites simply ignored or tolerated the black medical world until something occurred to bring their attention to it—either a great medical discovery or a slave death caused by abuse.

Because blacks practiced medicine in virtually every portion of the Old Dominion and because their methods were based partially on magic, problems occasionally arose. The main source of trouble was usually not the misuse of home remedies, but the "prescriptions" and activities of so-called conjure doctors, whose system existed in the South only because slaves brought it with them from Africa and the West Indies. These men and women used trickery, violence, persuasion, and medical proficiency to gain their reputations among local black communities. They were viewed as healers of illnesses that white doctors could not touch with their medicines and as perpetrators of sicknesses on any person they wished—all through "spells."

Superstition was a powerful force within the slave community, and a difficult one for white nonadherents to understand or overcome. For instance, the older brother of a slave patient of Dr. A. D. Galt of Williamsburg observed to the doctor that his medicines were useless because Gabriel "had been tricked" and "must have a Negro Doctor" to reverse the progress of the illness. Galt soon claimed to have cured the man, though he did admit that Gabriel suffered frequent relapses, "probably from intemperance in drink."[35] In another case, a slave woman took sick and eventually died on a plantation near Petersburg from what her fellow bondsmen believed were the effects of a conjurer. Some slaves speculated that the young man whom she had refused to marry "poisoned or tricked" her, though the overseer attributed her death to consumption.[36] Virginia Hayes Shepherd, a former slave interviewed at age 83 in 1939, described an incident to illustrate how

34. Richard S. Cauthorn, "A New Anti-Periodic and a Substitute for Quinia," *Monthly Stethoscope and Medical Reporter*, II (1857), 7–14.

35. A. D. Galt, *Practical Medicine: Illustrated by Cases of the Most Important Diseases*, ed. John M. Galt (Philadelphia, 1843), 295–96.

36. [William McKean to James Dunlap], July 17, 1810, in Roslin Plantation Records, Virginia State Library, Richmond.

superstitious her stepfather had been: "He believed he had a bunch something like boils. White doctor bathed it. After a few days it burst and live things came out of the boil and crawled on the floor. He thought he was conjured. He said an enemy of his put something on the horse's back and he rode it and got it on his buttocks and broke him out."[37]

Whites did permit blacks to fulfill certain medical functions. Some planters assigned "trusted" slaves to the task of rendering medical assistance to all ailing blacks on the farm. In most cases, these people simply dispensed white remedies and performed venesection and cupping as learned from the master. Though not complete black self-care, this activity did represent a transitional stage in which slaves had the opportunity to apply some of their own knowledge of herbs and so forth gained from elders, in addition to white remedies. These nurses, predominantly women, usually won the respect of both blacks and whites for their curative skills. "Uncle" Bacchus White, an eighty-nine-year-old former slave interviewed in Fredericksburg in 1939, attested: "Aunt Judy uster tend us when we uns were sic' and anything Aunt Judy couldn't do 'hit won't worth doin."[38] A white lady writing at about the same time provided a similarly romantic view of the black plantation nurse: "One of the house-servants, Amy Green—'Aunt Amy' we children called her—was a skilled nurse. My father kept a store of medicines, his scales, etc. So with Aunt Amy's poultices of horseradish and plattain-leaves and her various cuppings and plasters the ailments of the hundred negroes were well taken in hand."[39] Given such high testimony and devotion from plantation folk, one could hardly dispute the novelist Louise Clarke Pyrnelle's depiction of Aunt Nancy, a fictional antebellum household nurse, who claimed, while dosing several young slaves, "Ef'n hit want fur dat furmifuge [vermifuge—worm medicine], den Marster wouldn't hab all dem niggers w'at yer see hyear."[40]

To Negro women often fell another task: prenatal and obstetrical

37. Interview of Virginia Hayes Shepherd, 1939, in WPA Folklore File, University of Virginia.

38. Interview of Uncle Bacchus White, 1939, in WPA Folklore File, University of Virginia.

39. White Hill Plantation Books, I, 8, Southern Historical Collection. See also White, *Ar'n't I a Woman?*, 125.

40. Louise Clarke Pyrnelle, *Diddie, Dumps, and Tot; or Plantation Child-Life* (New York, 1882), quoted in Blanton, *Medicine in Virginia in the Eighteenth Century*, 49.

care of whites and blacks, especially in rural areas.[41] At least one slave on most large Virginia plantations learned and practiced the art of midwifery, not only at home but also throughout the neighborhood. Masters perferred to employ these skilled accoucheurs in uncomplicated cases rather than pay the relatively high fees of trained physicians. Doctors, remarked one member of the medical profession, attended at less than half of all births in the state. He estimated that nine tenths of all deliveries among the black population (another physician set it at five sixths) were conducted by midwives, most of whom were also black. He further asserted that midwives attended half the white women. Physicians often saw obstetrical cases only when problems arose. As a result of this demand for competent nonprofessional obstetrical services, Negro midwives flourished in the countryside.

Blacks did play a significant role in the health-care system of the South. They assisted whites and blacks in delivering children, letting blood, pulling teeth, administering medicines, and nursing the sick. The techniques and drugs they used were overtly derived from white medical practices. But unknown to masters, overseers, health officers, or physicians, blacks did also resort to their own treatments derived from their own heritage and experience. Occasionally the white and black medical worlds merged or openly clashed, but usually they remained silently separate.

The health and medical needs of slaves added an important dimension to the antebellum South's distinctiveness from the rest of the nation. Whites were legally required to see to the proper medical care of, by 1860, some four million enslaved people who, these same whites believed (sometimes accurately, sometimes not), differed physically and medically from themselves. Whites focused on these differences both to understand the best treatments of "black diseases" and to justify slavery to the rest of the nation and to the world. Furthermore, the living and working conditions of slaves, dictated in the main by whites and by the South's agricultural economy, directly affected the health of these blacks. Southern blacks received medical care from white masters, mistresses, overseers, and physicians of several sects, but also used various healing practices on each other, some of which found their way into common usage. In these ways, slave medical affairs contributed to the region's distinctiveness.

41. See also White, *Ar'n't I a Woman?*, 111–24. Free black women also practiced midwifery in parts of the Old South. See, for example, Suzanne Lebsock, *The Free Women of Petersburg: Status and Culture in a Southern Town, 1784–1860* (New York, 1984).

CONTRIBUTORS

James H. Cassedy received his Ph.D. in American civilization from Brown University in 1959. Since 1968 he has been historian in the History of Medicine Division of the National Library of Medicine, where he edits the annual *Bibliography of the History of Medicine*. A former president of the American Association for the History of Medicine, he is the author of *Charles V. Chapin and the Public Health Movement* (1962), *Demography in Early America* (1969), *American Medicine and Statistical Thinking, 1800–1860* (1984), and *Medicine and American Growth, 1800–1860* (1986).

Charles B. Dew received his Ph.D. in history from the Johns Hopkins University in 1964. Since 1977 he has taught at Williams College, where he is currently Class of 1956 Professor of American Studies and chairman of the Department of History. His publications include *Ironmaker to the Confederacy: Joseph R. Anderson and the Tredegar Iron Works* and a number of essays on industrial slavery. His most recent work on slavery in the American South is "The Slavery Experience," in *Interpreting Southern History: Essays on the Recent Historical Literature in Honor of S. W. Higginbotham* (1986).

Thomas G. Dyer received his Ph.D. in American history from the University of Georgia in 1975. He is presently professor of history and higher education at the University of Georgia and editor of *The Georgia Historical Quarterly*. He is the author of *Theodore Roosevelt and the Idea of Race* (1980) and *The University of Georgia: A Bicentennial History* (1985) and the editor of *"To Raise Myself a Little": The Diaries and Letters of Jennie, a Georgia Teacher, 1851–1866* (1982).

ELLIOTT J. GORN is associate professor and director of American Studies at Miami University, Oxford, Ohio. He received his Ph.D. in American Studies at Yale University in 1983. He is the author of *The Manly Art: Bare-Knuckle Prize Fighting in America* (1986), as well as articles on the history of fighting and on black folklore in the *American Quarterly* (1984), the *American Historical Review* (1985), the *Journal of American Studies* (1985), and the *Journal of American History* (1987).

E. BROOKS HOLIFIELD received his Ph.D. in church history from Yale University in 1970. He is currently the Charles Howard Candler Professor of American Church History at the Candler School of Theology, Emory University. A recipient of two research fellowships from the National Endowment for the Humanities, he is the author of *The Covenant Sealed: The Development of Puritan Sacramental Theology in Old and New England, 1570–1720* (1974), *The Gentlemen Theologians: American Theology in Southern Culture, 1795–1860* (1978), *A History of Pastoral Care in America: From Salvation to Self-Realization* (1983), *Health and Medicine in the Methodist Tradition: Journey Toward Wholeness* (1986), and *Era of Persuasion: American Thought and Culture, 1521–1680* (1989).

ELIZABETH B. KEENEY received her Ph.D. in the history of science from the University of Wisconsin-Madison (1985), where she submitted a dissertation entitled "The Botanizers: Amateur Scientists in Nineteenth-Century America." A Smithsonian Institution Fellow in 1980–1981, she is currently lecturer in the Department of the History of Science at Harvard University and Allston Burr Senior Tutor at Harvard College. She has coauthored an article on sectarian medicine in Wisconsin (1981) and *Sources in the History of American Pharmacology* (1982).

JANET S. NUMBERS received her Ph.D. in psychology from the University of Wisconsin-Madison in 1983 and subsequently spent two years as a postdoctoral fellow at the Menninger Foundation in Topeka, Kansas. She currently serves as head of the psychology division, Department of Psychiatry, Dean Medical Center, Madison, Wisconsin. In addition to several articles in psychology, she has coauthored, with Ronald L. Numbers, "The Psychological World of Ellen White" (1983) and "Millerism and Madness: A Study of 'Religious Insanity' in Nineteenth-Century America" (1985).

RONALD L. NUMBERS received his Ph.D. in history from the University of California at Berkeley in 1969. Since 1974 he has taught at the University of Wisconsin-Madison, where he is professor of the history of medicine and the history of science. A recipient of fellowships from the Macy and Guggenheim foundations, he has written or edited numerous books, including most recently, *God and Nature: Historical Essays on the Encounter between Christianity and Science* (1986, with David C. Lindberg), *Caring and Curing: Health and Medicine in the Western Religious Traditions* (1986, with Darrel W. Amundsen), *Medicine in the New World: New Spain, New France, and New England* (1987, and *The Disappointed: Millerism and Millenarianism in the Nineteenth Century* (1987, with Jonathan M. Butler). He was recently appointed the editor of *Isis*.

K. DAVID PATTERSON received his Ph.D. in history from Stanford University in 1971 and a master's degree in public health from the University of North Carolina at Chapel Hill in 1982. A specialist in African medical history, he is professor of history at the University of North Carolina at Charlotte. In addition to a number of articles, he has co-edited *History and Disease in Africa* (1978), compiled a bibliography entitled *Infectious Diseases in Twentieth Century Africa* (1979), and written *Health in Colonial Ghana: Disease, Medicine, and Socio-Economic Change, 1900–1955* (1981).

TODD L. SAVITT received his Ph.D. in history from the University of Virginia in 1975. Before joining the faculty of East Carolina University, where he holds a joint appointment in the School of Medicine and the Department of History, he was a postdoctoral fellow at Duke University (1974–1976) and a faculty member at the University of Florida (1976–1982). In addition to co-editing the *Dictionary of American Medical Biography* (1983, with Martin Kaufman and Stuart Galishoff) and *Disease and Distinctiveness in the American South* (1988, with James Harvey Young), he has written *Medicine and Slavery: The Diseases and Health Care of Blacks in Antebellum Virginia* (1978) and articles on the medical history of blacks and on blacks as health-care professionals.

WILLIAM K. SCARBOROUGH received his Ph.D. in history from the University of North Carolina in 1962. A specialist in antebellum southern and Civil War history and a former president of the Mississippi Historical Society, he is currently professor of history and department chair at the University of Southern Mississippi. In addition to numerous articles, essays, and reviews, he has written *The Overseer: Plantation Management in the Old South* (1966, rpr. 1984) and has edited *The Diary of Edmund Ruffin*, three volumes (1972–1989).

LESTER D. STEPHENS received his Ph.D. from the University of Miami in 1964. In 1963 he joined the faculty of the University of Georgia, where since 1981 he has been the chairman of the Department of History. Presently conducting research on the history of science in the American South, he is general editor of the University of Alabama Press series on the history of American science and technology. In addition to numerous articles, he has written *Probing the Past* (1974), *Historiography: A Bibliography* (1975), *Joseph LeConte: Gentle Prophet of Evolution* (1982), and *Ancient Animals and Other Wondrous Things: The Story of Francis Simmons Holmes, Paleontologist and Curator of the Charleston Museum* (1988).

SAMUEL B. THIELMAN received his M.D. from Duke University in 1980 and his Ph.D. in history from the same institution in 1986. In private medical practice in Asheville, North Carolina, he also currently serves as senior research scientist, University of Georgia, and clinical assistant professor of psychiatry and family medicine, University of North Carolina School of Medicine. He has published historical essays in the *American Journal of Psychiatry* and the *Bulletin of the History of Medicine* (1987) and is completing a book on madness and medicine in antebellum America.

JOHN HARLEY WARNER received his Ph.D. in the history of science from Harvard University in 1984, where he held a Charlotte W. Newcomb Dissertation Fellowship. Following a two-year appointment at the Wellcome Institute for the History of Medicine in London, supported in part by a NATO Postdoctoral Fellowship in Science, he joined the faculty at Yale University in 1986 as an assistant professor of the history of medicine. His many publications include "The Selective Transport of Medical Knowledge: Antebellum American Physicians and Parisian Medical Therapeutics," which won the Richard H. Shryock Medal of the American Association of the History of Medicine, and *The Therapeutic Perspective: Medical Practice, Knowledge, and Identity in America, 1820–1885* (1986).

MARGARET H. WARNER received her Ph.D. in the history of science from Harvard University in 1983 and her M.D. from Harvard Medical School in 1987. She is currently a resident in internal medicine at Brigham and Women's Hospital in Boston and lecturer in the Department of the History of Science at Harvard University. In addition to articles in the *Journal of the History of Medicine* (1981) and the *Journal of Southern History* (1984), she has written *Public Health in the New South: Government, Medicine and Society in the Control of Yellow Fever* (forthcoming).

INDEX

Abbey, Richard, 80, 84
Abbott, Simon, 283, 286–87
Academy of Natural Sciences of Phila-
delphia, 59–76 *passim*, 92
Accidents. *See* Injuries
Acclimatization: to disease, 233, 234; to
humid heat, 334
Acoustics, taught, 42, 45
Africa: diseases from, 152, 158–63; as
source of folk beliefs, 298–322 *passim*;
diseases in, 330, 332–33; heat toler-
ance in, 334; medical practices from,
351, 353. *See also* Hookworm; Malaria;
Yellow fever
Agassiz, Louis, 34, 49, 57–58, 65, 93,
136, 139
Aging, 155, 156
Agricultural chemistry. *See* Chemistry
Agricultural societies, 81, 84–85, 86, 87,
93, 96–97, 98, 100, 102
Agricultural surveys, 93, 96, 99, 105
Agriculture: deters scientific activity, 18,
20; taught, 43, 50–51, 93, 96–97, 101;
scientific, 52, 80–106; papers on, 69; in
North and South, 83, 84–86, 104; state
bureaus of, 96; technology and, 107;
spreads malaria, 160–61
Alabama: scientists in, 21; soil survey in,
96; diseases in, 164, 170–71, 196, 230–
31; asylum in, 266; mentioned, 11, 39,
81, 100, 112, 137, 138, 201, 208, 214,
215, 281, 293, 337

Alabama, University of, 53, 101
American Association for the Advance-
ment of Science, x, 12–13, 15n, 19–20,
21, 33, 33n, 58, 71, 78
American Medical Association, 172, 218,
225
American Philosophical Society, 55, 88
Anatomy, 45, 183, 215, 217, 220
Animal husbandry, 79, 102
Anticontagionism, 172, 173, 228–29,
238–55
Appalachians, as disease subregion, 163
Arthritis, 156
Association of Medical Superintendents
of American Institutions for the In-
sane, 256, 268, 273
Astronomy: interest in, x–xi, 34, 54, 68,
87–88, 103; taught, 40, 42, 43, 44, 51,
137–38; religion and, 127, 137–38
Asylums (for insane), 256–75 *passim*
Athens, Ga., 21, 24, 47, 49, 132
Atlanta, Ga., 112, 217–18
Audubon, John J., 24, 93, 139, 174
Augusta, Ga., 81, 218, 248

Bachman, John, 6, 11, 19, 21, 24, 58, 60,
101, 132, 139–40
Baltimore, Md., 109, 252, 259, 268
Baptists, and science, 34, 131, 136, 137
Barnard, Frederick A. P., x, 19–20, 21,
23, 25, 30, 34, 53, 54